PSYCHOLOGICAL ISSUES
OF HUMAN-COMPUTER INTERACTION
IN THE WORK PLACE

Edited by

Michael FRESE

Department of Psychology
University of Munich
Munich, FRG

Eberhard ULICH

Work and Organizational Psychology Unit
Swiss Federal Institute of Technology
Zürich, Switzerland

Wolfgang DZIDA

Society for Mathematics and Data Processing
St. Augustin 1, FRG

1987

NORTH-HOLLAND
AMSTERDAM · NEW YORK · OXFORD · TOKYO

ISBN: 0 444 70318 7

Published by:
ELSEVIER SCIENCE PUBLISHERS B.V.
P.O. Box 1991
1000 BZ Amsterdam
The Netherlands

Sole distributors for the U.S.A. and Canada:
ELSEVIER SCIENCE PUBLISHING COMPANY, INC.
52 Vanderbilt Avenue
New York, N.Y. 10017
U.S.A.

Library of Congress Cataloging-in-Publication Data

Psychological issues of human-computer interaction in
    the work place.

    Includes indexes.
    1. Computers--Psychological aspects. 2. Man-machine
systems. I. Frese, Michael. II. Ulich, Eberhard,
1929-   . III. Dzida, Wolfgang.
QA76.9.P75P76 1987   004'.019   87-22229
ISBN 0-444-70318-7 (U.S.)

PRINTED IN THE NETHERLANDS

PSYCHOLOGICAL ISSUES
OF HUMAN-COMPUTER INTERACTION
IN THE WORK PLACE

PREFACE

The human-computer interaction area is increasingly becoming an important area in computer science, in engineering, and in psychology. One result of this is that there is a great variety of books in the area (plus new journals appear). The editors of this book have decided to add yet another book to this variety because this book stands for a different approach. The idea behind it is to present an analysis of human computer interaction *in the work place*. This approach implies that work place issues are more prominent than in other volumes on human-computer interaction and that the interplay between organizational aspects, task problems and software ergonomics is emphasized. Thus, molar, integrative, and practical issues for using software in the work place are emphasized in this book.

This book is meant to be read by the computer scientist, human factor specialist, the professional working on practical issues of training, introducing computers and adapting software, and by the psychologist. It is useful as a supplementary text for courses on the graduate level in the field of human-computer interaction.

Our approach in this book is different from the many other ones in the area that have been rather narrowly experimental, either within a cognitive science or a narrow human factors tradition.

There is even a tendency to develop something like a new cognitive Taylorism in the field of human-computer interaction (cf. e.g. the book by Card, Moran & Newell, 1983. This means that performance in the work place is seen as a simple addition of processing operators and the task of the human factors specialist consists of reducing the number of operators. There is little thought on the allocations of tasks between human and computer within this tradition except in terms of a short term gain in performance times (usually examined within narrow experimental settings).

Although we find congenial the precise laboratory work that underlies some of these concepts, we think that the area of human- computer interaction has to be considerably broadened (and we have tried to do this in this book). Therefore, this book emphasizes non-Tayloristic perspectives in which organizational conditions and concrete working conditions are seen in interrelation with traditional software ergonomics problems.

In short, this book takes a work and organizational psychology perspective. It is mainly integrative and oriented to practical problems of integrating computer systems into the work place. Integration means that organizational issues, work place issues, and software ergonomics are brought together. This integrative perspective should be theoretically spelled out and developed -- another goal that we have tried to achieve with this book.

The Content of the Book

The book is organized into 6 sections: The section on "Organizational conditions and the use of computers in the work place" analyzes the organizational problems when introducing computers and the interplay between the computer system and the organizational conditions. The next section "The fit between the work place and the human" asks the question, how the work place and the dialogue should be constructed to fit human needs. The section on "Cognitive optimization of human-computer interaction in the work place" discusses some specific issues of how software design can enhance human productivity. In the section on "Training for human-computer interaction skills" suggestions for optimizing training are given. The final two sections ("Conceptual issues in the psychology of human-computer interaction" and "Methodological issues in the psychology of human-computer interaction") discuss various conceptual and methodological issues in the area that appear when taking an integrative and work place oriented perspective.

We do not attempt here to given a short overview on each article. Rather, we want to shortly discuss some key issues that appear in this book and that we think are particularly important.

The Taylorist perspective can be shown to be theoretically and empirically not quite adequate because it does not take into account individual differences (Greif & Gediga in this book). These individual differences should be encouraged at the work place rather than muted (Ackermann & Ulich).

Moreover, this narrow approach leaves out all those aspects that are important when working with a computer not in the laboratory but at work (cf. Landy, Rastegary & Motowidlo): the danger of increasing monotony with this kind of approach (cf. Hacker), the question of dealing with errors (Arnold & Roe, Long & Buckley), the problem of control over one's activities (Corbett, Frese, Spinas), the problem of stress and stress-reactions (Boucsein, Landy), fun and joy in the use of computers (Katz), and the problem of organizational conditions that have an impact on even small level movements (Hacker, Nullmeier & Rödiger, Spinas, Sydow).

The real problems in using computer systems in the work place are usually not so much concerned with a particular design of a system (although we do not deny the importance of a better design), but they are a result of the organizational and work place conditions which determine how the systems are used. Organizational conditions shape the behavior of computer users and software ergonomics has to have a subservient function to these organizational issues (cf. Landy et al., Corbett, Nullmeier & Rödiger, Sydow, and Katz).

The fit between the work place and the human is emphasized as well. One way to do this is to individualize work procedures. This can be done with computers and has great potential both for performance and for well-being and personality enhancement (Ackermann & Ulich, Boucsein, Hacker, Spinas). This is, of course, a radical departure from a Tayloristic conceptualization which emphasizes the one best way (Greif & Gediga).

The traditional approach underrates the importance of the task. But it is the task (usually something outside the computer system) that needs to be done with the computer. There is no "computer-job" per se but only jobs in which computers are used. Therefore, the tool character of the computer is accentuated in this book (Carroll, Dzida, Dirlich et al, Frieling et al., Hacker, Helmreich, Landy et al., Long & Buckley).

The perspective of considering organizational conditions and the tool character of computer systems shows up even when approaching apparently traditional problem areas of cognitive optimization of systems (cf. practically all articles in this book do this, but particularly Cakir, Dzida, Frieling et al., Dirlich et al., Long & Buckley).

When designing an adequate work place in which computer systems are used, it is necessary to consider not only criteria of performance but also human criteria of well-being, prevention of stress, and personality enhancement. This issue comes up in several papers (most notably in Ackermann & Ulich, Boucsein, Frese, Hacker, Nullmeier & Rödiger, Sydow). In the long range, emphasizing these "soft" human criteria will pay off even in terms of productivity at the work place.

Qualifying and training has long been an important area of work and organizational psychology. That is also reflected in this book (Carroll, Dutke & Schönpflug, Waern, Moll's methodological article).

Specific theoretical problems loom behind the issues discussed so far. These have been taken up in a separate section. One problem area has already been alluded to, the theoretical and empirical critique of Taylorism (Greif & Gediga, cf. also Landy et al., Nullmeier & Rödiger). Another theoretical question is concerned with task orientation and the tool character of computer systems (Dzida, cf. also Briggs). Thereby, it is a conclusion of many articles in this book that the user should be able to master his or her machine. Thus, the issue of control is discussed in this book (Frese, cf. also Cakir, Corbett, Spinas, Sydow).

Since this book is concerned with work place applications, there is a need to develop adequate methods (Briggs, Long & Buckley, Moll). The work place orientation of these methods means that additionally to the usual criteria of reliability and validity, they have to be robust and usable in a practical setting.

There is final difference of this volume to many other books in the area of human-computer interaction. Most of the contributors of this volume are from Europe (although a few well-known American authors are included, as well). We think in all modesty that there is a longer tradition in Europe of emphasizing ergonomics in the work place, and even more importantly, of integrating ergonomics into some larger work place and organizational context. It is within this tradition that we edited this book and we hope that this tradition can be enhanced with this book.

Words of Thanks

There are a great many words of thanks that have to be said at the end of editing a book of this kind: The first editor's secretary Mrs. Kneffel has helped tremendously in dealing with some administrative problems and in doing and redoing some of the figures. Ms. Altmann was responsible for retyping a large part and adapting the manuscripts to our laser printer so that this book has a rather unitary print. Without her, we would still brood over the difficulties of using the laser printer. Ms. Brink has edited the English of the non-English speakers. Thanks a lot to them and to the authors who have kept to a very tight time schedule so that this book will still be timely when it arrives on the market.

Michael Frese, Eberhard Ulich, Wolfgang Dzida

Munich, Zürich and St. Augustin, May 1987

CONTENTS

ORGANIZATIONAL CONDITIONS AND THE USE OF COMPUTERS IN THE WORK PLACE

Psychological Issues of
Human Computer Interaction in the Work Place
M. Frese, E. Ulich, W. Dzida (Editors)
© Elsevier Science Publishers B.V. (North-Holland), 1987

3

HUMAN-COMPUTER INTERACTIONS IN THE WORKPLACE: PSYCHOSOCIAL ASPECTS OF VDT USE

Frank J. Landy, Haleh Rastegary, and Stephan Motowidlo

Department of Psychology, The Pennsylvania State University, University Park, Pa., USA, 16802

VDT use has substantially increased among clerical workers. This increase in use has been accompanied by an increase in complaints related to VDT work. Initially, complaints were related to vision and muscular fatigue. More recently, the complaints have become more general and seem to be associated with perceived stress in VDT work. This chapter explores the various points of view that are representative of those studying human computer interactions in VDT work. The general theme of the chapter is that there is widespread disregard for the process of sociotechnical change that characterizes transition to VDT work. It is suggested that careful longitudinal studies of the changes in work tasks plus a traditional examination of operator individual differences may help to explain the continuing high levels of VDT operator complaints in spite of advances in ergonomic design.

INTRODUCTION

The last decade has seen an explosion of desktop computing and word processing devices. The development of the personal computer has revolutionized both work and education. Rafaeli and Sutton (1986) estimate that there are currently over 13 million information processors in U.S. offices. It is not surprising, then, that there has been substantial debate about the extent to which this revolution has been "good". Proponents suggest that the gains in efficiency clearly overwhelm the modest and temporary discomfiture of technological change. It has been suggested that the office of the future will see improved productivity, customer satisfaction and worker satisfaction as a direct result of the introduction of computer-based office operations (Guiliano, 1982). Further, there were some early apologists who felt that the only "victims" of the revolution would be women and elderly clerical workers who were second class citizens in work settings (Mumford and Banks, 1967). In spite of (or possibly because of) this utopian and chauvinist view of the possible effects of massive technological change on workers and work, critical examinations of the effect of computer use at the workplace began to appear. Many of the critics expressed reservations based on broad historical, philosophical or political issues. For example, Cohen (1984) suggested that clerical work had *never* been a source of satisfaction for workers and that the revolution simply exaccerbated an already difficult situation. Glenn and Feldberg (1977) were more strident and suggested that computerized office work had been "proletarianized" by the new technology. Workers were under tighter control, work was less meaningful and most workers saw more fragmentation of work.

Kling (1980) clearly recognized this philosophical split between the protagonists and antagonists of the computer revolution. He termed those favorable toward the revolution the "systems rationalists" and those opposed, the "segmented institutionalists". As Foster (1986) suggests, however, a great deal of the early debate was carried out in the popular press rather than in serious and scholarly outlets.

From the scientific perspective, the early debate revolved around issues of safety. There were questions about the extent to which VDT use would cause eye strain and permanent damage, the possible effects of VDT use on reproductive systems of the users and the effects of VDT work station design on musculo-skeletal abnormalities. As a result of these specific concerns, a number of studies were undertaken in several different countries to consider these issues. Excellent reviews of this research can be found in various sources (e.g. Committee on Vision, 1983; Frese, 1987; Smith, 1984). These early studies did reveal some clear problems in workplace design and work arrangement (e.g. Stammerjohn, Smith and Cohen, 1981). As a result of these early studies, handbooks were developed to govern the design of VDT jobs and work locations (e.g. Cakir, Hart and Stewart, 1979) and countries such as Sweden developed rules to protect workers from the possible dangers to visual and reproductive systems from prolonged VDT use.

Nevertheless, when the ergonomic issues were resolved, complaints of VDT users did not disappear. It is this phenomenon that is the focus of the present chapter. We will consider both the nature of VDT work and the process by which a workplace is transformed from a non-VDT to a VDT environment. For the most part, we will limit our interest to clerical type activities for two reasons. First, the bulk of VDT systems are operated by those whose jobs would be categorized as clerical rather than professional or managerial. In addition, it is the clerical worker, by and large, who seems to experience the most extensive discomfort with VDT systems. The theme of the chapter will be socio-technical change. More specifically, we will argue that in spite of the fact that there is widespread general recognition that technological changes are accompanied by psychosocial changes, the implications of this relationship are not yet fully integrated into the research designs or conclusions of those who study human-computer interactions in clerical work settings.

As indicated above, there are many good reviews of specific issues. For example, Frese (1987) reviews over 300 published works on human-computer interactions. His review is particularly detailed with respect to mental model and the cognitive architecture of the computer user. Similarly, reviews by Smith and his colleagues (Smith, 1984; Smith, Cohen, Stammerjohn, and Happ, 1981) and the National Research Council Committee on Vision (1983) do an excellent job of describing the potential effects of VDT systems on physiology and performance. Nevertheless, there are staggering holes in the research picture that need to be considered. As an example, the appreciation for differences among users in terms of cognitive and affective characteristics is almost non-existent. Similarly, a good taxonomy of VDT activities is yet to be developed. Finally, and most importantly, there seems to be little appreciation for the differences in *learning to use a system* and using a system *after it has been learned*. These are some of the issues that we will address in this chapter.

Industrial and Organizational Psychology and VDT Use

It is interesting to note the disciplinary loyalties of those conducting research on the VDT user. There is a split between the computer scientist, the educational/cognitive psychologist and the industrial and organizational psychologist. Each of these researchers approaches the problem in a very different way. Although we will see these differences in some detail in the material to follow, it may be useful to briefly touch on these differences at the outset.

Computer science literature

Many of the articles that appear in the professional literature of VDT use appear in computer science publications. An examination of recent reviews of this literature (e.g. Frese, 1987) show that over 50% of the publications were in computer journals. This percentage was considerably higher in the early stages of VDT research. Moran (1981) is representative of this approach and suggests that there is an emerging field of the "psychology of the computer user" that is a subfield of computing science. This approach has emphasized the functional characteristics of commands and generalized software. In addition, there has been some attention paid to the ergonomic issues of workplace design by the computer science journals.

Educational/cognitive literature

The educational/cognitive psychologist has studied issues of training and learning as well as the issue of operator efficiency. This approach depends heavily on the development of "expert" systems and mental models of the learner or user of the computer system. The mental model approach emphasizes the development of *the* best hardware/software configuration in terms of ease of learning or efficiency of operations. It is tempting to see this as a modern form of Taylorism (Taylor, 1911). Instead of the "best" shovel and range of motion, we are now asked to use the "best" interactive training system, or manual, or command structure.

Industrial and organizational literature

Finally, the industrial and organizational psychologist is represented in two types of approaches. The first approach is a straightforward human engineering/ergonomics one. Recent books in workplace design emphasize various sensory-motor and anthropometric characteristics of the human operator (e.g. Kantowitz and Sorkin, 1983). The second approach relates more closely to the issue of psychosocial adjustment of the worker as well as sociotechnical changes embodied in the introduction of computers to the workplace. In this latter category, we are presented with studies related to participation in system design, frustrations encountered in learning to use computers and stress related to VDT use. These articles are likely to appear in traditional psychology journals.

Missing links

Individual differences. There are two links that seem to be missing among these perspectives. The first link is any apparent appreciation for individual differences in human computer interaction. To be sure, there are those who caution that one must allow for individual differences in learning rates or learning styles. As an example, Robertson (1985) suggests that because of differences among individuals in terms of cognitive strategies, if one expects to use a single model for teaching new systems to operators, careful selection and or preparation of those learners must occur. Salvendy (1984) cautions that handedness and prevalence of red-green color blindness should be considered when designing work systems. Van Der Veer, Tauber, Waern, and Muylwijk (1985) suggest that the importance of individual differences in cognitive strategies and personality variables is substantial for the occasional and beginning computer user. Nevertheless, these cautions are widely ignored by the computer scientist and the educational/cognitive scientist. Even when these cautions are attended to, it is usually in the form of an obstacle to be overcome rather than as a strength or unique capacity of the operator. This is in contrast to

recent work by Hacker (1985) suggesting that work systems should be designed with sufficient flexibility to allow for an optimizing accomodation
of the worker to the system demands. In other words, Hacker argues that
the system design should be malleable rather than rigid and universal.

The sociotechnical approach. A second link that is missing in this
literature is any genuine appreciation for the importance of a sociotechnical approach to system design. That is not to say that the issue of
sociotechnical design is not mentioned in the literature. Pava (1983),
Buchanan and Boddy (1982), Kalimo and Leppanen (1985), among others,
identify sociotechnical issues in their research. Nevertheless, the typical
research study conducted by the computer scientist or cognitive scientist
addresses only a small part of this larger sociotechnical system. This is all
the more startling in light of the fact that the concept of sociotechnical
change and its impact on psychosocial adjustment has been widely recognized and effectively used in industries in transition (Trist and Bamforth,
1951; Trist, Susman and Brown, 1977; Landy, 1985).

VDT use and the perception of stress

The fact is that the industrial and organizational psychologist has
barely scratched the surface of the VDT domain. Traditional areas such as
job analysis have received little attention to this point. Individual
differences research in cognitive, motor and perceptual-motor areas is
virtually non-existent. Finally, the research that deals with the extent to
which VDT use produces stress is parochial. For example, NIOSH (Smith,
1984) and the Committee on Vision (1983) seem to have uncritically
adopted the Michigan P-E Fit model of stress. That model and its exten-
sions are often cited as the underlying theoretical foundation for claiming
that social support systems are damaged by the introduction of VDT use
(Cobb, 1976; Smith, 1984). Turner and Karasek (1984), on the other hand,
invoke the model of demands and constraints suggested by Karasek (1979)
to account for the stress associated with VDT use. The work of Glenn and
Feldberg suggests still another possible stress model -- the Type A/Type B
distinction of Friedman and Rosenman (1974). One final model of stress
that is implicit in much of the VDT research (although it has not been
explicitly invoked) is the Life Change Unit model of Holmes and Rahe
(1967). In the area of stress research, we are blessed with too many good
models and too little good data. Further, there have been few parametric
studies designed to assess the relative advantages of one of these models
over the others. Thus, even in the area of VDT use and stress, the research has been constrained by the adherence to one or another model as
accepted doctrine.

A PRELIMINARY AGENDA FOR NEEDED RESEARCH

Our review of extent literature in VDT use brings good news and bad news. The good news is that many of the early concerns regarding physical well being have been resolved. Further, a great deal of substantial work has been done on identifying effective training systems and models of computer use. The bad news is that many traditional and obvious areas of research have been largely ignored. In the following sections, we will consider some of the issues that need greater attention. As such, we are suggesting that certain gaps be filled by the research community. We believe that in filling these gaps, we will come closer to realizing the full sociotechnical impact of VDT use.

Job Analysis

It is clear that there are many different types of clerical work that can be performed on VDTs. Several brief taxonomies can be inferred from the research literature. For example, Smith (1984) suggests that tasks be broken down into data entry tasks, data acquisition tasks, interactive tasks and word processing tasks. Salvendy (1984) emphasizes cycle time as an important characteristic of the VDT task. Dainoff (1982) is broader in approach and, in addition to task variables, suggests that environmental variables and VDT system characteristics become defining characteristics of VDT work.

It seems clear from the heterogeneous nature of the VDT tasks studied by researchers that there is no such thing as a VDT job. Instead, it is likely that there are clusters of jobs that share some common characteristics. For example, Smith's preliminary taxonomy might be a good one. One cluster of VDT jobs might be word processing in nature; another cluster might involve CAD/CAM duties; still a third might relate to data acquisition duties. But it is equally clear that *within* those broad clusters there are other characteristics that could lead to further refinement of cluster membership. For example, it is possible that there are differences in cycle time within word processing tasks. It may also be that in some word processing tasks, the system is a "stand alone" system and unaffected by mainframe characteristics. Still further, there may be differences within clusters in terms of the "friendliness" of the system to the new or occasional user.

If we are interested in isolating *which* variables of VDT interaction are associated with stress or well being, the first step is a clear articulation of what these potential variables are. A model for use with this approach might be the Position Analysis Questionnaire (PAQ) developed by McCormick and his colleagues for job analysis (McCormick, Jeanneret and Mecham, 1972). This structured questionnaire deals with nature of tasks from an information processing standpoint as well as the conditions under which these tasks are performed. As a preliminary step, a wide range of VDT jobs might be described using the PAQ. A cluster analysis of the results of these descriptions would produce homogeneous clusters of VDT jobs. The cluster analysis would also highlight the most important parameters on which VDT jobs differ. It is likely, however, that additional parameters will be needed in the PAQ. Since the questionnaire was not developed specifically for VDT type work, many of the issues already implicated in earlier research (e.g. cycle or response time, friendliness of the system, etc.) would not be directly addressed in the questionnaire. It would be a simple matter to add additional parameters.

It is our belief that a taxonomic approach to the description of the full range of VDT activities would be illuminating. Further, it can provide the first set of working hypotheses for examining important issues of user efficiency and perceived stress. We are recommending that basic work be done in determining the varieties of VDT work. Real progress in understanding the interactions between VDT activities and worker behaviors and responses will not occur until and unless a disaggregation of VDT jobs is accomplished. In our minds, the *nature* and *scope* of the VDT tasks that comprise any single job may substantially moderate all other relationships of interest. To return to the issue of stress in VDT work, once various VDT jobs are segregated into homogeneous subgroups, it would be a simple matter to contrast the reported levels of stress among and between the various groups. It is not unreasonable to hypothesize that higher levels of stress would be reported in those jobs that are characterized as having short cycle time, interdependence on other parts of the operating system outside of the VDT operators control, and an emphasis on data entry rather than more truly interactive operations.

Another important aspect of the job analytic approach to understanding the effect of VDT technologies on behavior is the extent to which a job is characterized by VDT tasks. As an example, the typical secretary may use the VDT for 3 hours per day in the production and editing of documents. The other working hours are spent answering the telephone, making photocopies, filing, etc. On the other hand, the accounts clerk might use the VDT for 7 hours per day in creating and updating files, paying bills, receiving payments, etc. Finally, the purchasing agent may use the VDT for less than one hour per day to check on bids or current production demands. Thus, each of these jobs has a different "VDT saturation index". It would be very useful to arrange jobs along a continuum from those with little VDT saturation to those with heavy concentrations of VDT interaction. This will help us to understand the extent to which saturation plays a role in perceived stress. There is a clear anomaly in the literature involving the issue of use or saturation. Numerous studies have failed to find a linear relationship between VDT use and user complaints (Howarth and Istance, 1985; Laubli, Hunting and Grandjean, 1981; Smith, Cohen, Stammerjohn, and Happ, 1981; Smith,

1984). This is puzzling since most of the underlying ergonomic and physiological models (including the stress models) would predict that higher levels of use would lead to higher levels of complaints. It may very well be that the saturation index or extent of use has meaning only within the context of a moderating variable such as type of task, response or cycle time, or opportunity for social interaction. With a well articulated taxonomy, it would be possible to examine the relationship between extent of use and severity of complaints in a more sophisticated manner.

An even more useful avenue for research would be to use a standard job analysis questionnaire to track the changes imposed by a switch from a non-VDT to a VDT system. The design is a simple pre-post analysis of job descriptions. As an example, Bell Labs has compared the jobs of directory assistance operators who use hard copy vs. those who use VDTs to answer customer queries (Starr, Thompson and Shute, 1982). They found no negative effects associated with the use of VDTs. They attributed this to the fact that the jobs with and without VDT use were not appreciably different. Although they did not use a pre-post design, they assumed that when the VDT was introduced, the important aspects of the job remained the same. In contrast, research by Buchanan and Boddy (1982; 1983) and Argote, Goodman and Schkade (1983) clearly describes the substantial changes that can occur as a result of the introduction of computers and robots in the workplace. Much would be learned by contrasting duties and responsibilities before and after a transition to a VDT-based work system.

Operator Attributes

Cognitive characteristics

There is a rich history in differential psychology that attests to the pervasiveness of differences among individuals in terms of both cognitive capacities and cognitive styles (Landy, 1985). Historically, these differences were thought to be on a single continuum called intelligence. More recently, there has been a growing appreciation for the complexity of intellectual behavior. It is now generally recognized that intellectual behavior consists of differences in cognitive capacities as well as differences in cognitive operations (Sternberg, 1982). Individuals might differ in their capacity to reason inductively, to reason deductively, to recall information, to recognize information, to order steps in a multi-step sequence, or to comprehend verbal instructions. All of these are independent aspects of cognitive activity (Fleishman, 1975; Fleishman and Quaintance, 1984). It would seem reasonable to expect that individuals with greater or lesser amounts of these basic abilities would experience greater or lesser amounts of success with systems that demand particular ability profiles. As an example, word processing systems would seem to require high levels of memory (both recall and recognition), high levels of deductive reasoning (i.e. rule application) and moderate to low levels of inductive reasoning (rule derivation). On the other hand, interactive systems (such as CAD/CAM use or directory assistance for telephone operators) might require higher levels of inductive reasoning and only moderate to low levels of deductive reasoning and recall/recognition memory. There is little serious research on these issues. As mentioned earlier, there are frequent references to individual differences in cognitive strategies of learners (Rich, 1983; Robertson, 1985; Van Der Veer, Tauber, Waern and Muylwijk, 1985) but no serious discussion of what these differences might be and how they might be measured and used to advantage in developing a system. Although Frese (1987) discusses the issue of individual operator differences, he deals predominantly with motivational/ personality differences such as goal orientation, planfulness and impulsivity.

We would suggest that some careful attention be given to traditional validation models and designs in examining the human-computer interaction. Much is to be learned from a simple correlation matrix illustrating the extent to which standard cognitive and perceptual-motor abilities are implicated in "success" in VDT use.

Affective characteristics

Glenn and Feldberg (1977) provide a rich collection of quotes from clerical workers using VDT technology. One of these workers is quoted as follows:

> *You need a lot of patience. You need to be more or less good natured, easy going. Sometimes the tension gets really bad. Some people look on it as boring. If you go on saying 'Oh, God - another day' you wouldn't last long. (p.57)*

This is a description of an affective style. The style is easy going and unexcited. It appears close to the concept of the Type B personality as articulated by Friedman and Rosenman (1974). In contrast, the Type A pattern of behavior is characterized as hard driving, competitive and time urgent. There is good reason to believe that there will be an interaction between the affective characteristics of users and the nature of the system being used. As an example, Turner and Karasek (1984) argue that many operators become frustrated with down time or long response time from the system. It is thought that this frustration results from high levels of arousal that are associated with action delays. It is a reasonable extension to suggest that some people (e.g. those displaying Type B behavior patterns) are more able to tolerate these delays than others (e.g. those displaying a Type A behavior pattern). This is just what the worker quoted by Glenn and Feldberg is saying. Frese (1987) has suggested other variables of interest. These might include locus of control, self-esteem, and impulsivity. The point is that these differences are likely to play a role in the extent to which an individual experiences stress from inter-action with VDT systems.

Training and Learning

By far, the most frequent topic addressed in the human computer interaction literature is that of training and support systems for computer use. As a result of the commercial pressures experienced by computer manufacturers from potential buyers, there has been an extensive and well documented effort to develop systems that can be learned easily. The concept of "friendliness" is integral to this training and support arena.

Frequently, the research question addresses the mode of learning or training. Thus, the extent to which real instructors present a learning advantage or handicap to the learner when compared to manuals and com-puter based learning systems is considered. The educational/cognitive typically approaches the problem as a modeling exercise. Attempts are made to discover how people interact with a training system in order to develop a system that will be maximally efficient (e.g. Carroll, Mack, Lewis, Girschkowsky and Robertson, 1985; Hammer and Rouse, 1982; Kieras and Bovair, 1984; Newell and Card, 1985).

These optimizing training systems frequently are built on the notion that the most efficient way for a novice to learn is with some form of programmed instruction. This instruction is delivered either by the com-puter itself, in a self-contained training module, or by a user's manual that accompanies the computer. It is interesting to note that these optimizing systems stand in contrast to how people actually learn these computer based systems. They typically learn by asking other, more experienced, users.

The "local expert" concept

Scharer (1983) suggests that in every learning situation, there is a "local expert". This is an individual who is an incumbent in the work unit that is learning the new system. This individual learns quickly and is motivated to help others to learn. Scharer goes so far as to suggest that this person is central to the ultimate success of the training effort. Other research illustrates why this local expert is so important. Eason (1984) showed that computer users try to minimize costs and maximize benefits. He suggested that people will expend as little effort as possible in solving a problem. As a result, it is infinitely easier to ask another person how to solve a problem than it is to page through a poorly written and indexed document full of unfamiliar terms. In an earlier study of computer users, Lang, Auld, and Lang (1982) discovered a clear preference for colleagues over computer center personnel in solving problems. They attributed this preference, at least in part, to the proximity of colleagues. They noted that convenience often won out over competence when advice was being sought. Bannon (1986) and O'Malley (1986) confirm this preference for human help over system or manual based help in learning new systems.

There seem to be several parameters involved in the choice of who will be solicited for help. These characteristics include variables such as rank, expertise, sociability, accessibility, status and organizational role (Lang, Auld, and Lang, 1982; Bannon, 1986). This would suggest that the local expert be carefully selected as well as oriented toward the facilitating and supporting role that he or she will play. For example, many learners may believe that asking for help is a sign of ignorance or failure (Bannon, 1986). Brown (1986) suggests that it is important for learners to understand that even experts ask for help on occasion. This would suggest that the local expert not adopt an air of omniscience but instead an empathic demeanor in interacting with learners.

Social learning.

All of this discussion of human/human interactions in the context of training suggests a substantial role for social learning theory and modelling. It has been widely recognized that social learning models are effective alternatives to the more traditional classical and operant conditioning models of training and learning (Landy, 1985; Landy, 1987). Models may have unique learning advantages over paper or computer based training programs. This may account for the ubiquity of the local expert (Scharer, 1983) and the preference for interacting with other users in an attempt to solve problems. In any event, the literature contains virtually no references to or designs that explicitly include variables related to social learning and modeling. It would seem that the early work of Bandura on social learning (Bandura and Walters, 1959; Bandura, 1971) as well as more recent work by others on modelling (Decker and Nathan, 1985; Latham and Saari, 1979) would be an important addition to the VDT research agenda. As an example, one might prepare a videotape of a new computer user encountering a problem and contacting a "local expert" to solve that problem. Similarly, the modelling tape might show the "local expert" seeking advice from another knowledgeable person. Brown (1986) suggests that if novices see local experts seeking help, they will be more willing to seek help. Many of the current training techniques for orientation and skill learning have yet to make an appearance in the VDT literature.

Meaningfulness of the material.

There are some advantages of the local expert system that may not be so obvious to the non-psychologist. Many new users of computer-based systems complain that there is too much information to process and that they can't remember everything necessary to use the system efficiently (Mack, Lewis and Carroll, 1983). There are several solutions to that problem. The first is to reduce the amount of information to be processed. This was exactly what Eason (1984) found in a study of the use of computers by bank personnel. They used a small number of command functions to do everything. They used these functions in spite of the fact that they were not always the most effective ways to solve the problem. They preferred to use old codes that they knew rather than new codes that had to be learned.

Another way to deal with the problem of information overload is to make that information more meaningful. It is generally accepted that memory can be described as a process of coding. This coding can occur at several levels. Craik and Lockhart (1972) introduced the notion of levels of processing to describe the memory coding process. They suggested that one could code information to be retrieved structurally, phonemically or semantically. Structural and phonemic coding are related to orthographic and labelling processes for stimuli. Semantic coding, on the other hand, is related to the meaningfulness of the information. It is distinctly possible that information gained through interactions with others is coded at the deeper, semantic level than information received from manuals or computer screens.

It seems clear that other individuals are salient in the learning process. It is not completely clear why that is the case. It may be because learning situation imply stress and stress can be buffered by social support. It may be that the principle of least effort controls the actions of the learners and it simply is the easiest solution to their problem. It may be that there is a prepotency for social learning because of the special properties of social reinforcement or because of an inchoate realization that meaningfulness can be enhanced and information load reduced by interacting with others. For whatever reason, it seems clear that human to human interactions are common and effective in computer learning environments. Research is warranted into discovering why that is the case. The continual search for the "best" computer based or manual based training system may be less fruitful than a search for an explanation of the preference for human interaction.

Expectations

There is little doubt that expectations play a role in all motivated behavior. This is just as true of learning environments as other environments. Expectancy theory, equity theory, and goal setting theory place great emphasis on the role of expectations in determining satisfaction and, ultimately, effort expenditure (Landy, 1985). Much of the training literature in VDT use also recognizes the importance of expectations of learners and users. As an example, Shneiderman (1984) suggests that user expectations regarding system response time will affect user performance. Dzida, Herda and Itzfeldt (1978) imply that the extent to which a system is deemed "friendly" will depend on the extent to which user expectations are met. Hiltz (1983) also suggests that the extent to which expectations are met will determine the extent to which a new system is accepted by potential users. In the area of robotics and automation, two studies clearly delineate the role of expectations on acceptance and ultimate efficiency. Argote, Goodman and Schkade (1983) demonstrated that many of the expectations of skilled workers in a steel fabricating plant about the impact of a robotic addition were in error. Similarly, the work of Buchanan and Boddy (1983) on the computerization of biscuit making also suggests a substantial discrepancy between reality and expectations. In contrast, Rafaeli (1986) has asserts that familiarity breeds acceptance. He shows that the frequent user is more positive in attitudes toward the computer than the occasional or new user. By implication, then, it is the group that needs the most attention that has the least positive attitude. This may be because of expectations about skills required, about the elimination of jobs, about the pace of work, etc.

In other instances where new users or employees harbor inappropriate expectations about work, realistic job previews have been effective in discounting these incorrect expectations (Dean and Wanous, 1984). The realistic job preview might prove equally effective in the introduction of computer systems. The preview might built on the experiences of frustrated new users. These users might be interviewed to determine which expectations were least and most likely to be met. For example, it might be that new users expect quicker response times from the system or less down time. Whatever the inaccurate expectation, they could be easily addressed in an orientation session.

Interference theory

One thing that seems clear in considering the manner by which most VDT systems are introduced is that there is ample opportunity for proactive interference or negative transfer (Waern, 1985). The clerical employee who is asked to learn to use a new VDT system finds that many old responses are competing with new ones. In word processing, there is the tendency to hit the return key at the end of every line. Similarly, there is the temptation to simply turn off the machine when you walk away from it. Both of these responses are counterproductive in a computer-based word processing environment. Nevertheless, when the new system is being learned, the old system (e.g. the typewriter) is still available as an alternative response mechanism. The effects of both proactive and retroactive interference need to be better understood if the introduction of a new work technology such as a VDT is to be accomplished efficiently. It is interesting to note that new users have fewer problems of interference than experienced users, particularly in the use of commands although the new user does have a slightly more difficult time dealing with command jargon (Scapin, 1981).

Participation in System Development and Implementation

If there is one area that seems to have largely eluded the discussion of the computer science community, and to some extent the educational/ cognitive psychologist community as well, it is the potential role for participation in decision making regarding the introduction of a new or replacement VDT system. The general belief seems to be that one simply needs to model the cognitive system of the new user to ensure ease of use and acceptance (e.g. Carroll, Mack, Lewis, Girschkowsky and Robertson, 1985). If one can discover the most common mistakes of the new user, a training system can be developed that will circumvent those problems. In fact, a very important part of stress reduction may involve the perception of control and involvement. Davidson and Cooper (1981) imply that participation in decision making can diminish perceptions of stress. This follows directly from the early work by Glass and Singer (1972a; 1972b) on perceptions of control and perceptions of stress. In two case studies of the introduction of computer systems in clerical work, Mumford (1980) illustrated the ameliorating effects of this participation on resistance to change. Yet the hypothesis that involving employees in the choice of hardware and software systems and in the general system architecture remains untested in any substantial way and the system designers continue to search for the best method of introduction to impose on the learner or user. It is distinctly possible that the best system architecture is developed with the active participation of the ultimate user of that system.

Considering the Sociotechnical System

It seems clear that when a VDT is introduced to the workplace, a substantial alteration occurs on many levels. If we consider the typical clerical position and the introduction of computer based word processing and record keeping, the most immediate change that occurs is in the pattern of social interaction. There is no longer any necessity to walk to and from file cabinets (Salvendy, 1984). This can have the effect of radically reducing the extent of social interaction that occurs in workday. If this social interaction was serving the role of a buffer against various stressors in the environment, that buffering mechanism is neutralized and stress undiminished. Similarly, several studies have shown that work patterns change as an accomodation to a system prone to failure. Clerical VDT workers in a study in at Saab/Scania in Sweden (Johansson and Aronsson, 1984) worked harder and felt more pressure in the morning than in the afternoon. This was the result of rushing to get work done before the system broke down or became inaccessible for other reasons. In contrast, non-VDT users felt no more pressure in the morning than in the afternoon. This certainly suggests that there was an alteration of the pattern of work to match the characteristics of the system. This alteration of work schedules and styles must have similarly affected the social pattern of the office.

Numerous studies suggest substantial changes in many different aspects of work as a result of the introduction of VDT technology. Buchanan and Boddy (1982) examined the jobs of typists as they were altered by VDT technology and found changes in task variety, work cycle, feedback of results, and skill/knowledge demands. Kalimo and Leppanen (1985) found that the introduction of VDT technology had differential effects on various jobs. As an example, the jobs of proofreaders and photocompositors remained complex but the jobs of perforator typesetters become less complex and more fragmented. Glenn and Feldberg (1977) assert that the VDT clerical worker experiences less autonomous, less meaningful and more fragmented work. Smith, Cohen and Stammerjohn (1981) suggest one additional variable that is part of the sociotechnical change that accompanies VDT introduction -- there is an increased capacity for monitoring the activity of the worker through the VDT system. In many organizations, the employee is fed back specific information about productivity rate, errors, and response times. For example, in the Plymouth office of Blue Shield of Massachusetts, the introduction of a computer-based claims adjustment procedure led to the development of a standard for productivity for claims personnel. Each employee's performance was compared to this standard and pay was adjusted depending on whether the employee was under or over the standard. In effect, the method of payment was changed from salary to piece rate (Landy, 1985).

It seems clear that we are still in the beginning stages of understanding the sociotechnical changes that accompany the transition from non-VDT to VDT environments. Nevertheless, it is equally clear that there is an excellent possibility that the complaints that are heard from VDT workers are most likely associated with many of these sociotechnical changes. We are well past the stage of poor ergonomic design of the physical workplace and VDT equipment. To use a term suggested by Brown (1986), perhaps the time has arrived for a consideration of the social ergonomics of the VDT environment. By the use of the term social ergonomics, Brown suggests that it is possible to develop socialstructures within the work setting in such a way that information exchange can occur in an environment that encourages experimentation, collaborative learning and the sharing of knowledge.

A CONCLUDING COMMENT

Seventy years ago, the industrial revolution produced scientific management (Taylor, 1911). Taylorism, in turn, set the stage for the Hawthorne studies. These classic field experiments illustrated with dramatic clarity that the expectations and emotions of workers played a major role in the ultimate effectiveness of production systems. It is time to remember the lessons of the Hawthorne studies and consider the implications of VDT technology on psychosocial structures at the workplace. The most effective way to operationalize this consideration is through systematic longitudinal studies of the changes in work that occur with the introduction of VDT technologies. It is our hope that many of the ideas presented in this chapter will be incorporated into an appropriate longitudinal design and will result in an enhanced understanding of the interaction between VDT users and the VDT technology in the workplace. Perhaps it will then be possible to directly address the complaints that surround VDT work.

FOOTNOTE

Stephan Motowidlo is now at Personnel Decisions, Incorporated In Minneapolis, Minnesota.

REFERENCES

Argote, L., Goodman, P., & Schkade, D. (1983). The human side of robotics: How workers react to a robot. *Sloan Management Review*, *24*, 31-41.

Bandura, A. (1971). *Principles of social learning theory*. New York: General Learning press.

Bandura, A., Walters, A. H. (1959). *Adolescent aggression*. New York: Ronald press.

Bannon, I. J. (1986). Helping users help each other. In D. A. Norman & S. W. Draper (Eds.), *User centered system design* (pp. 399-410). Hillsdale, NJ: Lawrence Erlbaum Associates.

Brown, J. S. (1986). From cognitive to social ergonomics and beyond. In D. A. Norman & S. W. Draper (Eds.), *User centered system design* (pp. 357-486). Hillsdale, NJ: Lawrence Erlbaum Associates.

Buchanan, D. A., & Boddy, D. (1982). Advanced technology and the quality of working life: The effects of word processing on video typists. *Journal of Occupational Psychology*, *55*, 1-11.

Buchanan, D. A., & Boddy, D. (1983). Advanced technology and the
     quality of working life: The effects of computerized controls on
     biscuit-making operators. *Journal of Occupational Psychology,*
     56, 109-119.
Cakir, A., Hart, D. J., & Stewart, T. F. M. (1979). *The VDT manual:*
     Ergonomics, workplace design, health and safety, task organi-
     zation. Darmstadt: IFRA.
Carroll, J. M., Mack, R. L., Lewis, C. H., Grischkowsky, N. L., &
     Robertson, S. R. (1985). Exploring exploring a word processor.
     Human-Computer Interaction, 1, 283-307.
Cobb, S. (1976). Social support as a moderator of life stress.
     Psychosomatic Medicine, 38, 300-314.
Cohen, B. G. F. (1984). Organizational factors affecting stress in the
     clerical worker. In B. G. P. Cohen (Ed.), *Human aspects of*
     office automation (pp. 33-42). Elsevier, Amsterdam: Oxford.
Committee on Vision. (1983). *Video displays, work and vision.*
     Washington, C: National Academy Press.
Craik, P. I. M., & Lockhart, R. S. (1972). Levels of processing: A
     framework for memory research. *Journal of Verbal Learning and*
     Verbal Behavior, 11, 671-684.
Dainoff, M. J. (1982). Occupational stress factors in visual display
     terminal (VDT) operation: A review of empirical research.
     Behaviour and Information Technology, 1, 141-176.
Davidson, M. J., & Cooper, C. L. (1981). A model of occupational stress.
     Journal of Occupational Medicine, 23, 564-574.
Dean, R. A., & Wanous, J. P. (1984). Effects of realistic job previews on
     hiring bank tellers. *Journal of Applied Psychology, 69*, 61-68.
Decker, P. J., & Nathan, B. R. (1985). *Behavior modeling training.* New
     York: Praeger.
Dzida, W., Herda, S., & Itzfeldt, W. D. (1978). User-perceived quality of
     interactive systems. *IEEE Transactions on Software Engineering,*
     4, 270-276.
Eason, K. D. (1984). Towards the experimental study of usability.
     Behaviour and Information Technology, 3, 133-143.
Fleishman, E. A. (1975). Toward a taxonomy of human performance.
     American Psychologist, 30, 1127-1149.
Fleishman, E. A., & Quaintance, M. K. (1984). *Taxonomies of human*
     performance. Orlando, FL: Academic press.
Foster, K. R. (1986). The VDT debate. *American Scientist, 74*, 163-168.
Frese, M. (1987). The industrial and organizational psychology of human-
     computer interaction in the office. In C. L. Cooper & I. T.
     Robertson (Eds.), *International review of industrial and*
     organizational psychology. London, New York: Wiley.
Friedman, M., & Rosenman, R. H. (1974). *Type A behavior and your*
     heart. New York: Alfred Knopf.

Giuliano, V. E. (1982). The mechanization of office work. *Scientific American, 24*, 149-165.

Glass, D. C., & Singer, J. E. (1972a). *Urban stress*. New York: Academic Press.

Glass, D. C., & Singer, J. E. (1972b). Behavioral aftereffects of unpredictable and uncontrollable aversive events. *American Scientist, 60*, 457-465.

Glenn, E. N., & Feldberg, R. L. (1977). Degraded and deskilled: The proletarianization of clerical work. *Social Problems, 25*, 52-64.

Hacker, W. (1985). Activity: A fruitful concept in industrial psychology. In M. Frese & J. Sabini (Eds.), *Goal directed behavior* (pp. 262-283). Hillsdale, NJ: Lawrence Erlbaum Associates.

Hammer, J. M., & Rouse, W. B. (1982). The human as a constrained optimal editor. *IEEE Transactions on Systems, Man, and Cybernetics, 12*, 777-784.

Hiltz, S. R. (1985). A study of the determinants of acceptance of computer-mediated communication systems (Research-in-Progress Report). *Sigchi Bulletin, 14*, 16-17.

Holmes, T. H. & Istance, H. W. (1985). The social readjustment rating scale. *Journal of Psychosomatic Research, 11*, 213-218.

Howarth, P. A., & Istance, H. W. (1985). The association between visual discomfort and the use of visual display units. *Behaviour and Information Technology, 4*, 131-149.

Johansson, G., & Aronsson, G. (1984). Stress reactions in computerized administrative work. *Journal of Occupational Behavior, 5*, 159-181.

Kalimo, R., & Leppanen, A. (1985). Feedback from video display terminals, performance control and stress in text preparation in the printing industry. *Journal of Occupational psychology, 58*, 27-38.

Kantowitz, B. H., & Sorkin, R. D. (1983). *Human factors: Understanding people-system relationships*. New York: Wiley.

Karasek, R. A., Jr. (1979). Job demands, job decision latitude, and mental strain: Implications for job redesign. *Administrative Science Quarterly*, 285-308.

Kieras, D. E., & Bovair, S. (1984). The role of a mental model in learning to operate a device. *Cognitive Science, 8*, 255-273.

Kling, R. (1980). Social analyses of computing: Theoretical perspectives in recent empirical research. *Computing Surveys, 12*, 61-110.

Landy, F. J. (1985). *The psychology of work behavior*. Homewood, IL: Dorsey Press.

Landy, F. J. (1987). *Psychology: The science of people*. Englewood Cliffs, NJ: Prentice Hall, Inc.

Lang, K., Auld, R., & Lang, T. (1982). The goals and methods of computer users. *International Journal of Man-Machine Studies, 17,* 375-399.

Latham, G. p., & Saari, L. M. (1979). Application of social learning theory to training supervisors through behavioral modeling. *Journal of Applied Psychology, 64,* 239-246.

Laubli, T., Hunting, W., & Grandjean, E. (1981). Postural and visual loads at VDT workplaces II. Lighting conditions and visual impairments. *Ergonomics, 24,* 933-944.

Mack, R. L., Lewis, C. H., & Carroll, J. M. (1983). Learning to use word processors: Problems and prospects. *ACM Transactions on Office Information Systems, 1,* 254-271.

McCormick, E. J., Jeanneret, P., & Mecham, R. C. (1972). A study of job characteristics and job dimensions as based on the position analysis questionnaires. *Journal of Applied Psychology, 56,* 347-368. (Monograph)

Moran, T. P. (1981). An applied psychology of the user. *Computing Surveys, 13,* 1-11.

Mumford, E. (1980). The participative design of clerical information systems two case studies. In N. Bjorn-Anderson (Ed.), *The human side of information processing* (91-107). Amsterdam: North Holland.

Mumford, E., & Banks, 0. (1967). Some problems of office automation. *The computer and the clerk* (pp. 9-18). London: Routledge and Kegan Paul.

Newell, A., & Card, S. K. (1985). The prospects for psychological science in human-computer interaction. *Human Computer Interaction, 1,* 209-242.

O'Malley, C. (1986). Helping users help themselves. In D. A. Norman & S. W. Draper (Eds.), *User centered system design* (377-398). Hillsdale, NJ: Lawrence Erlbaum Associates.

Pava, C. H. P. (1985). The office in the future. *Managing new office technology* (122-144). New York, NY: The Free Press.

Rafaeli, A. (1986). Employee attitudes toward working with computers. *Journal of Occupational Behaviour, 7,* 89-106.

Rafaeli, A., & Sutton, R. I. (1986). Word processing technology and perceptions of control among clerical workers. *Behaviour and Information Technology, 5,* 31-37.

Rich, E. (1983). Users are individuals: Individualizing user models. *International Journal of Man-Machine Studies, 18,* 199-214.

Robertson, I. T. (1985). Human information-processing strategies and style. *Behaviour and Information Technology, 4,* 19-29.

Salvendy, G. (1984). Research issues in the ergonomics, behavioral, organizational and management aspects of office automation. In B. G. F. Cohen (Ed.), *Human aspects in office automation* (ll5-126). New York, NY: Elsevier Pub.

Scapin, D. L. (1981). Computer commands in restricted natural language: Some aspects of memory and experience. *Human Factors, 23,* 365-375.

Scharer, L. L. (1983). User training: Less is more. *Datamation,* 175-236.

Shneiderman, B. (1984). Response time and display rate in human performance with computers. *Computing Surveys, 16,* 265-285.

Smith, M. J. (1984). Ergonomic aspects of health problems in VDT operators. In B. G. F. Cohen (Ed.), *Human aspects in office automation* (87-114). Amsterdam: Elsevier.

Smith, M. J., Cohen, B. G. F., Stammerjohn, L. W., Jr., & Happ, A. (1981). An investigation of health complaints and job stress in video display operations. *Human Factors, 23,* 387-400.

Stammerjohn, L. W., Smith, M. J., & Cohen, B. F. G. (1981). Evaluation of work station design factors in VDT operation. *Human Factors, 23,* 401-412.

Starr, S. J., Thompson, C. R., & Shute, S. J. (1982). Effects of video display terminals on telephone operators. *Human Factors, 24,* 699-711.

Sternberg, R. J. (Ed.) (1982). *The handbook of human intelligence.* Cambridge: Cambridge University Press.

Taylor, F. W. (1911). *The principles of scientific management.* New York: Harper and Row.

Trist, E. L., & Bamforth, K. W. (1951). Some social and psychological consequences of the long-wall method of coal getting. *Human Relations, 4,* 3-38.

Trist, E. L., Susman, G. I., & Brown, G. R. (1977). An experiment in autonomous working in an American underground coal mine. *Human Relations, 30,* 201-236.

Turner, J. A., & Karasek, R. A., Jr. (1984). Software ergonomics: Effects of computer application design parameters on operator task performance and health. *Ergonomics, 27,* 663-690.

Van Der Veer, G. C., Tauber, M. J., Waern, Y., & Van Muylwijk, B. (1985). On the interaction between system and user characteristics. *Behaviour and Information Technology, 4,* 289-308.

Waern, Y. (1985). Learning computerized tasks as related to prior task knowledge. *International Journal of Man-Machine Studies, 22,* 441-455.

Psychological Issues of
Human Computer Interaction in the Work Place
M. Frese, E. Ulich, W. Dzida (Editors)
© Elsevier Science Publishers B.V. (North-Holland), 1987

COMPUTER AIDED MANUFACTURING AND THE DESIGN OF SHOPFLOOR JOBS: TOWARDS A NEW RESEARCH PERSPECTIVE IN OCCUPATIONAL PSYCHOLOGY

J. Martin Corbett

MRC/ESRC Social and Applied Psychology Unit,
University of Sheffield, Sheffield, S10 2TN.

The relationship between Computer Aided Manufacturing (CAM) technology and the design of shopfloor jobs is examined in relation to research findings in occupational psychology. It is argued that the theories and methods used in this research are too general and ill-defined to assess the role of CAM technology as a discrete independent variable in the shaping of shopfloor jobs. The need for occupational psychologists to take a more direct, proactive role in the design and development of CAM technology is discussed and illustrated through a case study example.

INTRODUCTION

This chapter discusses the relationship between Computer Aided Manufacturing (CAM) technology and the design of jobs on the shopfloor. This discussion is in four parts. The first part of the chapter examines some of the research literature which argues the case for the technological determination of job design. In this view, CAM technology is socially shaped during design in such a way as to overly constrain the subsequent choices of job design. The historical trend identified by these researchers is toward job simplification and fragmentation and the shifting of control and decision competence from operator to machine.

The second part critically examines occupational psychology research into the design of jobs with CAM. Findings from this research suggest that there is no unique connection between CAM and the design of jobs. However, it is argued that both the definitions of technology and the levels of analysis utilised by these job design researchers are too broad to permit a valid analysis of the role played by CAM technology as a discrete independent variable in shaping the design of shopfloor jobs.

In the third part of the chapter research into the design of CAM technology is discussed. These findings indicate that the design of technology may indeed overly constrain the subsequent design of operator tasks. The discussion then considers the role of psychologists in the shaping of CAM design and implementation to enhance operator control and job satisfaction.

The final part of this chapter presents a case study example of CAM design involving psychologists and engineers working together on a project to develop a flexible manufacturing system in which operators are not subordinate to technology. Problems arising during this project are discussed and recommendations are made for further research and development in the social shaping of CAM technology and work

COMPUTER AIDED MANUFACTURING TECHNOLOGY

The advent of the digital computer and the development of micro-processing technology is creating a revolution in manufacturing organisations, according to a number of commentators (e.g. Forester, 1980). This 'revolution' stems from the use of computers to support and control information and mechanical systems throughout an organisation, from design through to customer delivery. These computer and micro-processor based systems will be described here under the generic term of Computer Aided Manufacturing or CAM technology.

Stand alone Computer Numerically Controlled (CNC) machine tools may be regarded as the first generation of these CAM systems, and are the building blocks for further innovation. Such machines, like the manual and semi-automatic machines they are designed to replace, enable a skilled metal-worker to cut or form metal to a high level of precision and quality. The main difference between CNC and manual machines lies in the use of computer programs in the former, which make it possible for metal to be cut or formed much faster than before. This innovation en-ables manual manipulation and control of machining operations (through the use of hand wheels) to be largely replaced by automatic computer manipulation and control.

However, the next generation of technology enables several such machines to be linked to create a Flexible Manufacturing System (FMS). These systems comprise several CNC machines, some automatic transfer capability between them, and the use of computers to integrate the functioning of the system (e.g. work scheduling and pacing).

The third generation of CAM incorporates additional activities and functions into the integrated computer control system. Computer Aided Design (CAD), the ordering and re-supply of parts and materials, and scheduling are integrated to form Computer Integrated Manufacturing (CIM) systems.

The penetration of CAM into industry, at the present time, is very low, although the rate of uptake is accelerating. CNC machines tools, for example, accounted for less than five percent of the British machine tool population in the early 1980's (Metal Working Production, 1983), and worldwide there are probably less than 200 fully operational FMS and only a handful of CIM installations.

THE SOCIAL SHAPING OF CAM TECHNOLOGY

There is a theoretical and research perspective in the organisational studies literature which argues the case for the technological determination of job designs on the manufacturing shopfloor. The writers sharing this perspective view CAM as an artefact which has essentially political qualities (Winner, 1985). CAM technology, in this view, is socially shaped during design in such a way as to heavily constrain subsequent opportunities for socially shaping the work environment into which it is placed.

Although this group of writers fundamentally agree about the important determining role played by technology in the design of shopfloor work, they differ in their emphasis on the causes or reasons for this process. For Marxist commentators, such as Braverman (1974), Gouldner (1976) and Zimbalist (1979), the historical trend in CAM technology design towards the removal of the control of work processes from the shopfloor to the machine reflects a wider political and economic rationality aimed at the subordination of labour by capital.

Noble (1979), for example, traces the development of Numerical Control (NC) machine tools and argues that this technology gained ascendency over Record-Playback technology owing to the greater opportunities for managerial control over shopfloor production offered by NC. "There is no question but that management saw in NC the potential to enhance their authority over production and seized upon it despite questionable cost effectiveness" (Noble, 1979; 34). Similarly, Braverman (1974) argues that "machinery offers to management the opportunity to do by wholly mechanical means that which it had previously attempted to do by organisational and disciplinary means" (p.174).

For other commentators sharing this radical perspective, such as Habermas (1971), Weizenbaum (1976) and Rosenbrock (1982), this trend reflects the uncritical application of scientific rationality and methodology to essentially social concerns. In other words, the centralisation of control and fragmentation of human skills associated with manufacturing technology generally, has not come about through a conscious political act. In this view, it stems from a preoccupation with predictability, quantifiability and repeatability - the three major tenets of western scientific rationality (Cooley and Crampton, 1986).

Despite this difference in emphasis, there are two common strands to the technological determinancy argument. Firstly, there are social choices available as to how manufacturing technologies are designed and developed. Despite these choices, the argument goes, the technological designs that have been developed are those which encapsulate shopfloor machining and discretionary skills into the machine, despite the availability of designs which utilise such skills and make them more productive. Secondly, this trend is continuing as CAM develops, and the application of powerful digital computers now makes possible the almost total subordination of shopfloor personnel to the dictates of the CAM system.

An important aspect of computer technology in general is that it "substitutes for or complements people's mental and clerical capabilities, in contrast to mechanical technology which substitutes for people's physical capabilities" (Child, 1984; p 245). CAM technology thus offers the potential to displace both the physical and the mental component of jobs, and therefore reduce shopfloor jobs to routine monitoring and machine minding. These types of simplified jobs are recognised by occupational psychologists to be strongly associated with low job satisfaction and poor mental health (Wall, 1987).

OCCUPATIONAL PSYCHOLOGY RESEARCH INTO CAM

Occupational psychology empirical research examining the impact of CAM on the design of jobs does not appear to support the proposition of technological determinism. The assertion that CAM technology leads directly to the removal of shopfloor control and skill is strongly resisted by researchers and commentators in the field of occupational psychology. Often in reaction to the technological determinism espoused by the commentators discussed in the previous section, it is argued that social variables rather than technological variables are of primary importance in shaping work (e.g. Buchanan and Boddy, 1983). A key phrase in this literature is 'strategic choice' (Child, 1972).

Research focusing on CAM and work, such as that by Jones (1982), Sorge et al. (1983), Kemp and Clegg (1986), and Wall et al. (1987), support the contention that there is no unique connection between first generation (CNC) CAM and the design of jobs.

Clegg, Kemp and Wall (1984), for example, compared the use of CNC machine tools in two British engineering companies making components for aerospace applications. In both companies the CNC part programs were prepared away from the machines by specialist programmers. In one company, these specialists were also responsible for proving out and editing the part programs, specialist tool and machine setters prepared the equipment and operators were reduced to monitoring the machines and calling upon engineers in the event of malfunction. In this company, therefore, operators' jobs were simplified in the manner described by commentators supporting a technological determinist perspective. In the other company, however, operators were responsible for

program proving and editing, as well as tool setting and machine preparation. In other words, the design of the operators' jobs was 'shaped' by
organisational, rather than technological, factors.

CNC machine tools are primarily used as stand-alone systems at the
present time, that is they are not usually linked to other machines or
computers. Therefore, choices as to how the machines are operated are not
constrained by how such choices would affect other parts of the production process. As Burnes and Fitter (1986) point out; "not only does this
allow greater flexibility in the design of shopfloor jobs ... but it also
allows modifications of the work organisation to take place after the
machines have been installed" (p.3).

However, Wall (1987) argues that the research findings supporting
this contention should be regarded as tentative, as they arise largely "from
atheoretical and exploratory studies of technology which in itself and its
application is at a very early stage of development" (p 22). It is pertinent
to note that a majority of CAM case studies whose results support a technological indeterminist interpretation of CAM and job design focus on
stand-alone CNC machine tools. Such studies are studying the basic
building blocks of CAM. "They are all sampling organisations/firms at a
particular historical point, one in which the form of the technology has
not been closed off by a series of decisions and technical developments
which, in combination, constitute sunk costs such that unwinding them,
making a series of different choices, becomes an impossible cost burden"
(Littler, 1983; p.144).

This argument is difficult to evaluate empirically owing to the small
number of second generation CAM systems in operation. The pattern that
is emerging, however, suggests that, in an effort to exploit the full
benefits of Flexible Manufacturing Systems (such as increased machine
utilisation, reduced inventories and lead times), user organisations are
striving to achieve a high degree of cross-functional integration. Such
aspirations, argue Jalinek and Golher (1983), "suggest the pending demise
of older, functionally specialised structures - or, perhaps, their radical
revision" (p.35).

Despite the availability of choice in this radical revision of work
organisation, in terms of upgrading or downgrading the role of system
operators, the dominant trend identified by empirical case studies of FMS
is toward job designs which involve increased task demands on operators
associated with less control and autonomy (e.g., Jones, 1982; Ingersoll
Engineers, 1983; Blumberg and Gerwin, 1984; Corbett, 1987a; Seppala et
al., 1987). The extent to which these job characteristics can be directly attributed to technology is difficult to determine, primarily because research
findings are predominantly based on FMS installations in which operator
roles are narrowly defined. In other words, it may be that this pattern of
job design derives from organisational, rather than technological, factors.

At the present time, however, there is no indication that mainstream occupational psychology is theoretically or methodologically prepared to undertake a detailed analysis of CAM technology and its relationship to social variables, such as job design. The methodologies most frequently used in occupational psychology research do not make a clear distinction between technological and organisational determinates of job design, and therefore cannot realistically be expected to prove or disprove the proposition of technological determinism (Corbett, 1987a).

In studies where such a distinction has been attempted (e.g. Woodward, 1958; Pugh et al., 1969; Pierce, 1984), technology has been defined so broadly as to include factors which refer to organisational techniques for operating and supporting technology (Gerwin, 1979; Fry, 1982; Winner, 1985). In this view it is possible to conceive of "technology beyond machines" (MacDonald, 1985) and to include factors such as degree of work role specialisation as a 'social technology'. To make matters worse, researchers differ in their assignment of such factors to either a technological or organisational category, making comparisons between case studies very difficult (Stanifield, 1976; Rousseau, 1979).

Whilst shopfloor work with CAM can undeniably be socially shaped to afford opportunities for the removal or enhancement of shopfloor control and skill, there seems to be no valid reason to reject the hypothesis that developments in CAM design may constrain these opportunities. In other words, although CAM work may be socially shaped by an organisation, the organisation of work may also be shaped by CAM design. The extent to which one dynamic may constrain or pre-empt the other is an empirical question that occupational psychologists have been slow to address.

STRATEGIC OPTIONS FOR PSYCHOLOGICAL RESEARCH ON CAM TECHNOLOGY

Two strategic options are available to occupational psychologists concerned to understand the impact of CAM technology on job design. One strategy is based on the view that psychological researchers should observe and analyse technological progress and monitor its effects on jobs more systematically than at present. This will involve the generation of theories and analytical methods which make a clear distinction between technological and organisational variables. A recent study of the relation between telephone exchange technology and job design by Rose and co-workers (1986) offers an excellent example of this kind of endeavour. A further example is offered by Corbett (1987a).

A second strategy for psychological research on CAM technology is based on a more proactive orientation and involves psychologists in the actual process of technological design, in a similar role to that adopted by ergonomists. This strategy also serves as a counter to the determinists' implicit assumption that technological design and development is somehow an autonomous process, possessing an inner logic that is divorced from social relations. The two strategies are clearly complementary. As particular aspects of CAM design which contribute to, or diminish, operator control and job satisfaction are identified, this information may then be fed back to inform CAM designers.

The remainder of this chapter concentrates on the illustration of how these two complementary strategies may be utilised in the design of jobs with a Flexible Manufacturing System (FMS). To begin with, a conceptual framework is outlined which enables CAM technology to be analysed in terms of the relationship between technological design and the design of jobs. The use of this framework in the design of an FMS in which operators' are not subordinate to machines is then outlined.

The concept of "strategic choice", discussed earlier in this chapter, is typically related to the choices open to an organisation once a particular CAM system has been chosen; in other words, the choices that are available during the *implementation* of technology. However, the concept of choice may also be related to the *design* of technology in order to examine how technology is socially constructed during the design stage, and to examine the choices that are available during design.

This analysis is described below and is used as a basis for an examination of the relationship between design and implementation, with particular focus on the ways in which early design choices may constrain the choice of job designs (and restrict operator control) once a CAM system is implemented on the shopfloor.

SOCIAL CHOICE IN CAM DESIGN

The development of CNC technology has produced a shift in decision competence from shopfloor worker to machine, whereby the operator of a CNC machine tool, for example, is not alone in the control of the machine but, owing to the decisions and choices taken by the designer and stored in the computer, is forced to co-operate intimately with the designer.

The number of design decisions and choices open to a designer is almost infinite, but research in the field of ergonomics points to three key choice points in the design of CAM which have the most impact on operator control (see Clegg and Corbett, 1987). To these three choice points can be added a fourth, organisational, choice. The four key choices are:
(1) Allocation of functions between human and CAM system technology
(2) The control characteristics of the human–system interface
(3) The informational characteristics of the human–system interface
(4) The allocation of responsibilities between system personnel.

With regard to the first of these choice points - the allocation of function - ergonomists stress that there are choices over what humans do and over what machines do in any automated system (Jordan, 1963; Singleton, 1971; Price, 1985). These choices will inevitably affect the extent of human operator control, and will have implications for the design of operating tasks. The conventional engineering approach to the allocation of function involves the practice of human-machine comparability: functional requirements are typically realised with respect to the technological state-of-the-art, where the human takes over those functions that are technically not yet solved. As Rasmussen (1979) argues, "The fact that all control functions which can be formally described also can be automated by means of computers leads to the danger that the role of the system operator will be to plug the holes in the thoroughness of the designer's work. On the one hand as a convenient, movable manipulator, he will have a category of trivial, infrequent actions for which automation is unfeasible; on the other hand, as an intelligent data processor he will be expected to respond to ill-structured and unforeseen tasks" (p.2).

A second key choice point in CAM design concerns the control characteristics of the human-system interface. Design decisions here concern how the control of the system is to be shared between human and machine (Rouse, 1981). For example, CNC machine tool software can be designed to enable operators to interrogate data bases in order for them to take important controlling decisions (such as determining tool path geometry, work scheduling and pacing). On the other hand, the software may contain complex algorithms which enable the computer to take all the controlling decisions, thus restricting the operator's role to that of machine minder.

Control characteristics of second and third generation CAM systems may fundamentally differ from those of stand-alone CNC machines owing to the integrated nature of their computer system architectures (Winch, 1983). In such systems there are design choices to be made concerning the apportionment of control between the different technological components of the overall system. For example, an FMS which is designed so that CNC part programs may be automatically generated at the CAD work stations and directly transmitted to the CNC machines on the shopfloor will have a direct impact on the design of the machine operators' jobs. Their control over the planning of work will be reduced and their freedom to edit part programs may be overly constrained by the potential 'knock on' effects of program changes to other parts of the FMS (unless sophisticated real time scheduling aids are provided). An alternative, network system architecture may be chosen to promote a more decentralised control system.

The third key choice point in CAM design concerns the informational characteristics of the human-machine interface. The invisibility of many software functions means that an operator must rely heavily on information and data that is transmitted or generated by computer in order to structure his or her work behaviour (Edwards and Lees, 1974). Software which only presents machine-specific information to an operator in the event of system malfunction, for instance, will not enable the operator to see the overall consequences of his or her actions for system performance. Restricting information in this manner inevitably restricts operator control as one can never fully control a system without understanding it.

The interaction between human and machine may thus be viewed as a social interaction, between operator and software designer, in which the designer predefines the situation through the type and scope of the information given to the operator. Because of this, the designer has a further means to restrict or increase an operator's control. One has only to recall Milgram's (1974) dictum: "Control the manner in which a man interprets the world, and you have gone a long way toward controlling his behaviour" (p.145).

The argument so far is that key design choices are open to CAM designers and that these have implications for what one may term the 'balance of control' between human operator and CAM. The fourth key design choice point concerns the allocation of responsibilities between personnel. It is at this point that the concept of strategic choice is focused in the occupational psychology literature, but it is clear from the above discussion that this choice can be overly constrained by earlier CAM design choices.

HUMAN CENTERED CAM SYSTEMS DESIGN

The awareness of the relationship between CAM technological design and the resultant shopfloor job design lies at the heart of the recent development of the 'human centered systems' perspective (Brodner, 1982; Corbett, 1985; Rosenbrock, 1985; Cooley and Crampton, 1986). In this view, shopfloor jobs are shaped predominantly by the choices made by the system designers. The wider the scope available to the operators and support personnel using the resultant CAM system to shape their own working behaviour and practices, the more 'human centered' the system. This idea is more easily envisaged when juxtaposed against the prevailing 'technology centered' second and third generation CAM systems, which aim at the elusive 'people-less' system. The table below illustrates the difference between these two approaches to CAM system design in relation to the four key design choice points identified above.

In the final part of this chapter we turn our attention to how such a conceptual framework may be used proactively to inform the design of a human centered Flexible Manufacturing System (FMS).

*Table: A Comparison of Technology Centered and Human Centered CAM
          System Design Choices*

DESIGN CHOICE POINT	TECHNOLOGY CENTERED SYSTEM	HUMAN CENTERED SYSTEM
Allocation of Function	Operator carries out those functions which cannot be automated	Operator allocates functions depending upon particular circumstances during production
Control characteristics of human-system interface (human-machine)	Operator's actions paced and regulated by directives stored in the computer system	Actions at the operators' discretion. Where possible the computer system protects against major error of judgement
Control characteristics of human-system interface (machine-machine)	Centralised control system. Production machines controlled at highest possible level, e.g. part program generated at CAD level	Decentralised control system. Machines controlled at lowest possible level, e.g. part programms generated at shopfloor level
Informational characteristics of human-system interface	System status information displayed at highest possible information level. Restricted access for shopfloor personnel	System status information available at all machines. Data bases accessible to all personnel
Allocation of personnel responsibilities	Work controlled by functional specialists, e.g. programming, setting, maintenance, monitoring carried out by individual specialists	Work controlled by shopfloor operators, e.g. operator is responsible for programming, setting, micro-scheduling and monitoring

THE ROLE OF OCCUPATIONAL PSYCHOLOGY IN THE DESIGN OF CAM TECHNOLOGY:
A CASE STUDY

In 1982, work began at the University of Manchester Institute of Science and Technology (UMIST), on the design and development of an FMS in which operators are not subordinate to machines. The project team comprised two engineers, a computer scientist and an occupational psychologist, under the guidance of a steering group made up of experts from the social and engineering sciences as well as representatives from the manufacturing industry. The FMS hardware was already in situ and the principle objective of the project was to develop human centered software which would enable operators to program the FMS in order to make the first of a batch of parts.

Of particular interest to the present discussion is the project's secondary objective: to develop a methodology for the simultaneous consideration of social and technical criteria during the design of CAM technology. Whilst the conceptual framework for human centered design offers an important starting point for such a project, it requires a methodology in order to make it workable in practical, proactive research. The research question that derived from this objective was thus: how can the concept of human centeredness be operationalised in order to influence or direct the process of engineering design?

Decisional Structure and Design

Lanzara (1983) argues that design carried out by a team is difficult, not because of any internal technical complexity of a given problem, but because people do not agree about what to do. What is often lacking, and needs to be created, is a decisional structure within which to create an appropriate representation of the design problem. The UMIST team therefore devised a decisional structure based on the maximisation of user's freedom of choice over work methods and procedures.

The experience of freedom of choice in the operation of a CAM system can be related to decisions and alternatives that the system designers either allow or deny. Hence, if the structure of choices within the proposed system design can be identified in terms of the number, valency and similarity of the options available at choice points, these alternatives may be restructured to increase operator freedom of choice and control. The discussion that follows illustrates the use of choice point analysis in the design of the CNC lathe software. The reader is referred to Corbett (1985) for a more detailed account.

The first choice point (see table) concerns the allocation of functions between human and machine/computer. In contrast to the 'technocentric' approach, which involves the allocation of as many functions as possible to the machine or computer, the UMIST team utilised the concept of human-machine complementarity to aid their decision-making. In this view, the human is given responsibility for all functions and work tasks which are prone to disturbance or uncertainty, and therefore difficult or impossible to accurately pre-plan or program within a machine or computer. Such tasks require the use of discretionary skill and the interpretation of information arising during (and not prior to) task execution. Those tasks and functions which are predictable, i.e., not prone to disturbance or uncertainty, are better suited to the power of the computer which is fast and reliable but totally uncreative.

The second key choice point (see table) concerns the control characteristics of the human-computer interface. In contrast to the either-or allocation of function choices, the allocation of control between human and computer is based on the recognition that the development of CNC now places the human operator in a position of shared or concurrent control with the computer. Using the concept of complementarity, the UMIST team decided that routine (certain) functions should be placed under computer control, whilst uncertain functions and tasks should be under operator control with the option of software support. In other words, an operator of the CNC lathe component of the system is given control over the choice of tooling, for example, but can be warned automatically if the chosen tool is inappropriate for the machining task at hand.

The third key choice point concerns the informational characteristics of the human-machine interface. An operator cannot control a machine without comprehending its functioning. It is therefore important that the human-computer interface should support the operator's cognitive model of the machining process so that knowledge which is needed during infrequent task activity is obtained during general activity.

Complementarity of human and computer control relies on the design of the interface between them, on the medium and type of information and operating strategies that the two must exchange. For efficient system functioning, information should be utilised as near as possible to the point where it is generated and, in the case of uncertain tasks, this information is almost exclusively generated at the CNC lathe on the shop-floor. It was therefore agreed by the design team that interaction between operator and machine should be maximised for uncertain tasks. This entails giving the operator control, to enable data and object manipulation to be changed to fit actual, rather than normative, demands. These tasks include machine set-up, the determination of metal cutting sequences and the determination of cutting feeds and speeds. Those tasks which are routine may be software-activated (e.g. tool files, primitive mathematical functions) and only require an interactive screen editing facility.

Human-Centered Design Criteria

Whilst the decisional structure formed the framework for design decisions and choices, there was an awareness within the design team that a list of criteria was needed to enable design choices to be evaluated. Therefore, all tasks and functions that were designed during the lathe system design process were negotiated, analysed and evaluated with regard to the following three criteria:

1. COMPATIBILITY - Operation should not require skills unrelated to existing skills but should allow existing skills to evolve. The operator should input and receive information which is compatible with conventional shopfloor practice. In this way, the interface will conform to the user's prior knowledge and skill.

2. TRANSPARENCY - One cannot control a system without understanding it. Therefore, the operator must be able to 'see' the internal processes of the software in order to facilitate learning. A transparent system makes it easy for users to build up an internal model of the decision-making and control functions that the system can perform.

3. MINIMUM SHOCK - The system should not do anything which operators find unexpected in the light of the information, detailing the present state of the system, available to them.

In addition, all tasks containing a degree of uncertainty involved a further four design criteria:

1. DISTURBANCE CONTROL - Uncertain tasks (as defined by the choice structure analysis) should be under operator control with computer decision-making support.

2. FALLIBILITY - Operators' tacit skills and knowledge should not be designed out of the system. They should never be put in a position where they helplessly watch the software direct an incorrect operation.

3. ERROR REVERSIBILITY - Software should supply sufficient feedforward of information to inform the operator of the likely consequences of a particular operation or strategy.

4. OPERATING FLEXIBILITY - The system should offer operators the freedom to trade-off requirements and resource limits by shifting operating strategies, without losing software support. This criterion is discussed in detail in Corbett (1985).

Using Design Criteria

Although the decisional structure and design criteria proved a valuable guide to the design engineers, as technical questions grew in complexity, they proved of more limited value and uncertainties of interpretation typically arose in the face of particular technical problems. A number of factors may account for this. Firstly, engineering design is not simply a matter of applying criteria (technical, economic or psychological) to a design problem - there appear to be strong aesthetic and tacit knowledge elements in the design process that play an important role in the representation of a design problem within the designer's mind. Hence, good human work design criteria do not guarantee good design.

A second factor stems from the nature of the design criteria. Largely because of the absence of a coherent body of research findings relating CAM technology to the design of shopfloor jobs, it is impossible to prove, for example, that a flexible allocation of functions between human and machine necessarily contributes to the design of non-subordinate roles for system operators. In the event of a conflict between technical and work design criteria, it proved difficult to formulate a strong case for the inclusion or exclusion of a particular design solution when so little supportive empirical evidence is available. During the UMIST project, such conflicts were often resolved through the participation of prospective users.

A third factor contributing to the weakness of the criteria in influencing design stems from their generality. Even the 580 seemingly highly specific, human-computer interface design criteria developed by Smith and Aucella (1983) are not immune to this problem (Mosier and Smith, 1986).

CONCLUSION

The UMIST project experience indicates that CAM technology can be socially shaped during the design process to overcome the predominantly 'technocentric' approach to technological design. It also reveals that, whilst occupational psychology can have a role in the design and development of CAM technology, there is a pressing need for a coherent and usable methodology to make such a role more effective. As Rosenbrock (1985) has pointed out, the psychologist's model of the ideal behaviour of a design engineer "may not include the effective practice of engineering design, and the problems which arise may then be attributed to a lack of right-thinking by the engineer" (p.6). The participation of users in technical design projects does not seem to have overcome this methodological problem (see Briefs et al., 1983) and it therefore seems opportune for the research literature on the psychology of the design process to be explored and addressed to this issue. Ravden et al., (1987) and Corbett (1987b) offer examples of this approach. The experiences of human factors experts are also clearly relevant to this research endeavour.

Proactive research also requires a theoretical base from which to develop. Unfortunately, mainstream occupational psychology research into CAM technology and work is negatively defined in reaction to theories of technological determinism. Hence research findings typically reject determinism as a theory without offering an alternative. There is not yet a psychological theory of CAM technology and work which directly addresses the role of technology as a discrete independent variable in shaping the design of jobs.

This chapter has argued the case for the development of a proactive research strategy which involves both the development of theory and of method in order to critically evaluate the impact of CAM technology and to use this accumulative knowledge and understanding to inform the design and development of subsequent generations of CAM technology. Such a strategy reflects a concern that, by failing to examine the range of technological options open to us, we are permanently closing off technological options and alternative forms of work organisation. As Norbert Wiener, the founder of modern cybernetics, cautioned in a seminal paper: "Although machines are theoretically subject to human criticism, such criticism may be ineffective until long after it is relevant" (1960; p.1355).

REFERENCES

Blumberg, M. and Gerwin, D (1984). Coping with Advanced Manufacturing Technology. *Journal of Occupational Behaviour,5*, 113-130.

Boddy, D. and Buchanan, D. A. (1986). *Managing New Technology*, Oxford: Basil Blackwell.

Braverman, H. (1974). *Labor and Monopoly Capital*. New York: Monthly Review Press.

Briefs, U., Ciborra, C. and Schneider, L. (1983). Systems design for, with, and by the users. Amsterdam: North-Holland.

Brodner, P. (1982). Humane work design for man-machine systems. A challenge to engineers and labour scientists. *Proceedings of IFAC Conference on Analysis, Design and Evaluation of Man-Machine Systems*. Baden-Baden.

Buchanan, D. A (1983). Technological Imparatives and Strategic Choice. In G. Winch (Ed) *Information Technology in Manufacturing Processes*. London: Rossendale.

Buchanan, D. A and Boddy, D. (1983). *Organisations in the Computer Age*. Aldershot: Gower Press.

Burnes, B. and Fitter, M. (1986). Control of Advanced Manufacturing Technology: Supervision without Supervisors?. University of Sheffield: *SAPU Memo*. No. 801.

Child, J. (1972). Organisation structure and strategies of control. *Administrative Science Quarterly, 17*, 1-17.

Child, J. (1984). *Organisation*. London: Harper Row.

Child, J. (1987). Organisational design for Advanced Manufacturing Technology. In T. D. Wall, C. W. Clegg and N. J. Kemp (Eds.),*The Human Side of Advanced Manufacturing Technology*. Chicester: Wiley.

Clegg, C. W. and Corbett, J. M.(1987). Research and development in 'humanising' Advanced Manufacturing Technology. In T. D. Wall, C. W. Clegg and N. J. Kemp (Eds). *The Human Side of Advanced Manufacturing Technology*. Chichester: Wiley.

Clegg, C. W., Kemp, N. J. and Wall, T. D. (1984). New technology: Choice, control and skills. In G. C. van de Veer, M. J. Tauber, T. R. G. Green and P. Gorny (Eds.) *Readings on Cognitive Ergonomics: Mind and Computers*. Berlin: Springer-Verlag.

Cooley, M. and Crampton, S. (1986). Criteria for Human-Centred Systems. *Paper presented at CIM Europe Working Conference on Production Systems,* Bremen, West Germany.

Corbett, J. M. (1985). Prospective work design of a human-centred CNC lathe. *Behaviour and Information Technology, 4,* 201-214.

Corbett, J. M. (1987a). A psychological study of advanced manufacturing technology: the concept of coupling. *Behaviour and Information Technology* (in press).

Corbett, J. M. (1987b). Human work design criteria and the design process: The devil in the detail. In P. Brodner (Ed.) *Skill-Based Automated Manufacturing*. Oxford: Pergamon Press.

Dickson, D (1974). *Alternative technology and the politics of technical change*. London: Fontana.

Edwards, E. and Lees, F. P. (Eds.) (1974). *The Human Operator in Process Control*. London: Taylor and Francis.

Forester, T. (Ed) (1980). *The Microelectronics Revolution*. Cambridge, Mass: MIT Press.

Fry, L. W. (1982). Technology-Structure research: Three critical issues. *Academy of Management Journal, 25,* 532-552.

Gerwin, D. (1979). The comparative analysis of structure and technology: A critical appraisal. *Academy of Management Review, 4* 41-51.

Gouldner, A W. (1976). *The dialectic of ideology and technology*. London: MacMillan.

Habermas, J. (1971). *Toward a Rational Society*. London: Heinemann.

Ingersoll Engineers (1983). *The FMS Report*. London: IFS publications.

Jalinek, M. and Golher, J. D.(1983). The interface between strategy and manufacturing technology. *Columbia Journal of World Business*. Spring, 26-36.

Jones, B. (1982). Destruction or redistribution of engineering skills? The case of numerical control. In S. Wood (Ed.), *The Degradation of Work?*. London: Hutchinson.

Jordan, N. (1963). Allocation of functions between man and machines in automated systems. *Journal of Applied Psychology, 47,* 161-5.

Kemp, N. J. and Clegg, C. W. (1986). Information technology and job design: A case study on CNC machine tool working. University of Sheffield: *SAPU Memo. No. 716.*

Lanzara, G. F. (1983). The design process: Frames, metaphors and games. In U. Briefs, C. Ciborra and L Schneider (Eds.), *Systems Design for, with, and by the users*. Amsterdam: North Holland.

Littler, C. (1983). A history of new technology. In G. Winch (Ed.), *Information technology in manufacturing processes*. London: Rossendale.

MacDonald, S. (1985). Technology beyond machines. In E. Rhodes and D. Wield (Eds.), *Implementing New Technologies*. Oxford: Basil Blackwell.

Metal Working Production (1983). *The Fifth Survey of Machine Tools and Production Equipment in Britain*. London: Morgan-Grampian.

Milgram, S. (1974). *Obedience to Authority*. London: Tavistock publications.

Mosier, J. N. and Smith, S. L.(1986). Application of guidelines for designing user interface software. *Behaviour and Information Technology*, 5, 39-46.

Noble, D. F. (1979). Social choice in machine design: The case of automatically controlled machine tools. In A. Zimbalist (Ed.) *Case Studies on the Labour Process*. New York: Monthly Review Press.

Pierce, J. L. (1984). Job design and technology. *Journal of Occupational Behaviour*, 5, 147-154.

Price, H. E. (1985). The allocation of functions in systems. *Human Factors*, 27, 33-45.

Pugh, D., Hickson, D. and Turner, C. (1969). The context of organisational structure. *Administrative Science Quarterly*, 14, 91-114.

Rasmussen, J. (1979). Notes on human system design criteria. Invited paper for IFAC/IFIP Conference on Socio-technical Aspects of Computerisation. Budapest. *mimeo*, Riso: Danish Atomic Energy Commission.

Ravden, S. J., Johnson, G. I., Clegg, C. W. and Corbett, J. M. (1987). Human factors in the design of a flexible assembly cell. In P. Brodner (Ed.), *Skill-Based Automated Manufacturing*. Oxford: Pergamon Press

Rose, H., McLoughlin, I., King, R. and Clark, J. (1986). Opening the black box: the relation between technology and work. *New Technology, Work and Employment*, 1, 18-26.

Rosenbrock, H. H. (1982). Technology Policies and Options. In N. Bjorn-Andersen, M. Earl, O. Holst and E. Mumford (Eds.), *Information Society: For richer, for poorer*. Amsterdam: North-Holland.

Rosenbrock, H. H. (1985). Engineering design and social science. Discussion paper for ESRC/SPRU Workshop on New Technology in Manufacturing Industry, Windsor. *UMIST Project Discussion Paper 175*, University of Manchester.

Rouse, W. B. (1981). Human-computer interaction in the control of dynamic systems. *Computing Surveys, 13*, 71.

Rousseau, D. M. (1979). Assessment of technology in organisations: Closed versus Open system approaches. *Academy of Management Review, 4*, 531-542.

Seppala, P., Tuominen, P. and Koskinen, P.(1987). Job structure in a Flexible Manufacturing System. In P. Brodner (Ed.), *Skill-based Automated Manufacturing*. Oxford: Pergamon Press.

Singleton, W. T. (1971). Systems design. *Applied Ergonomics, 2*, 141-163.

Smith, S. L. and Aucella, A. F.(1983). Design guidelines for the user interface to computer-based information systems. *Technical report ESD-TR-83-122*, U.S.A.F, Hanscom, Massachusetts.

Sorge, A., Hartmann, G., Warner, M. and Nicholas, I. (1983). *Microelectronics and Manpower in Manufacturing: Applications of CNC in Great Britain and West Germany*. Aldershot: Gower.

Stanifield, G. G. (1976). Technology and structure as theoretical categories. *Administrative Science Quarterly, 19*, 183-197.

Wall, T. D. (1987). New technology and job design. In P. B. Warr (Ed.), *Psychology at Work*. (3rd Edition) Harmondsworth: Penguin.

Wall, T. D., Clegg, C. W., Davies, R. T., Kemp, N. J. and Mueller, W. S. (1987). Advanced manufacturing technology and work simplification: an empirical study. *Journal of Occupational Behaviour* (in press).

Walton, R E. (1982). Social choice in the development of advanced information technology. *Human Relations, 35*, 129-148.

Wiener, N. (1960). Some moral and technical consequences of Automation. *Science, 131*, No. 3410.

Weizenbaum, J. (1976). *Computer power and Human Reason*. San Francisco: W. H. Freeman.

Wilkinson, B. (1982). *The shopfloor politics of new technology*. London: Heinemann.

Winch, G. (1983). Organisation Design for CAD/CAM. In G Winch (Ed.), *Information Technology in Manufacturing Processes*. London: Rossendale.

Winner, L (1985). Do Artefacts have Politics? In D. A MacKenzie and J. Wajcman (Eds.), *The social shaping of technology*. Milton Keynes: Open University press.

Woodward, J. J. (1958). *Management and Technology*. London: Her Majesty's Stationery Office.

Zimbalist, A (Ed.) (1979). *Case studies of the labour process*. London: Monthly Review Press.

Psychological Issues of
Human Computer Interaction in the Work Place
M. Frese, E. Ulich, W. Dzida (Editors)
© Elsevier Science Publishers B.V. (North-Holland), 1987

THE LIMITATIONS OF TASK COMPLEXITY THROUGH INFORMATION TECHNOLOGIES: RESULTS OF A FIELD STUDY

Erhard Nullmeier and Karl-Heinz Roediger

Technical University of Berlin, Dept. of Computer Science, Sekr. FR 5-6, Franklinstr. 28/29, D-1000 Berlin 10

An interdisciplinary research project, entitled "The Structuring of Dialogue Interfaces" and sponsored by the Technical University of Berlin has developed guidelines for the design of dialogue systems based on the action-regulation theory. A tool - VERA/B - was built to analyze task complexity and the mental regulation required when a task is executed by a skilled worker using a dialogue system. VERA/B classifies tasks according to the required mental regulation and provides guidelines as to how the tasks and the dialogue system might be improved. VERA/B was evaluated in a field study by investigating 247 tasks. This paper presents the results of the study with respect to the usefulness of the tool and contains some empirical observations on the use of dialogue systems.

AIMS OF THE PROJECT

The project "The Structuring of Dialogue Interfaces" began in 1981, the year in which Moran (1981) called for an "Applied Psychology of the User" and presented his Keystroke-Level Model as the only example of what he understands by a psychology of the user. We feel that Moran's approach is not the right way to tackle the problem of human-computer interaction (Floyd, Keil & Nullmeier, 1981). Moran selected a given technology, namely existing editors, and investigated how users adapted their behaviour to this given system. The results of such studies may be considered as improving the interface of the system under investigation, but the kernel of what human-computer interaction means is not touched upon at all.

Moran stated that his model was only a beginning, and that others should build better, more appropriate models. However, we consider his point of departure to be wrong in itself. Our approach proceeds from the task to be performed by the worker. This means analyzing the task requirements and the user's actions when performing the task. Only then it is possible to design the dialogue system so as to support the performance of tasks by humans.

VERA/B - THEORETICAL BACKGROUND

Task analysis from a psychological point of view is, to begin with, an extremely difficult undertaking. We have considered only one psychological aspect of human action in the work context: the mental regulation demanded by the task. When executing a task, the worker must decompose the task's complexity and generate actions. This requires a certain degree of mental regulation.

The number, sequence, and importance of the decisions inherent in a skilled worker's task - are a measure of the quality of working life. Our concept of mental regulation requirements is based on the action-regulation theory (cf. Volpert, 1982; Frese & Sabini, 1985). One important proposition of this concept is that "action is objective; it brings about changes in the objective conditions of the environment and is at the same time in part determined by them. Action is directed neither by reaction alone nor by thought alone" (Oesterreich & Volpert, 1986, p. 508). The regulation requirements of a given task are attributable to objective conditions inherent in the task. Our project is intended to structure work and provide guidelines for the design of software systems. Thus, our interest focusses primarily on the objective conditions inherent in the task, and not the idiosyncrasies of individuals. Therefore, in structuring tasks and the use of dialogue systems in industrial and administrative work, we proceed from the psychological characteristics of the tasks involved, and not from a given technology.

VERA/B, a tool designed for analyzing clerical work (Roediger, Nullmeier, & Oesterreich, in print), is based on VERA (Volpert, Oesterreich, Gablenz-Kolakovic, Resch, & Krogoll, 1983), a tool developed for analysing industrial work. Neither VERA nor VERA/B claims to undertake a comprehensive psychological analysis of the work activity in question. Reduction to one psychological aspect only and neglect of all others - for example, communication, motivation, and mental stress - can be justified by reference to empirical studies that stress the overwhelming importance of the decision latitude (i.e. mental regulation) for the workers' health (cf. Karasek, 1979).

When designing work for specific individuals, consideration of objective requirements, such as mental regulation, does not suffice. The individual qualification of the worker as well as his own particular manner of performing a task should be taken into account (cf. Ulich, 1981). Objective requirements may be seen as a minimal criterion for the structuring of tasks, to be complemented by individuals' subjective criteria.

Our intention in developing VERA/B was to elaborate guidelines for structuring work and for designing and using dialogue systems. Our main concern was to integrate psychological criteria into the analysis and definition of system requirements (cf. Roediger, 1985). Software engineers are in great need of such a tool. Analysis and design techniques used by software developers have the advantage that they describe the necessary flow of information for executing a given task in a complete, consistent, and unequivocal way. However, these methods neither take into consideration psychological characteristics of the workers' activities, nor can they be used to structure tasks that, in some cases, do not exist when the software requirements must be determined.

The evaluation of regulation requirements in VERA/B is based on a five-level model describing the working activity in general terms (Oesterreich, 1981). This model has been further refined by the introduction of a restrictive step for each level. The model is briefly outlined in Table 1.

The examples given directly after Table 1 serve to illustrate the different levels. A field study failed to yield any example of level five. It is conceivable that heads of the departments planning the organizational development of institutions regulate their activities at level five.

Table 1: Five Level Model of Regulation Requirements

Level 5: PLANNING NEW ACTION SPACES
New interactive working processes are to be introduced and coordinated; the material conditions are to be created for them.
Level 4: COORDINATING SEVERAL ACTION SPACES
Several sub-goal plans (in the sense of level 3) for interacting parts of the working process are to be coordinated with one another.
Level 3: SUB-GOAL PLANNING
Only a roughly determined sequence of sub-activities can be planned in advance. The worker has to make plans for each sub-activity (in the sense of level 2). Only after completion of a sub-activity can further action be considered.
Level 2: ACTION PLANNING
The sequence of work-steps can be planned in advance; the planning process can be determined up to the final result.
Level 1: SENSORY-MOTOR REGULATION
No conscious planning is required for the projection of the sequence of actions to be regulated, although different tools (e.g. software systems) have to be used occasionally.

Examples:

Level 4: In an insurance company, some programmers have to adapt standard software to the requirements of the various departments. The analysis as well as the discussion of these requirements are constituent parts of their activities.

Level 3: Workers in a warehouse have to plan whether requested parts should be delivered by train, by truck, or by aircraft. They have to take into consideration changing external conditions, such as weather, the possibility of new requests from the same client, or changing discount rates.

Level 2: Workers in public administration have to respond to comprehensive inquiries of citizens. Each inquiry demands many simple sub-activities; the correct sequencing of these sub-activities determines the success of the whole activity.

Level 1: Workers have to read hand-written letters and to input some of the information, for example, the names and the corresponding insurance numbers, into a computer.

In contrast to VERA, which is designed to investigate industrial work, i.e. the processing of material, which can, to a large extent be observed directly, VERA/B requires the investigator to obtain his information mainly by interviewing the individual worker. In addition to the interview, one can observe the manipulation of data - with or without computer - that serves to represent the information being processed. Normally, the user selects a specific menu and fills out masks; he stores and manipulates data. The problem is to deduce mental regulation requirements from the observations and the interview (Roediger & Nullmeier, 1987).

EXECUTION OF THE FIELD STUDY

VERA/B was applied and evaluated by investigating 247 clerical tasks at 179 computer-aided workplaces. These workplaces were chosen from 19 companies corresponding to the following six branches (Table 2).

The field study was carried out during 1984 - 1985. More than 90 % of the analyses were done by four persons, one a psychologist, two computer scientists, and the other an engineer. Hence, they had a very similar understanding of the workplaces under investigation. This is not a disadvantage in view of the claim of VERA/B to serve as a tool for software requirements analysis and definition.

The investigation of each company took an average of two hours for obtaining general information, and about three hours for each workplace, depending on the complexity of the task to be investigated. On completion

Table 2: Number of Companies, Workplaces, and Corresponding Branches

Branch	Number of Companies	Number of Workplaces
Industry	5	50
Banking Houses	2	41
Public Administration	5	29
Insurance Companies	3	24
Pension Offices	2	24
Public Utilities	2	11
	------------	------------
	19	179

of the analysis, approximately one hour was needed to evaluate the information and to assess each workplace. Once investigation of a particular company was completed, discussions were held with - where possible - all those involved in the investigation. A number of principal areas proved to be weak-points in all the companies examined:

- Hardware Ergonomics
- Software Ergonomics (screen design, interactive techniques)
- Users' qualification gap
- Work-oriented changes of organizational structures related to the workplaces under investigation.

This list is not exhaustive, but the areas mentioned represent a good cross-section. In most cases, company executives accepted criticism of hardware and software ergonomics. To explain deficiencies, they stated that the systems were developed and implemented some years ago. The lack of user qualification and the need for organizational changes to improve work processes were much more controversial issues. Often, representatives of central departments responsible for data processing or organizational structures agreed with us, whereas the heads of specialized departments tended to defend existing organizational structures.

RESULTS OF THE FIELD STUDY

Usefulness of VERA/B as a Tool for Software Requirement Analysis

The objectivity of VERA/B is measured by keeping regulation requirements independent of both the investigator and the person under investigation. An analysis was made of 65 tasks identical both from the point of view of the organizational plan and according to the statements made by the heads of the corresponding departments.

Table 3: Results of Classifying Identical Tasks

	IR	1	2R	2	3R	3	4R	4
IR	10	2	0	0	0	0	0	0
1	2	2	3	4	0	0	0	0
2R	0	1	7	3	2	0	0	0
2	0	1	4	6	5	1	0	0
3R	0	1	0	2	0	0	0	0
3	0	0	0	1	0	5	0	0
4R	0	0	0	0	0	0	3	0
4	0	0	0	0	0	0	0	0

The deviations in classifying the required regulation levels are very small (Table 3). Most of the deviations are caused by the difficulties encountered in defining a common task as compared with several different tasks. The strict definition of a common task is as follows: a given number of work units belong together to form a common task if, and only if, one single person can process these work units at the same time. When investigating clerical work, where the main thing being processed is information, this criterion is difficult to apply: using modern information technologies, it is often possible to share information and tasks which would no doubt be single tasks without these technologies. Therefore, the expression 'can process' must be interpreted pragmatically as 'normally does process'.

When talking about VERA/B, it is sometimes objected that a high degree of concurrence can be obtained in the classification by making the different classes so large that sufficient differentiation is not possible. Thus, the results look perfect, while the real regulation levels nevertheless differ. Let us look at an extreme example: If one has only one class, no deviation can occur in classifying tasks. This objection cannot be refuted without taking into consideration the function of VERA/B: namely, to serve as a tool for the analysis and definition of task requirements with a view to improving the workplaces under investigation.

Therefore, the classification of the regulation requirements must be detailed, so as to enable isolation of certain characteristics of the task belonging strictly to this class. In addition, it must be possible to find characteristics of the task, and of neighbouring tasks, which can be modified in order to increase the regulation level of the task under investigation. This latter criterion has been tested, and in about two thirds of the cases we have discovered possibilities of improving the task by job enrichment. In a lot of cases, especially at the lower levels, we pleaded for dissolving the analyzed workplace as there was little prospect of improvement. This is caused by the extreme division of labour that is normally accelerated by the introduction of computer systems. We felt it would be better - for reasons of job satisfaction - to integrate those tasks into more demanding ones. Since tasks of lower complexity are then dissolved, the remaining tasks must be regulated at higher level. This can cause problems when the qualification of the existing workers cannot be increased to the necessary level. Then, the tasks must be adapted to existing qualifications. In nearly every case, we were able to make a lot of suggestions for improving the system interface.

Analysis of Tasks

The central idea behind VERA/B is to analyze the regulation requirements of a task. Therefore, the main result is the classification of tasks according to this criterion (Figure 1). About 80 % of the tasks investigated require a regulation level equal to, or below, two; these routine tasks can be processed by action planning or even at the sensory-motor level.

If we distinguish between tasks according to whether the worker uses the dialogue system more or less than 50 % of his working time (Figure 2), we obtain the expected result that the tasks of workers who use the system continuously have lower regulation requirements than those of workers who use their system only sporadically. There are at least two different groups of permanent users: One in computer departments, e.g. application programmers and system analysts. We have found specialists of this sort, who execute complex tasks, in banking houses and insurance companies. However, the majority of permanent users have nothing in common with these computer specialists: They simply execute tasks that cannot as yet be performed automatically by computer systems (at least not at a reasonable cost). If one considers only the latter workplaces, the situation looks even more hopeless.

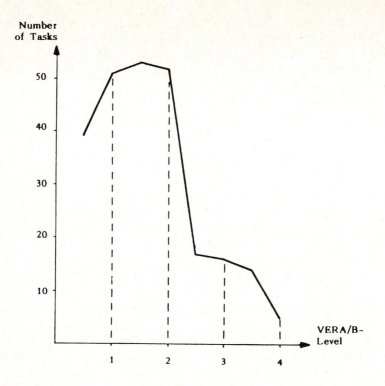

Figure 1: Classification of 247 Tasks Using VERA/B

Similarly, if we distinguish between male and female workers, we obtain the expected result that women are required to perform tasks with lower regulation levels (Figure 3).

According to Hacker (1986), "subjects prefer tasks of medium complexity. Simultaneously their efficacy proves optimal: Performance is highest without increased perceived fatigue" (p. 459). Following these results, for the majority of workers using dialogue systems, especially for female users who are working continuously with the system, the work content should be changed to increase the level of regulation.

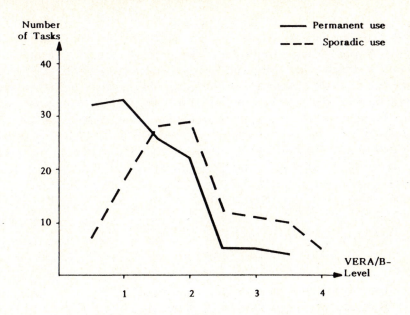

Figure 2: Permanent and Sporadic Use of Dialog Systems

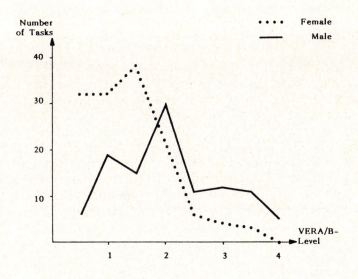

Figure 3: Classification of Male and Female Workers

We have distinguished between tasks of different branches: for example, industrial administrations as compared with insurance companies and banking houses. When carrying out the investigations, we gained the impression that tasks in industrial administrations were much more demanding than those in insurance companies, where, today, a high degree of automation has already been realized. However, as Figure 4 shows, this impression is incorrect. The discrepancy between our hypothesis and the results of the VERA/B analyses can be explained by the fact that it was more difficult for us as investigators to understand the tasks in industrial administrations than those in insurance companies. This is because the former showed greater variation in content, but not in the regulation level, which is an indicator of general planning processes, quite independent of task content.

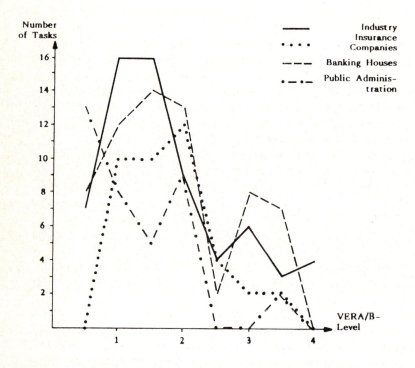

Figure 4: Classification of Tasks According to Branches

Analysis of Dialogue Systems

One section of VERA/B was used to analyze the interaction between the user and the dialogue system. This was done after analysis of the tasks. Thus, we are able to judge whether the interaction is appropriate to the task, or whether the system interface is more of a hindrance to execution of the task. We investigated the interfaces of dialogue systems in accordance with the proposal for "Principles of Dialogue Design" published by the German Institute of Standards (Deutsches Institut für Normung, 1986). Five criteria are listed in this proposal:

- Suitability for the task
- Self-descriptiveness
- Controllability
- Correspondence to user expectations
- Error tolerance

We have added one further criterion: the adaptability of the system interface by the user himself. In doing so, we have made allowences for the flexibility of recent developments as well as the unbridgeable gap between two individuals as a result of their interindividual differences. One may wish to have all the information needed simultaneously on a (perhaps) overcrowded and unstructured screen, while the other prefers page-turning. Adaptability of the interface will be helpful for both.

According to the Standards Institute's proposal, each of these criteria should be applied independently of the others. Formulation of the criteria is abstract so as to stimulate system designers to use their imagination in realizing the intentions of the proposal. The examples given for each criterion reflect the state of the art and should not prevent the development of new techniques supporting the underlying ideas, though perhaps at variance with the wording of the proposal. This cautious approach was taken so as not to hinder new developments, e.g. desktop interfaces, which were already developed at the time when the proposal was being discussed.

Many deficiencies of dialogue interfaces were observed. Their number, however, in no way indicates their importance for performing a given task. Thus, a quantitative comparison would be pointless. Nevertheless, we hope to give some idea of the most frequent problems encountered when carrying out our analyses.

First of all, it is a noteworthy fact that we have only looked at companies with their own DP department and which produce their own software. Most of the analyzed software was therefore tailor-made. Only a small part was standard software, such as word processing systems, editors, data base systems etc. We assume that the companies willing to submit to our analyses hoped to gain some quick ideas for their own software development.

On the question of suitability for the task, the German Standards Institute's proposal states: "A dialogue is fit for the task it has to perform if it supports the user in the job he is actually doing without an unnecessary additional strain being placed on him by the system itself" (p. 3). The predominant problems encountered in this respect are response time, divergence between screen design and written forms, and the necessity for inputting data which could be generated by the system itself.

"A dialogue is self-descriptive if, on request, the user can obtain an explanation of the purpose and the capabilities of the dialogue system and if each step of the dialogue is immediately comprehensible..." (p. 5). The main problem here is that nearly half of the analyzed software systems does not have any help system; the only source of explanatory notes is a handbook; sometimes, not even this is available.

"A dialogue is said to be controllable if the user can influence the speed of operation as well as the selection and sequence of the tools or type and scope of inputs and outputs" (p. 6). The deficiencies encountered here are: the lack of a general UNDO-statement; system-driven sequencing of dialogue steps; difficulties in returning back to the point where the dialogue was ceased.

A dialogue is said to be adaptable if the user can freely select tools, which are adequate for the job he is actually doing, according to his individual talent and wont. The only problem here is that we did not find any system fulfilling these requirements.

"A dialogue corresponds to user expectations if the system's dialogue behavior is based on user's experience with work processes as well as experiences formed in the course of using the system" (p. 8). Deficiencies according to this criterion are: non-homogeneous command languages, non-homogeneous messages, and changing screen-partitioning.

"A dialogue is error-tolerant if the intended result is obtained despite recognizably faulty input without or with only minimal correction effort" (p. 10). Main problems with this category are missing directions for fault correction, no tolerance with typing errors, and unspecific error messages.

All individual considerations apart: the more demanding the task, the worse was the dialogue interface. The most simple tasks were found to be supported by the best dialogue interfaces. This does not mean that all the criteria listed in the proposal were fulfilled, but nearly all the criteria appropriate to the task in hand. One reason for this fact may be that it is simpler to implement a good interface for such tasks. Another, even more important, interpretation is that problems of dialogue interfaces are the most evident deficiencies, and can be removed the most easily without tackling the kernel of the job: the content of the task itself.

WORK-ORIENTED DIALOGUE SYSTEMS - DESIGN AND USE

The use of dialogue systems was investigated in companies with extensive and little experience in computer systems. We feel that the amount of experience is less important than the generation of a software system; a new generation is a totally new software system implemented on the basis of prior experience with at least one former system. Some companies that were still using the first software generation for one specific application had already made profound advances in other application areas. The experiences gained here have proved to be of great benefit for further applications.

As a result of a distinction between software systems of the first generation and newer ones (experienced) we have perceived that newer generations of software offer a greater range of resulting workplaces and tasks both with very high and very low regulation requirements (Figure 5).

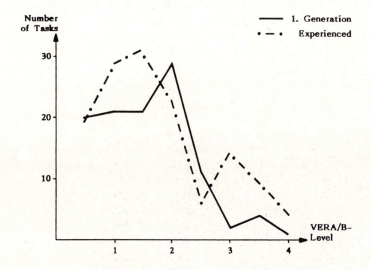

Figure 5: Classification of Tasks and Software Generations

In another context, we have analyzed software systems for production planning and control (Nullmeier & Roediger, 1986). Here, the philosophy behind computer-aided work was vital for the resulting systems. Older systems, and, unfortunately, also many new systems, are based on the principle that as many human activities as possible should be performed by the system. Computer scientists as well as engineers have internalized this view; and this is the point that we (Floyd et al., 1981) have criticized.

In the late seventies, this view changed a little: Some computer scientists and psychologists realized that humans are at their best, not when doing as little as possible, but when they are offered a challenge. All tasks that cannot, or should not, be totally computerized, thus calling for qualified human actions, can profit from human capabilities and flexibility, but are susceptible to human errors, too. The development of human capabilities and the avoidance of errors is highly dependent on human activities. This change of view - known as the principle of the active operator - did not come from scientists themselves, but was a result of severe failures of man-machine systems, for example in aircraft (Lomov, Ponomarenko, & Saverlowa, 1971) and nuclear power plants such as Three Miles Island.

Figure 6 illustrates the qualitative effects of the classical system-oriented philosophy on mental regulation requirements. In the case of badly designed systems permitting the user to perform his task without using the system, it could be said that the more elaborate the system, the lower the regulation level.

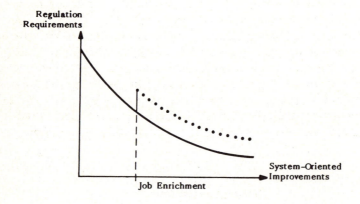

Figure 6: Influence of a System-Oriented Design on Regulation Requirements

If one wishes (as is the professed aim of the German Government Programme for the Humanization of Working Life) to enrich work by adding new tasks to the existing ones, the positive effect is likely to be only transient, enduring, at best, only as long as government support is available. We have looked at a number of German banking houses which have combined previously isolated tasks - investments, credits, saving accounts and deposit accounts - to form one common task. The underlying idea behind this organizational change came from advertizing: The aim was to have as many services as possible, which might be required by a particular client performed by one and the same employee. This is desirable from the point of view of industrial psychology, too, since the resulting tasks demand higher regulation levels. However, there is a danger that all the important decisions are transferred to the software system and that the regulation level consequently drops to the initial one.

To avoid this drawback, two things are necessary: to enrich work as was done by the banking houses; and to design systems in such a way that they truly support their users and do not make human judgement superfluous. This was the design philosophy behind a still experimental production planning system (Jahn & Kalb, 1985): Here, not a single decision is performed by the system, but the effects of each user action are directly visible on the screen; also, all actions can be cancelled by a general UNDO-statement.

In contrast to the classical system-oriented approach of rationalization, the work-oriented approach does not affect the regulation level: it remains constant. The required regulation level cannot be seen as an isolated criterion: it must correspond to an appropriate qualification level in order to ensure perceptible job satisfaction. Otherwise, a high regulation level can result in unresolved strain (Kasarek, 1979). A certain qualification gap can be compensated by human capabilities (coping processes). However, if the gap exceeds this level, stress normally remains. This stress can be reduced by a work-oriented system whose features can be used to retrieve the information necessary to perform the task and which can stimulate learning by simulating experimental steps. In other words: The information and simulation features of the system enable the objectively required regulation level to be transformed into perceptible job satisfaction.

CONCLUSIONS

In the field study, we looked at a number of unsatisfactory computer-aided workplaces which did not allow high mental regulation. People were seen as mere appendages of computer systems,, and not as intelligent beings. However, by applying modern software technology in a work-oriented manner, it is possible to improve tasks not only at the level of human-computer interaction, but at a more fundamental level, i.e. the division of labour between human beings as well as between human and computer. As we were able to observe in many companies, modern technologies provide opportunities for significantly improving work, but also for dissolving jobs.

There are a number of ways of influencing the development and application of software: By laying down standards; by participation in the software development process; or by calling for more challenging tasks. VERA/B is a tool which can be used to anticipate some of the effects of definitive design decisions and can therefore be applied in a participative development process even before building prototypes.

REFERENCES

Deutsches Institut für Normung e.V. (1986). *DIN 66 234 - VDU work stations, Part 8: Principles of dialogue design* (Second editorial draft). Berlin: Beuth-Verlag.

Floyd, C., Keil, R. & Nullmeier, E. (1981). Letter to the Editor-in-Chief. *ACM Computing Surveys, 13,* 491-492.

Frese, M. & Sabini, J. (Eds.) (1985). *Goal Directed Behavior.* Hillsdale: Lawrence Erlbaum Ass.

Hacker, W. (1986). What should be computerized. In: F. Klix & H. Wandke (Eds.) (pp 445-461), *MACINTER*-1. Amsterdam: Elsevier.

Jahn, S. & Kalb, H. (1985). Arbeiten am PPS-Facharbeitsplatz: Interaktion mit Werkzeugen. In: H.-J. Bullinger (Ed.), *Software-Ergonomie '85* (pp. 260-269), Stuttgart: Teubner

Karasek, R.A. Jr (1979). Job Demands, Job Decision Latitude, and Mental Strain: Implications for Job Redesign. *Administrative Science Quarterly, 24,* 285-311.

Lomov, B.F., Ponomarenko B.A., & Saverlowa, N.D. (1971). Das Prinzip des aktiven Operateurs und die Funktionsverteilung zwischen Mensch und Maschine. *Wosprosni Psychologii, 5,* 1-21.

Moran, T.P. (1981). An Applied Psychology of the User. *ACM Computing Surveys, 13,* 1-11.

Nullmeier, E. & und Roediger, K.-H. (1986). Arbeitsorientierte Anforderungen an die Gestaltung von PPS-Systemen. In: H. Hirsch-Kreinsen & R. Schultz- Wild (Eds.), *Rechnerintegrierte Produktion* (pp. 111-142), Frankfurt: Campus.

Oesterreich, R. (1981). *Handlungsregulation und Kontrolle.* München: Urban & Schwarzenberg.

Oesterreich, R. & Volpert, W. (1986). Task Analysis for Work Design on the Basis of Action Regulation Theory. *Economic and Industrial Democracy, 7,* 503-527.

Roediger, K.-H. (1985). Beiträge der Softwareergonomie zu den frühen Phasen der Softwareentwicklung. In: H.-J. Bullinger (Ed.), *Software-Ergonomie '85* (pp. 455-464), Stuttgart: Teubner.

Roediger, K.-H. & Nullmeier, E. (1987). Work Design instead of System Design. In: K. Fuchs-Kittowski, P. Docherty, P. Kolm, & L. Mathiassen (Eds.), *Proceedings of the IFIP TC/WG9.1 Conference on System Design for Human Development and Productivity:*

Participation and Beyond. Berlin, GDR 12-15 May 1986, Amsterdam: North-Holland.

Roediger, K.-H., Nullmeier, E. & Oesterreich, R. (in print). *Verfahren zur Ermittlung von Regulationserfordernissen in der Arbeitstätigkeit im Büro (VERA/B)*.

Ulich, E. (1981). Subjektive Tätigkeitsanalyse als Voraussetzung autonomieorientierter Arbeitsgestaltung (pp. 327-347), In: F. Frei & E. Ulich (Eds.), *Beiträge zur psychologischen Arbeitsanalyse*. Bern: Huber.

Volpert, W. (1982). The Model of the Hierarchical-Sequential Organization of Action, (pp. 35-51). In: W. Hacker, W. Volpert, & M. von Cranach (Eds.), *Cognitive and Motivational Aspects of Action*. Amsterdam: North-Holland.

Volpert, W., Osterreich, R., Gablenz-Kolakovic, S., Krogoll, T. & Resch, M. (1983). *Verfahren zur Ermittlung von Regulationserfordernissen in der Arbeitstätigkeit (VERA)*. Köln: Verlag TÜV-Rheinland.

Psychological Issues of
Human Computer Interaction in the Work Place
M. Frese, E. Ulich, W. Dzida (Editors)
© Elsevier Science Publishers B.V. (North-Holland), 1987

OFFICE AUTOMATION - AN ORGANIZATIONAL PERSPECTIVE

Jörg Sydow

Institute of Management, Freie Universität Berlin,
Garystraße 21, D-1000 Berlin 33, Federal Republic of Germany

Typically, a psychologist's conception of office automation is restricted to human-computer interaction at the work place. Empirical evidence in this area focuses on technological features, and on the office worker. By defining office automation from an organizational perspective, this paper underlines the essentially organizational character of the use of a given technology. In order to exemplify this organizational perspective of office automation, recent technological developments are related to organizational strategies of implementation and usage. Particular reference is made to the organizational concept of the scope of choice. Theoretical approaches from industrial sociology and organizational theory are presented, which have been largely neglected by organizational and work psychologists. They offer a ground for a better understanding of the limits and possibilities of organizational design within automated office settings. These approaches, however, need to be complemented by psychological research on the subjective perception and meaning of a given scope of organizational choice to designers of sociotechnical systems.

THE PSYCHOLOGIST'S CONCEPTION OF OFFICE AUTOMATION

Office automation is a popular theme in psychological research to-day. While the bulk of psychologcial research on this matter is still carried out within the framework of human factors and cognitive science, there is an increasing amount of research paying attention to the organizational context of human-computer interaction.(1). This tendency is mainly evoked by the research of work, organizational and industrial psychologists.

Typically, the psychologist's conception of sociotechnical innovations such as office automation is by and large individualistic focussing on the office worker, as he or she perceives and evaluates them while neglecting the organizational context of this innovation. The results of this kind of *impact* research serve as a basis for recommendations on the design of hard- and software, of training programms, of work content. Besides impact research, psychologists more often conduct research related to the *process* of design. This process, in which managers, systems designers, organizational consultants, worker representatives, and not least the office workers themselves interact is also mostly conceptualized from an individualistic perspective. Although extensive psychological research has been carried out in the area of management (organizational behavior, leadership, organizational design), psychologists predominantly focusing on the individual interacting with the new technology seem largely to neglect the analysis of managerial behavior in their research on office automation.

The individualistic conception of office automation does not hold true for some British, German and Scandinavian psychologists who work close to the ideas of sociotechnical systems theory and related approaches (e.g. Ulich 1981, Baisch & Troy 1986, Westlander 1987).(2) In general, work and organizational psychologists are increasingly considering the organizational and socio-economic context of office automation and do not leave this to radical psychologists alone (e.g. Projektgruppe Automation und Qualifikation 1978). This tendency to recognize the importance of the organizational context of office automation can even be observed for some human-factor researchers (Knave & Widebäck 1987). This paper aims at encouraging psychologists to adopt even more of an organizational perspective. This could be achieved by starting with a definition of office automation from an organizational perspective.

DEFINING OFFICE AUTOMATION FROM AN ORGANIZATIONAL PERSPECTIVE

The *office* is considered as an organization of human beings (office workers) and machines (office technology) designed for processing information (Pirker 1962). *Automation* aims at the substitution of human work by technology and at the technological assistance of the remaining workers. Moreover, the notion of automation takes into account the conceptual interrelationship of technology and work organization as equally important strategies of work rationalization (Sydow 1985a). *Office automation*, hence, is a strategy comprising office technologies and organizational structures of different kinds in order to substitute office work carried out by office workers and to provide technological assistance to the remaining office workers. The latter aim usually being emphasized by the notion of Computer Aided Office (CAO).

Technological Aspects of Office Automation

In face of the permanent and short cycled innovation in the field of office technology, it is unsuitable to develop an appropriate definition of office automation which is bound to concrete technologies such as data terminals, personal computers, word processors or telecommunication technologies. This is of outstanding importance as some of these concrete technologies are often confounded with specific strategies of office automation such as individualized data processing or personal computing. The personal computer, for instance, may or may not be subject to an office automation strategy called personal computing. This is a matter of organizational choice.

It should be clear by now that office automation is *not* synonymous with text processing and telecommunication and, in this way supplementary to traditional electronic data processing used solely for automating well-defined routine tasks. Office automation is rather based on information technologies as it is on communication technologies and is applied to routine as it is to non-routine tasks.

Presently, and there is no indication that this will change in the future, the technological component of office automation may be characterized by *two integrative tendencies*: integration at the level of display units (either terminals or work stations) and integration at the level of communication networks and services. Both tendencies are concerned with the integration of different modes of communication such as data, text, voice, graphics and image.

Integration of office technology at the level of the visual display unit (VDU) is revealed by the usage of one single terminal/work station for data, text, graphics and finally voice and image processing. Currently available terminals/work stations do not as yet demonstrate this maximum level of integration. Office systems, personal computers and multifunctional terminals, however, are examples of office technologies utilizing a relatively high level of integration. The spread of multifunctional VDUs will certainly increase the scope of organizational choice and thereby the need for intentional organizational choices.

A parallel technological innovation aims at the *integration at the level of communication networks and services*. Communication networks such as the transport oriented local area network (LAN) and the host centered micro-mainfraim-connection (MMC) and traditional telephone networks (PABX) are currently and jointly used to integrate terminals and work stations into a communication network. In the 90s these networks will find a common denominator in the digitalization of telephone networks and the development of open communication networks according to international standards (ISDN). For the first time, this kind of communication network will provide different kinds of communication services such as Btx, Ttx, Fax, mailing and printing at any work place. It is open to question as to whether these two integrative tendencies of the development of office technology will be accompanied by an organizational integration.

Organizational Aspects of Office Automation

Technologies used for automation are inherently of an organizational character: "The true characteristic of automation is that the combination of technological means constitutes a process through technological integration where the human being, as a connecting link, is substituted. From that it can be derived that automation, being basically a manifestation of technology, exhibits organizational aspects. The substance of organization is the integrative structuring of entirities, which is also characteristic of the technological manifestation of automation. It follows that in automated systems specific organizational principles materialize through technological means" (Grochla 1964, p. 666). Automated systems furthermore make use of both a technological *and* an organizational concept. And both are not principally different, since they are "the result of complementary decisions on the productive use of industrial work made at different points in time and with a different time coverage... The technology installed may be conceived as being a materialized form of organizational regulations" (Fricke 1975, p. 33). Others consequently speak of information technology as a "quasi-organizational design parameter" (Kubicek 1975, p. 31) or even consider information technology to be a "technology of organization and control" (Brandt, Kündig, Papadimitriou & Thomae 1978; details on this are given below).

All these quotations demonstrate that information and communication technology used for the automation of office work is of an inherently organizational character. However, office automation also has a rather autonomous organizational dimension: the work organization which has not (yet) been done by software design. Due to the ongoing process of automation more and more structuring and organizing of office work is being done by software design, i.e. technology is amalgating more and more work organization. But the organization of office work still has to complement technology made up of hardware and software in order to form a complete sociotechnical system.

Many practitioners and scholars of organizational science seem to observe a tendency towards *organizational integration* accompanying the two kinds of technological integration stated above. Office systems and personal computers embodied into a communication network, for example, allow for a re-integration of formerly separated office procedures. They assume the (re-)appearance of the text-processing clerk and the spread of integrated clerical work. Some even expect the integration of office work with factory work (take the concept of Computer Aided Industry (CAI) comprising CIM and CAO as an example). However, this organizational integration of work is optional: whether office work is (re-)integrated or subject to a continuing Tayloristic design is a matter of organizational choice.

It is true that the re-integration of office work (content) is not (yet) very common in office automation. Rather organizational practice is characterized by organizational conservatism (Child, Ganter & Kieser 1986). "The technologies are employed far below their 'social potential'; that is, they are used socially in a far more 'conservative' way than it is technically possible" (Littek 1985, p. 66). Reasons for this organizational conservatism are, among others,

- the relative difficulty to change social systems (in contrast to mere technical ones) and to establish the most efficient organizational structure
- the resistance towards the redistribution of power and influence
- the general lack of appropriate methodologies for the analysis and design of offices as sociotechnical systems.

Despite this conservatism some organizational strategies comprising technological as well as organizational aspects may well be identified.

Strategic Aspects of Office Automation

The organizational aspect of office automation is of a twofold nature. Apart from office automation embracing organization as an autonomous aspect and as a phenomenon which is inherent to office technology, office automation is an *organizational strategy* in itself. In this context the notion of organization is used in its institutional rather than functional meaning. Office automation is considered to be an organizational strategy to enhance productivity but even more so to overcome the contradictory demands of production economics (mass production of information at low cost) and market economics (individual just-in-time production of strategically important information), i.e. to enhance organizational flexibility. As a strategy comprising technology and work organization it is a critical success factor and links organizational action to the turbulent environments of many organizations (Emery & Trist 1965).

Examples of such strategies are:

- host-centered computing accompanied by a rigid standardization of work
- personal computing allowing for more discretion at the work place
- office systems centered automation assisting integrated clerical work
- office communication via ISDN supplementing face to face communication in offices.

The *strategy of host-centered computing* and accompanying standardization of office work still is the most popular strategy of office automation, at least in large organizations. But it also is the strategy which contributes the least to organizational flexibility. In this case, the traditional computing facilities often based on the concept of distributed data processing (DDP) are also used for word and graphics processing applications. This allegedly out-dated strategy of office automation possesses advantages which no other strategy has: the broad utilization of existing resources and, most importantly, the central control over the use of these resources. Nevertheless, this strategy is criticized most with respect to its ability to respect the laws of market economics. But it has to be remembered that almost the same resources could also be used for individualized data processing, the possible outcome of a *different* organizational choice.

In contrast, the fashionable *strategy of personal computing* based either on individualized data processing applications on the host or on personal computers is somewhat under the control of the office worker, especially if he or she is able to develop his/her own applications. This strategy of personal computing is intentionally accompanied by a relatively wide scope of discretion by the office worker over his or her work organization. Personal computing as a strategy of office automation is therefore different from the disorganized spread of personal computers complained about by many computer department managers.

The *office system centered strategy* of office automation is often based on activities of the organization department in charge of the buying and implementation of traditional office technolgies such as type writers and word processors. The efficient implementation and usage of office systems presupposes a comprehensive re-organization of the office work process. The division of work between clerks and typists, for example, has to be reallocated as has the specialized work organization between different clerks (both aiming at the integration of clerical work). In any of these cases, a detailed analysis of the existing organization of the office seems to be indispensible.

Finally, the *office communication strategy* is often initiated by the technical department in charge of the servicing of the organizational telephone network. Only as long as the internal usage of ISDN compatible telecommunication facilities is not able to substitute for intensively used computer networks, this strategy is largely compatible with existing organizational structures.

In all these four cases both elements, technology as well as organizational design, are an outcome of largely independent but interrelated choices. The chosen strategy of office automation manifests itself in the kind of communication network. While the host-centered strategy of standardization is based upon MMC, the office system centered strategy as well as the strategy of personal computing make use of either MMC or LAN. The office communication strategy finally centers around ISDN. In all these cases, the work stations, by integration into the communication network lose their "organizational virginity" if they ever had any, when being used as stand alone systems. Electronic communication requires the adherance to specific standards and regulations.

Because of the long-term investment in these networks, the need to develop a true strategy of office automation is rapidly increasing. There seems to be some indication that the equal importance of organizational and technological aspects of office automation is recognized by management, sometimes climaxing in the request for putting organization ahead of technology when automating office work (Bullinger 1985).

THE RELEVANCE OF THE SCOPE OF ORGANIZATIONAL CHOICE TO OFFICE AUTOMATION

In the elaboration of the strategic aspects of office automation, it has been implicitly assumed that there is at least some scope of organizational choice. In fact, all practitioners of work and organizational design and most researchers agree that there is a scope of organizational choice, i.e. there is more than one optimum organizational design. The size of this scope, at least to some extent, is said to depend on the technology in use.

While there is little controversy that the scope of organizational choice is fairly small with traditional centralized computer systems, it is widely hoped that, in the face of advanced office technology systems designers will regain the scope they had at their disposal in times of manual-type office work. Moreover, Beinum (1981) claims: "Microelectronics offers us opportunities to design jobs and organise work in accordance with the values of the quality of working life in a way that no other technology in industrialized society has done in the past" (p. 6). The less deterministic character of new office technologies is said to result from the fact that (programmable) software makes up the core of these technologies and that, among other things, their economics are difficult to establish.

Actually, empirical studies of the impact of these technologies on the work situation of secretaries, typists and clerks have produced very diverse evidence, seeming to substantiate the alleged existence of a scope of organizational choice. A review of empirical studies on the change of clerical work due to the introduction of office technology carried out by the author shows that the results are particularly diverse as such dimensions of work organization as work content, time structure and human interaction are concerned (Sydow 1985a). However, this review also makes clear that the empirical evidence is less contradictory with regard to an intensification of work, a change of control structure, an increase of standardization and formalization, and a further abstractification of office work.

The assertion that there is a scope of organizational choice is not surprising for psychologists. In face of their individualistic orientation, psychologists in general and also most work and organizational psychologists have never doubted the potential of individuals to make organizational choices. Because of this more or less voluntaristic orientation they tend to overlook the structural limitations imposed on organizational choices. Precisely because of this voluntaristic orientation of much psychological research on office automation it seems useful to make some reference to the literature of organizational theory and industrial sociology which discusses many orientations lying on the bipolar continuum between voluntarism and determinism. Some psychologists already have recognized the importance of the notion "scope of choice" (3), depicting a concept which could bridge methodologically the gap between volunatrism and determinism in theories of organizations (Sydow 19895a).

Approaches from Organizational Theory and Industrial Sociology

All recent theories of organization thematize the scope of organizational choice. Either they simply assume some scope of choice without looking at it in more depth or they develop a theoretical understanding of the problem. The former group comprises pure behavioral approaches and concepts of the organizational culture debate (c.f. Jelinek, Smircich & Hirsch 1983, Schein 1985). The latter group of organizational theories includes such popular approaches as sociotechnical systems theory (Trist 1981), contingency theory (Woodward 1958, Burns & Stalker 1961, Thompson 1967), population ecology (Hannan & Freeman 1977, Aldrich 1979) and the resource dependence approach (Pfeffer & Salancik 1978) as well as most approaches from industrial sociology (4).

The contrasting of organizational theories of the 1980s such as the population ecology model on the one hand and the current interest in the concept of organizational culture on the other demonstrates clearly that the views on the scope of organizational choice continue to be diverse: while the former reduces organizational design to organizational adaption and consequently neglects the influence of proactive choices, the latter tends to deny the relevance of the hard-fact context and includes its reflection in terms of symbols, myths and values only.

Due to the limitations of space only two of these approaches will be discussed here in more detail: sociotechnical systems theory and contingency theory. Both theories may be refered to as dominant paradigms in organization theory (Van de Ven & Joyce 1981). Moreover, both specifically deal with the relationship between technology and work organization. It is interesting to note that sociotechnical systems theory was developed by industrial psychologists. Despite this, only few work and organizational psychologists make use of this concept in their research on office automation.

Contingency theory started with the assumption that technology determines organizational structure (Woodward 1958). This assumption of technological determinism was not seriously questioned by contingency theorists until the introduction of the concept of strategic choice by Child (1972). Child clarified that the inclusion of the organizational strategy as an outcome of strategic choice, which will improve the explanatory power of contingency theory. According to this concept, the organizational strategy mediates the relationship between the context and the structure of an organization. The contextual factors, such as the uncertainty and com-plextity of the environment or as the technology in use, are not entirely taken as given, they may themselves be the object of organizational strategies. Child succeeds in overcoming situational determinism, one of the features of traditional contingency theory which has been criticized most (e.g. Schreyögg 1980). He believes that much of the scope of organizational choice results from the minor impact of organization structure on organizational effectiveness and from the difficulties to assess this impact before choosing one design alternative. More recently the concept of organizational choice within the framework of contingency theory has been extended and specified. While Montanari (1978) and even more so Bobbitt & Ford (1980) introduced some behavioral constructs (perceived power, cognitive and motivational orientation of designers) into the framework developed by Child, Hage (1977) pointed to the importance of the time factor in developing a theory of organizational choice. Kubicek (1980), taking up this thought developed a concept of limited choice of structural choices which stresses the importance of socio-economic constraints on structural decisions in capitalist economies.

Sociotechnical systems theory, in contrast, dropped the assumption of a deterministic relationship between technology and work organization very early. The belief in the existence of structural equivalents, however, was not a theoretical supposition of the researchers at the Tavistock Institute for Human Relations, but an important outcome of their very early action research. The researchers at the Tavistock Institute agreed early on the existence of organizational choices (Trist, Higgin, Murray & Pollock 1963), however they have always differed on the assessment of the scope of this choice. Their assessment varies from a fairly voluntaristic approach to a very sceptical assessment of the flexibility of technology and organizational variables (Sydow 1985b). These differences can only in part be attributed to the various technologies under consideration. Sociotechnical systems theory does not state any other variable apart from technology (and here and there culture) which has to be explored in order to determine the scope of organizational choice available to the designer. In particular, the role of economic constraints is not stated very clearly (Sydow 1985b).

Surprisingly, much more about the role of economic constraints on the scope of organizational choice can be learned from industrial sociology than from these two organizational theories. Without going into detail into these approaches, some of their theoretical arguments will be taken up in the following discusssion of the implications for the debate of organizational choice in the context of office automation. This discussion will shed some light on the ambivalence of the theme, i.e. of the size of the given 'objective' scope of organizational choice in automated office settings.

Implications for the Debate of Organizational Choice in the Context of Office Automation (5)

Considering the scope of organizational choice in automated office settings at least two aspects of the problem have to be discussed in some detail. Both have been mentioned in the presentation of the two organizational theories dealing with the concept of organizational choice: the technological aspect and the economic aspect.

As stated above, the existence of a significant scope of organizational choice has almost always been expressed for new office technology. The above quotation of Beinum and the following one of Walton (1982) illustrate this attitude: "Information technology is less deterministic than other basic technologies that historically have affected the nature of work and people at work" (p. 1076). Many quotations of a similar kind could be added to these two. The less deterministic character of office technology, if substantiated at all, is mainly derived from the fact that
- computers are multi-purpose maschines made up of software which can easily be redesigned
- communication technology allows for a spatial as well as time decoupling of office work processes
- the economic costs and benefits of these technologies as applied in offices are difficult to determine.

Some scepticism about this reasoning seems to be called for. At least four technologically related arguments clarify that modern office technology is not characterized by an arbitrary flexibility with respect to organizational structures, but is fairly ambivalent in this respect.

Implications of Technology Related Reasoning

First, it is true that information and communication technology is multi-functional and mainly made up of software. However, it is less true that software can easily be (re-)designed in order to adapt it to a given work organization. One reason for this is the complexity of modern computer programmes, another, related reason, is the growing importance of standardized software, which is developed and very successfully marketed due to its relatively low price. The organization buying and using standard software is usually not able to adapt this to its organizational structures. Instead, it adjusts the structure to the technology, especially since organizational concepts are supplied together with the office technology. Another reason for this tendency to adapt the work organization to technology rather than vice versa is related to the spread of user-friendly computer programmes. This development makes the redesign and adaptation of software to organizational structures even more difficult and costly. On the other hand, the development of fifth generation programming languages may counteract these tendencies.

Secondly, and resulting from the fact that software takes over organizational functions, office technology is considered to be a "technology of organization and control" (Brandt, Kündig, Papadimitriou & Thomae 1978). This notion implies that information technology does not only form a framework within which work may be organized (so the common assertion of industrial sociology); this technology rather organizes and controls work and the whole production process. Modern information and communication technology serve the purpose of rational dovetailing of technology and organization, unifying formerly segmented information and control systems, and organizing the timely planned use of resources. Both features differentiate - according to Brandt et al. - this particular technology from conventional production and office technologies. Modern office technology is directly able to monitor not only the output of office work but also the work behavior. Even in the case of spatial and/or time decoupling of work processes, this technology increases the transparancy of the organization by passing the relevant information from the operating level directly on to management. Organizational regulations, mainly put into practice in reaction to pressure from unions or the works council, may delimit the use of the control function of office technology, but they cannot put it out of action. The potential of this technology to rationally dovetail technology and organization decreases the scope of organizational choice, as it makes the organization more autonomous of qualified employees, who had the function of the rational dovetailing of technology and organization in the past. Hence, there is less of an economic need to design work situations offering a high quality of working life for many where only a few remain in vital jobs. In consequence, conceiving information and communication technology as a technology of organization and control makes it - contrary to the cited assumptions - appearing fairly deterministic.

Thirdly, office automation leads to an abstractification of work. Office automation necessarily involves VDU work, and VDU work, it may be argued, offers to some extent no real alternative to the user regardless what the content of work is like. The strategy of job enrichment for example may lead to a delegation of decision making, but only to a form of decision making 'by pressing the key'. Furthermore, the office worker using a VDU cannot monitor any more the work process, its material inputs and outputs directly, but only its symbolic representation on the screen, which more often is "information taken out of its context" (Goodman & Perby 1985, p. 29). Symbolic representation is not necessarily bound to the use of modern office technology (take traditional office work as an example); but the use of this technology abstractifies office work once more. Zuboff (1982) expresses this tendency towards abstractification by his term of "computer-mediated work". Nevertheless, there are two phenomena counteracting this tendency towards abstractification: the development of self-explanatory software using icons depicting documents, files, records, services, and so forth, and the possible spread of VDU work combined with non VDU work ("Mischarbeitsplätze"). The influence of the former development on the process of abstractification has yet to be investigated by psychologists and cannot as yet be judged definitively. The possibly counteracting influence of the latter, in my view, seems to be very doubtful: The ongoing process of office automation and, hence, the spread of computer-mediated work will hardly leave any non VDU office work behind which might be combined with VDU work.

Forth, office automation based on complex information and communication technology tends to be irreversible. Organizations having entered the adventure of installing and using computers have hardly a chance of turning back the wheel of history (Weizenbaum 1976). This kind of automation assumes a thorough analysis of office work processes and incorporates a multitude of work process related knowledge substituting, at some point in time, the knowledge of employees. The resulting lack of qualification makes it almost impossible to withdraw this technology from the organization and to return to former organizational structures, even if the installation of the technology turned out to be inefficient. This irreversibility is less true for usage of micro computers and word processors as long as they represent stand alone systems. But when they become an element of an organization's wide communication system, the same reasoning may apply to these relatively low complex office technologies.

These four arguments, the argument of office technology being a technology of organization and control and the argument of this technology leading to a further abstractification of office work in particular, in some respect, seem to justify the notion of a "new technological determinism" (Sydow 1985a, p. 464). While modern office technology is in fact more flexible with respect to some dimensions of work organization such as space and time and richness of work content than any other technology that has historically affected the quality of working life, it is less flexible with respect to others such as control and the physical appearance of the work content. In any case, however, even this new technological determinism, like any situational determinism, may be reduced to economic considerations. Leaving economic considerations aside, office automation could be avoided completely or at least directed in a way that avoids a negative impact on the quality of working life.

Implications of Economic Based Reasoning

Office automation is an organizational strategy which is able to overcome the contradictory demands of production economics and market economics allowing for the simultaneous achievement of productivity and flexibility. The endeavour to increase productivity and flexibility, however, is not accomplished in a straigt forward manner. The reasons given below ensure that scopes of organizational choice arise from economic considerations where technological reasoning doubted their existence.

The *first* reason based on economics concerns the imperfect knowledge of management of the 'one best way' of organizational design. The novelty of many applications and the rapid innovation of information and communication technologies augment this lack of management knowledge. The current diversity of organizational arrangements with a given technology, however, does not necessarily prove the existence of a wide scope of organizational choice, due to the allegedly slight deterministic character of this technology. It may also perfectly illustrate this current lack of knowledge. If this is true the time will come when the economic optimum of technological *and* organizational design, the close interrelationship of which is typical of automation, will become more clear to the systems designer. Consequently, the size of the scope of organizational choice, which seems to be fairly wide today, may then be somewhat smaller.

A *second* related reason is of a methodological nature. There is no single appropriate and comprehensive technique to evaluate sociotechnical designs. The usage of a "total economic cost measurement" (Davis 1957) will certainly result in economically feasible design alternatives, which are entirely different to those produced if a very narrow concept of organizational efficiency is used. The inclusion of costs arising from absenteeism, employee turnover and sabotage, for instance, results in a different set of economically feasible solutions. Shortcomings of administrative theory contribute to a further aggravation of establishing the 'one best way' of organizational design. For administrative theory is not able to specify the economic benefits of additional information or the economic impact of information and communication technology, nor to include all relevant costs arising from a work organization, as required by the total economic cost measurement. Despite these and other theoretical deficiencies (see Sydow 1985a, pp. 494-516 for a comprehensive discussion), organizations will be able to use the experience they will gain with office automation in the near future. It will certainly take some years, but as in the past, systems designers at some stage will determine the economically most favourable forms of work organizations with a given technology. The scope of organizational choice, which seems to be fairly wide today, will then be somewhat smaller.

A *third* reason for the non-straight forward accomplishment of the organization's goals (that is productivity and flexibility) relates to the insight that these goals are neither definite nor accepted by all organizational members. For instance, while managers strive for the reduction of costs, systems designers follow principles of vocational ethics and optimize technical rather than economic efficiency, not to mention union representatives, members of the works council or the office workers themselves succeeding more or less in the inclusion of their specific interests in the sociotechnical design. The extent to which they succeed in this is not only dependent on the industrial relations system and the organizational power structure but also upon the design techniques used. It is true that more and more participative design techniques are used by systems designers, but most are still very restrictive and not likely to affect the scope of organizational choice significantly, although in general, this scope is not independent of those who make the choices.

A *fourth* and most fundamental reason relates to the goals of capitalist organizations in general. Increasing productivity and/or flexibility in capitalist economic systems just is a means of achieving long-term profit maximization. But despite this, there is no economic determinisim. On the one hand, most capitalist organizations are not exposed to perfect competition; current organized capitalism is rather characterized by imperfect competition (Robinson 1969). On the other hand, the mere existence of organizational strategies and of organizational science aiming at consulting management strengthens the impression that many capitalist organizations are provided with at least some scope of organizational choice. Hrebiniak & Joyce (1985) underpin this impression by showing that different markets or niches are characterized by different degrees of determinism or freedom. A theoretical argument forwarded by Altmann & Bechtle (1971) explains why capitalist organizations are exposed only to imperfect competition. Striving for long-term profit maximization, these organizations using managerial strategies (e.g. automation, cooptation) try and, to some extent, succeed in overcoming the market structures imposed on them by the economic system. The organization thereby gains a certain degree of autonomy in its product markets as well as in other markets. At first glance, this argument is similar to that of apologists of the idea of strategic management, which focuses on the potential of organizations to influence their environments. But it is more specific and takes into account the character of the capitalist economic system. In doing so, it grasps the argument of economic determinism at its roots. Managerial strategy, according to Altmann & Bechtle, is not a matter of free choice but is principally imposed on organizations by (imperfect) market structures and by the capitalist system.

These theoretical concepts borrowed from organizational theory and industrial sociology offer a ground for a better understanding of the 'objective' limits and possibilities of organizational design within automated settings. These approaches, however, need to be complemented by psychological research on the subjective perception and meaning of this given scope of organizational choice to designers of sociotechnical systems.

PERCEPTION OF THE SCOPE OF ORGANIZATIONAL CHOICE: THE NEED FOR FURTHER PSYCHOLOGICAL RESEARCH IN THE FIELD OF OFFICE AUTOMATION

There is an 'objective' scope of organizational choice in automated office settings even if this seems to be somewhat smaller than many believe. Nevertheless, this scope seems to be significant enough that systems designers perceive it. However, the organizational conservatism, which can be found in most organizations using modern office technology, suggests that systems designers in most cases do not make use of this scope of organizational choice. *One* reason for this may be the confined perception of the scope by systems designers. This confined perception may result from systems designers' education and professional socialization, their values and beliefs about the functioning of an organization and their lack of motivation in designing sociotechnical systems which pay regard to the interests of office personnel in terms of a better quality of working life.

Some Empirical Evidence on the Perception of the Scope of Organizational Choice

An empirical study by Bjorn-Andersen, Hedberg, Mercer, Mumford & Sole (1979), for instance, shows that the information technology installed (hardware and software) was not considered by systems designers to restrict the scope of organizational choice significantly (apart from the limited storage capacity in one case). So the authors of that study expected the systems designers to remember a certain number of design choices. In fact this expectation did not prove to be valid. The systems designers reported only a small number of technical design alternatives. The work organization had not been questioned at all. Reasons for this behavior being limited in scope may concern the technical orientation of systems designers, the lack of competence in the field of work organization, their wish not to stir up the office workers and not least the conditions under which systems designers usually work, i.e. the "design of the design process". These conditions may be well characterized by strict cost and time budgets (Kraft 1977, Greenberg 1979). They do not allow systems designers to consider work organization issues in depth and to put their theory Y view of office workers and organizational structures (Hedberg & Mumford 1975) into practice. Rather they offer one more explanation for the organizational conservatism in face of new office technologies.

Practitioners of work organization, according to a study of the introduction of word processors carried out by Weltz & Lullies (1983), show a more organizational orientation than a view dominated by technical efficiency. Simultaneously, they adhere to a theory X view of office workers; they tend to legitimize their rigid designs rhethorically since they cannot longer ignore the contradictions of their actions. Weltz & Lullies in their research find some indication that the contradiction between rationalization and humanization of office work is increasingly thematized in the design process. "However, it would be naive to derive a trend towards less rigid work designs from this re-orientation. This in fact would be to overvalue the weight of subjective orientations" (Weltz & Lullies 1983, p. 127). The given scope of organizational choice imposes some restrictions on their design behavior.

Implications for Psychological Research on Office Automation

More psychological research of the behavior of systems designers and practitioners of work organization, of their values and implicit theories could shed some light on these rather rough generalizations from two studies only. However, this research should recognize the importance of the given, 'objective' scope of organizational choice.

Using the catagory of design *behavior*, researchers could secure recognition of the subjectivity of sociotechnical design. It is true that the author of the present article assumes that the structural conditions prevail upon the subjective interpretations of design. Nevertheless, there is room for subjectivity of designers, for idiosyncratic perception, interpretation and attribution processes which affect the outcome of concrete design behavior significantly.

After one sided person-oriented and situational approaches have by and large been discarded within the situationism debate in psychology (Bowers 1973, Endler & Magnusson 1977), behavior today is considered by most psychologists to be an outcome of person-situation interactions. An interactionist's model, which may be applied for explaining organizational design behavior is the social learning theory (Bandura 1977). It has been applied to organizational problems by Davis & Luthans (1980) and Ginter & White (1982), for instance. The social learning theory includes three interacting elements:
- the person, including his/her cognitive processes
- the situation to which the person is exposed
- the behavior of the person
and conceptualizes interaction as "reciprocal determinism".

The inclusion of behavior not only as an outcome of person-situation interactions, but as one of the three components of the proposed interactionist's model, enables one to pay attention to

- the changing of situations due to the behavior and to
- the effect of behavior on the person and his/her cognitions (learning).
The cited theory is called *social* learning theory as it does not only explain learning by means of consequential experience of the person's own behavior, but also by the person's observation and interpretation of the behavior and behavior outcomes of others.

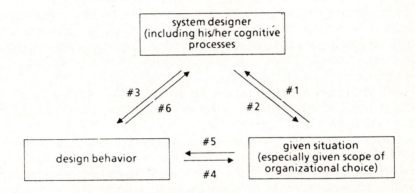

Fig. 1: An interactionist's model of organizational design

Applied to the explanation of (idiosyncratic) design behavior the social learning theory states (see fig. 1): The given scope of organizational choice - together with other features of the design situation such as power position and conditions of interaction with systems users - is actively perceived and interpreted by the designer (#1 and #2). The perception of a given scope of choice is cognitively integrated. Simultaneously cognitions such as
- the X and Y views of systems designers on office workers,
- their acquired views of how organizations function and
- their organizational philosophies (Shrivastva & Mitroff 1984) including the desired outcome of design behavior (e.g. the time structure) as well as incorporating views on the 'optimal' design process (e.g. the degree of user participation)
influence the perception process. Together with assumptions on cause-effect relationships, these cognitions are elements of naive or implicit organizing theories (c.f. Brief & Downey 1983) or subjective theories of organization (c.f. Frei 1985).

The active perception and interpretation of the design situation including the given scope of organizational choice influences the design behavior (#3). Systems designers may behave according to the given scope of choice, if their perceptions are congruent with this scope; or they may choose design alternatives, which - at least in the short run - may well lie outside the given scope of organizational choice.

Design behavior changes the situation, including the scope of organizational choice, as it will appear to the designer in the future (#4), for the chosen design alternative is considered to restrict future choices. The given scope of organizational choice does not only restrict design behavior via perceptual processes but also directly (#5). The design behavior practiced and its consequential influence on the situation initiate (social) learning by the designer, which may result in an increased competence to design future sociotechnical systems.

This interactionist's model of design behavior aims at the explanation of idiosyncratic choices made by the systems designer. Research on office automation in this line could, among other things, lead to the development of measures and instruments assisting those concerned with the design of sociotechnical systems in their perception and interpretation of the scope of organizational choice, and in their learning. At best such instruments would be able to help designers in discovering (or even enlarging) the scope of organizational choice and in stimulating sociotechnical experimentation (see Sydow 1987b, for an example). Not least they would assist them to satisfy the increased need for work and organizational design, where the scope of organizational choice has actually been enlarged in face of advanced office technologies. However, the development of such measures and instruments is not a sufficient condition to make systems designers use the scope of organizational choices; it is only *one* necessary step towards 'better' sociotechnical designs.

Psychological research on these themes must methodologically take into account the duality of 'objectivity' and subjectivity of organizational life and the overwhelmingly *processual* nature of sociotechnical design. Psychological research on office automation must also pay as much attention to the interaction of people with different values, interests and power positions within one organization as it currently does to human-computer interaction at the work place. Above all, there is need for more research in the area of human-computer interaction at the work place to be carried out by work, organizational and industrial psychologists.

FOOTNOTES

(1) See in addition to the contributions to this volume Frese (1987) for an impressive review of psychological research on human-computer interaction in the office.

(2) This description of the psychologist's conception of office automation requires some qualifying remarks. Changes are rapidly taking place in the area of psychological research on office automation, affecting research methods as well as theoretical frameworks. Secondly, the author is not a psychologist himself but only a vigilant observer of the Anglo-Saxon and German psychological research on this topic.

(3) For example, Ulich (1981), like many psychologists, assumes a growing scope of organizational choice due to micro-electronic based technologies. Neuberger (1984) mentions the scope of choice in his critical review of theories of leadership and Frei (1985) in building a subjective theory of organizing, which may explain as to why designers make a different use of a given scope of choice.

(4) For a summary and detailed discussion of these approaches see Sydow (1985a).

(5) This chapter has by and large been adapted from Sydow (1987a).

REFERENCES

Aldrich, H.E. (1979). *Organizations and environments*. Englewood Cliffs, N.J.: Prentice Hall.

Altmann, N. & Bechtle, G. (1971). *Betriebliche Herrschaftsstruktur und industrielle Gesellschaft*. München: Hanser.

Baisch, Ch. & Troy, N. (1986). Moderne EDV-Konzepte verlangen eine neue Organisation. In: *IO Management-Zeitschrift, 55* (10), pp. 418-420.

Bandura, A. (1977). *Social cognitive learning theory*. Englewood Cliffs, N.J.: Prentice-Hall.

Beinum, H. van (1981). Organizational choice and mirco electronics. In: *QWL Focus, 1* (3), pp. 1-6.

Bjorn-Andersen, N., Hedberg, B., Mercer, D., Mumford, E. & Sole, A. (1979). *The impact of systems change in organizations*. Alphen aan den Rhijn, The Netherlands: Sijthoff & Noordhoff.

Bobbitt, H.R. & Ford, J.D. (1980). Decision-maker choice as a determinant of organizational structure. In: *Academy of Management Review, 5* (1), pp. 13-23.

Bowers, K.S. (1973). Situationism in psychology: An analysis and critique. In: *Psychological Review, 80*, pp. 307-335.

Brandt, G., Kündig, B., Papadimitriou, Z. & Thomae, J. (1978). *Computer und Arbeitsprozeß*. Frankfurt & New York: Campus.

Brief, A. P. & Downey, H. K. (1983). Cognitive and organizational structures: A conceptual analysis of implicit organizing theories. In: *Human Relations, 36* (12), pp. 1065-1090.

Bullinger, H.-J. (1985). Organisation in der Krise. In: *Jahrbuch der Bürokommunikation*. Baden-Baden: FBO-Verlag.

Burns, T. & Stalker, G.M. (1961). *The management of innovation*. London: Tavistock.

Child, J. (1972). Organizational structure, environment, and performance: The role of strategic choice. In: *Sociology*, *6*, pp. 1-22.

Child, J., Ganter, H.D. & Kieser, A. (1986). *Organizational conservatism*. Working paper. Mannheim: Universtität.

Davis, L. E. (1957). Toward a theory of job design. In: *Journal of Industrial Engineering*, *8*, pp. 19-23.

Davis, T.R.V. & Luthans, F. (1980). A social learning approach to organizational behavior. In: *Academy of Management Review*, *5* (2), pp. 281-290.

Endler, D. & Magnusson, N.S. (1977). *Personality at the crossroads: Current issues in interactional psychology*. Hillsdale, Ill.: Erlbaum.

Frei, F. (1985), *Im Kopf des Managers ... Zur Untersuchung Subjektiver Organisationstheorien von betrieblichen Führungskräften - Eine Skizze*. Bremer Beiträge zur Psychologie. No. 44. Bremen: Universität.

Frese, M. (1987). The industrial and organizational psychology of human-computer interaction in the office. In: Cooper, C.L. & Robertson, I.T. (eds.): *International review of industrial and organizational psychology*. London & New York: Wiley.

Fricke, W. (1975). *Arbeitsorganisation und Qualifikation*. Bonn-Bad Godesberg: Neue Gesellschaft.

Ginter, P.M. & White, D.D. (1982). A social learning approach to strategic management: Toward a theoretical foundation. In: *Academy of Management Review*, *7* (2), pp. 253-261.

Goodman, S.E., & Perby, M.-L. (1985). Computerization and the skill of women's work. In: Oelrup, A., Schneider, L. & Monod, E. (eds.): *Women, work and computerization: Opportunities and disadvantages*. Amsterdam: North-Holland, pp. 23-41.

Greenbaum, J.M. (1979). *In the name of efficiency*. Philadelphia: Temple University Press.

Grochla, E. (1964). Zum Wesen der Automation. In: *Zeitschrift für Betriebswirtschaft*, *34* (10), pp. 660-666.

Hage, J. (1977). Choosing constraints and contraining choice. In: Warner, M. (ed.): *Organizational choice and constraints*. Farnborough, Hants.: Saxon House, pp. 1-56.

Hannan, M. & Freeman, J. (1977). The population ecology of organizations. In: *Amercian Journal of Sociology*, *82*, pp. 929-964.

Hedberg, B. & Mumford, E. (1975). The design of computer systems. In: Mumford, E. & Sackman, H. (eds.): *Human choice and computers*. Amsterdam: North-Holland, pp. 31-59.

Hrebiniak, L.G. & Joyce, W.F. (1985). Organizational adaption: Strategic choice and environmental determinism. In: *Administrative Science Quarterly*, *30*, pp. 336-349.

Jelinek, M., Smircich, L. & Hirsch, P. (1983)(eds.). Organizational culture. Special edition of the *Adminstrative Science Quarterly*, 28 (4).

Knave, B & Widebäck, P.-G. (1987)(eds). *Selected papers presented at the conference on work with display units*. Amsterdam: North-Holland.

Kraft, P. (1977). *Programmers and managers*. New York: Springer.

Kubicek, H. (1975). *Informationstechnologie und organisatorische Regelungen*. Berlin: Duncker & Humblot.

Kubicek, H. (1980). Perspektiven und Fragen zur Überwindung einiger Mängel des Situativen Ansatzes. In: Potthoff, E. (ed.): *RKW-Handbuch Führungstechnik und Organisation*. 6th part. August 1980. Berlin.

Littek, W. (1985). Administrative work and the impact of new information technologies - An overview of recent trends. In: International Sociological Association - Research Committee 30: Sociology of work (eds.): *Unattractive work*. Sofia, pp. 46-74.

Montanaari, J.R. (1979). Management discretion: An expanded model of organizational choice. In: *Journal of Management Studies*, 16, pp. 202-221.

Neuberger, O. (1984). *Führung. Ideologie, Struktur, Verhalten*. Stuttgart: Enke.

Pfeffer, J. & Salancick, G.R. (1978). *The external control of organizations*. New York: Harper & Row.

Pirker, Th. (1962). *Büro und Maschine*. Basel: Kyklos.

Projektgruppe Automation und Qualifikation (1978). *Theorien über Automationsarbeit*. Berlin: Argument.

Robinson, J. (1969). *The economics of imperfect competition*. 2nd edition. London: Macmillan.

Schein, E. (1985). *Organizational culture and leadership: A dynamic view*. San Francisco: Jossey-Bass.

Schreyögg, G. (1980). Contingency and choice in organization theory. In: *Organization Studies*, 1 (4), pp. 305-326.

Shrivastva, P. & Mitroff, I.J. (1984). Enhancing organizational research utilization: The role of decision makers' assumptions. In: *Academy of Management Review*, 9 (1), pp. 18-26.

Sydow, J. (1985a). *Organisationsspielraum und Büroautomation*. Berlin & New York: De Gruyter.

Sydow, J. (1985b). *Der soziotechnische Ansatz der Arbeits- und Organisationsgestaltung*. Frankfurt & New York: Campus.

Sydow, J. (1987a). Information technology and organizational choice. In: Child, J. & Bate, P. (eds.): *Organizations in transition*. Berlin & New York: De Gruyter.

Sydow, J. (1987b). Office automation and work organization: Making use of the scope of choice. In: Knave, B. & Widebäck, P.-G. (eds.): *Selected papers presented at the conference on work with visual display units*. Amsterdam: North-Holland.

Thompson, J.D. (1967). *Organizations in action*. New York: McGraw-Hill.

Trist, E. (1981). The evolution of sociotechnical systems. A conceptual framework and an action research program. In: Van de Ven, A.H. & Joyce, W.F. (eds.): *Perspectives on organization design and behavior*. New York: Wiley, pp. 19-75.

Trist, E., Higgin, G.W., Murray, H. & Pollock, A.B. (1963). *Organizational choice*. London: Tavistock.

Ulich, E. (1981). Möglichkeiten einer autonomieorientierten Arbeitsgestaltung. In: Frese, M. (ed.): *Streß im Büro*. Bern: Huber, pp. 159-178.

Van de Ven, A.H. & Joyce, W.F. (1981) (eds.): *Perspectives on organization design and behavior*. New York: Wiley.

Walton, R.E. (1982). Social choice in the development of advanced information technology. In: *Human Relations*, *35* (12), pp. 1073-1084.

Weizenbaum, J. (1979). *Computer power and human reason*. New York: Freeman

Weltz, F. & Lullies, V. (1983). Menschenbilder der Betriebsorganisatoren. In: Rammert, W., Bechmann, G., Nowotny, H. & Vahrenkamp, R. (eds.): *Technik und Gesellschaft. Jahrbuch 2*. Frankfurt & New York: Campus, pp. 109-128.

Westlander, G. (1987). Leadership styles in the implementation phase. In: Knave, B. & Widebäck, P.-G. (eds.). *Selected papers presented at the conference on work with display units*. Amsterdam: North-Holland.

Woodward, J. (1958). *Management and technology*. London: Her Majesty's Stationary Office.

Zuboff, S. (1982). Statement of concern. In: *Office: Technology & People*, *1* (1), pp. 66-70.

Psychological Issues of
Human Computer Interaction in the Work Place
M. Frese, E. Ulich, W. Dzida (Editors)
© Elsevier Science Publishers B.V. (North-Holland), 1987

CHANGING POTENTIAL USERS TO ACTUAL USERS:
AN EVOLUTIONARY APPROACH TO OFFICE SYSTEM ACCEPTANCE

Reinhard Helmreich

Siemens AG, Communications and Data Systems
Munich, Federal Republic of Germany

This paper outlines several issues which have proved critical in the discussion on office automation. The theses put forward are less concerned with theoretical considerations than with practical experience gained from investigations into the use of modern technology in the office. The main aspects examined are functional requirements, interface design, training and introduction strategy. Our findings confirm the assumption that participation is always worth supporting.

OFFICE TECHNOLOGY - FROM A NON-TECHNICAL VIEWPOINT

For a long time the use of technical resources was limited to the manufacturing sector. Nowadays, however, the office is being affected more and more by the spread of technology. New products from the world of communications engineering and information technology, such as data display terminals, word processing systems, and personal computers to name but a few, have already changed today's office environment. This development is continuing and accelerating. New systems, so-called 'office systems', are in hot pursuit.

The picture we can now form of the 'office of the future' is indeed impressive. Computer power will be made available at most workplaces and to nearly every office worker. Multifunction workstations will integrate such diverse services as voice communication, document handling and access to data bases. Communications systems will allow the exchange of information across the world (Johansen 1984, Uhlig, Faber & Bair 1979).

But what about the benefits of these possibilities? Will the user recognize the advantages offered by the new technology? And how should technical systems of this kind be structured and organized in the office so that they are accepted?

These questions indicate that it is not enough to look at office technology solely from the technical angle. Instead the extent to which technology can be applied profitably for the office worker, his working group and the organization as a whole must be examined.

Expectations and the demands at the workplace are to be considered during all phases of an innovative project - from design and development right through to the implementation of a new office system. Its usefulness only becomes apparent in application. And it depends on the acceptance of the user. In other words: It can't be forced - nothing can be achieved in the office without user cooperation.

It is therefore necessary to ensure that achievements in the technological sphere are accompanied by a program which views events from a non-technical angle. Everything centers around the term 'acceptance'. This term means the willingness of potential users to apply technology to support their work (Helmreich 1980, 1984a, 1984b).

ACCEPTANCE - A RESEARCH SUBJECT

The issue of acceptance of new office technology has been a subject for research in the Federal Republic of Germany for some years now. Manufacturers of office technology and scientific institutes have carried out a broad range of field studies, some with the support of the Federal Ministry for Research and Technology. A multitude of reports have been submitted (Kreifelts 1982, Picot & Reichwald 1984, Reichwald 1982).

They cover such aspects as
- user requirements with regard to functions, services and features of modern office technology
- user behavior in the handling of new office technology
- experiences in the introduction, training, learning support and organizational adaptation of office systems
- effects on people and the organization.

The studies are unanimous in the conclusion that three factors have a decisive influence on acceptance: (1) the user as a person, (2) the organization of work for the task that is to be performed with the aid of the technology, and (3) the technology itself, or more specifically its design and functional engineering.

These factors cannot be seen in isolation, of course, but are closely interrelated. The organization of work, for example, should always be geared to the qualifications of the user when new technology is put into application. Or: one-sided improvements in device ergonomics are of little help if the work sequence is incorrect.

RESEARCH STRATEGIES

In this field, as in others, it is true to say that the results of research are only as good as the methods with which they were obtained.

The numerous types of questions to be asked suggest that those research issues of acceptance should not limit themselves to a single research method. Only broadly based investigations using a variety of methods can provide the opportunity to pinpoint the relevant factors in this area and their effects. This paper gives a brief outline of two research strategies which are complementary to each other with regard to the results they achieve: the empirical/analytical method and the constructive method.

With an empirical/analytical approach, data on any aspects that appear relevant is collected by means of observation, written questionnaire and interview. In this way work structures, patterns of communication and opinions are recorded. The actual usage of the office system is logged and the user is questioned about his or her satisfaction with the new work tool. In many cases a long-term study with several inquiries being made at different points in time is a satisfactory form of investigation, so that changes in the interesting characteristics can be detected.

The relationship between the researcher and those involved in the study is characterized by distance. Care should be taken to ensure that the researcher as a person does not influence the findings submitted for measurement by the fact that he is carrying out research. The aim of empirical/analytical strategy is to gather extensive and largely objective findings on system utilization, personal assessments by the users and the effects of the application of technology.

With a constructive approach the researcher enters the field of investigation as an active partner. The aim of the research is to obtain not the most objective recording of phenomena defined in advance. Instead, the constructive approach aims to trigger and test changes in the field of practice.This is done in cooperation with the users of the new technology. In an iterative process the functions of the office system are adapted to the ideas of the users, which results in the technology being tailored to the user's needs. This means that the users, who are after all the experts in office processes, play a decisive role in the introduction and improvement of the systems. The objective of this kind of 'participatory system planning' is to bring human and technology closer together.

 ## LEARNING FORM THE MISFORTUNE OF MIS

Managers plan, make decisions, organize and control. To do this better they need reliable information, they need information systems. Question: Why is it that information systems appeal so little to executives?

This question was discussed by relevant trade journals years ago. The term 'management *mis*information systems' did the rounds (Keen 1981).

The assumption used to be that the reason for the lack of enthusiasm for information systems amongst managers lay primarily in the technology, in the data and its presentation. The technology was blamed with not functioning reliably and fast enough; the data entered were said to be out-of-date and the algorithms for prognoses and optimization too complicated.

Nowadays the reasoning has changed, in the wake of a new understanding of managers' tasks and their ways of tackling these tasks. Empirical studies have shown that a manager needs not only to think rationally but he may have the ability to handle informal, pliable and unstructured information.

The role of the manager is therefore a crucial hindrance to the acceptance of information systems because
- information systems do not make allowance for the pluralism of decisions or the connection between information and power
- information systems alter relationships, patterns of communication, influence and control
- information systems redistribute data and so break monopolies

System planners and developers therefore had to recognize that the demand was not for 'better' data, but for consideration to be given to the practices, styles and interests of people and groups. Implementation of information systems therefore should be understood not only as a technical process but also as a political process.

OVERCOMING THE ACCEPTANCE PROBLEM

As in the case of management information systems, the task of designing and applying office technology is not simply a technical matter. Technical misdevelopments which fail to take the needs of the users into account should be avoided. This also means preventing undesirable consequences in the economic and social sector.

Scientific analysis, however, is only the first step in mastering acceptance. The second step is translating empirical knowledge into a plan of action.

This does not mean belatedly curing symptoms, but setting up a planning process so that acceptance does not become a problem in the first place, if possible. This planning should incorporate all the phases of technological innovation in the office: the design, the development, the introduction and the evaluation. In other words we must shift from acceptance research to acceptance planning (Allerbeck & Helmreich 1984).

USER-ORIENTED SYSTEM PLANNING

What type of technology is needed in the office? What requirements does the user have? What tasks should be supported by technology? What necessities arise from the concepts of teamwork and specialization in the office?

An answer is to be found to these questions if we are to define and specify the features of office systems. However
- a system developer can seldom imagine where to find the problem areas in the office that can be eased with the help of a technical system;
- system analysis of scenarios and time-and-motion studies have thrown very little light on office activities to date. A considerable proportion of the tasks seems to defy formalization, and to a large extent the way in which they are performed is marked by the personality and style of those involved;
- there is no theory on the organizational structure of office activities from which it is possible to deduce convincingly what is required from the application of technology;
- even the future users of new office technology are hardly in a position to imagine what advantage they can draw from its application. At most they can appreciate that it will be easier to correct texts.

This means that it is not enough simply to provide a meticulous work analysis of the 'office make-up' before implementing the technology, or to ask the future users what their needs are, in order to find a suitable way of applying new office technologies. What is needed is rather an iterative strategy whereby the technical side offers functions which the user then tests, appraises and finally either accepts, rejects or modifies.

It should not be imagined that this modification can take the form of the user changing the system functions according to his own wishes. At this stage he still needs the system developer, i. e. the programmer. And he in turn should be prepared to go along with what he may often consider to be the 'naive' expectations of the user. So system developers and users must exhibit a high degree of willingness to cooperate.

All those involved should endorse the attitude that 'the user is always right', that operating errors reflect inadequacies in the technology and are not consequences of the user's 'incompetence' and that the user alone can set the standard for usefulness and acceptance.

'COMPUTER SERVICE FOR SECRETARIES AND EXECUTIVES'

An integrated office system with the label of 'Computer Service for Secretaries and Executives' has been the subject of wide-scale field studies by the Siemens corporation for some five years (Beckurts & Reichwald 1984, Helmreich & Wimmer 1982).

The functions of the system support elementary tasks common to all office jobs:
- text entry and word processing ('text system')
- correspondence ('electronic mail')
- filing and archiving ('electronic filing cabinet')

These core functions are offered in the Computer Service in an integrated form with a standard system interface. In January of 1979 the first workstation was installed. In the first two years the user community grew to over 100 people in five of the company's locations in Munich and Erlangen.

Empirical/analytical and constructive methods were used with equal emphasis. A research group was assigned to each of the two methods, with instructions to pursue their research goals independently. This separation of staff was intended to prevent mutual influencing and consequent blurring of the research objectives.

The introduction of the Computer Service was successful owing to the fact that both the user community and the functional power of the system were allowed to grow as they evolved. In cooperation with the users it was possible to improve and further develop the system continually. The research team following the empirical/analytical method was able to collect an enormous amount of data relating to the usage potential of the new technology, the communication structure and the communication activities of the users, and with respect to task and person-oriented acceptance factors.

Despite the strict separation of personnel in the two research groups it cannot be denied that the two methods could have adversely affected each other.

The dynamic growth of the user group, for example, did not allow a 'representative' sample to be taken which the empirical/analytical strategy would in fact require to specify the statistical evaluation methods and to justify generally applicable findings.

Added to this was the fact that the constructive approach was continually creating new conditions in the investigation field because of its constant intervention. This meant that particularly in the initial phase there were continuous improvements and additions to the system functions based on the suggestions of the users. This, no doubt, had a positive effect on the attitude and motivation of some users, but it made it considerably more difficult for the empirical/analytical researchers to define their inquiries and select the instruments of their survey.

THE ROLE OF THE 'CHANGE AGENT'

In the following section the Computer Service project will be considered from the point of view of the Change Agent. This should serve to make the methods and effectiveness of the constructive approach clearer.

The function of the Change Agent was 'innovation'. It consisted in promoting and assuring the adoption of the Computer Service in the daily office routine. More precisely it meant establishing initial contacts, presenting preparatory information, providing instruction and supporting the learning process. It was also necessary to promote the exchange of experiences between users and system developers and to encourage the users to exchange experiences between themselves. Finally the Change Agent was supposed to trigger new impulses for activities in the office.

Although the term used here is 'the' Change Agent, this does not refer to a single individual but to a common, innovation-oriented approach by all those involved. A social scientist who was supported by a colleague with secretarial experience, however, was at the center of all the activities.

The 'tool' used by the Change Agent was personal contact. Readiness to engage in trusting cooperation had to be built up both on the side of the system developers, to whom the Change Agent belonged organizationally, and on the side of the users.

One of the first actions was the publication of a brochure entitled 'Information for trial users'. This brochure provided information about the Computer Service project in a suitable form and in easy-to-understand terminology. It enabled everyone to identify to some degree with the goals of the application of technology and it can be assumed it had a positive influence on the motivation of users and developers alike.

A second action was the installation of the 'red telephone' on the desk of the Change Agent. All problems, questions, cries for help, etc. were addressed to this number. If possible assistance was given straight away, otherwise the relevant hardware or software specialist was alerted. Thus the users had one office to which they could always turn and where they could be sure that someone would always be willing to attend to their problems.

The motto for the Change Agent was: Be involved! This meant always appearing personally when decisions were being prepared. For example, in the initial discussions between executive and secretary about what they wanted to do with the technology. The Change Agent also took part in all the presentations which the accompanying researchers attended to express their concerns.

Training of the users was carried out by the Change Agent himself in the various offices. This gave him insight into the work methods and problems of these offices and was to the advantage of the users who joined the project later: good ideas could be passed on in the training phase.

Of course the Change Agent also included 'electronic mail' in his actions. Users could be reached quickly by memo and their questions in turn could be submitted by electronic mail. This proved to be extremely practical and efficient.

Finally, after the Computer Service had been running about one and a half years, the first user meeting to which not only users but also system developers and accompanying researchers were invited resulted in stimulating suggestions for further development of the technology, but also in a discussion of the problems that had occurred during use of the Computer Service.

From the viewpoint of the system developer the Change Agent was the 'first' user. He was included in designing and testing the system functions and the human-machine interface. System improvements were only passed on to the users after approval by the Change Agent. Certain so-called refinements were dispensed within the interests of easier operation.

UTILIZATION

Most users work with the Computer Service on a daily basis, although the time they spend varies considerably. It ranges from a quick glance into the mailbox to a number of hours on the system. A user's terminal is activated most of the time but is often placed on 'stand-by', ready to assist with the work at hand. In this way the computer services are used rather like a new set of tools tailored for office work.

Almost all the users create, maintain and make use of files. Files include text, tables and collections of data - directories, lists of leaflets to be contacted, calendars for appointments, travel arrangements, incoming and outgoing mail logs, letters, memoranda and address files - to mention only a few examples. Lists and tables tend to be structured in a customary form and their contents change continually. Some users maintain indexes and registers on subjects reports and books, which are themselves still stored in paper form outside of the computer system. Users benefit from its retrieval and sorting capabilities.

Users also entrust personal and sensitive data to the system. This would not be the case if data protection against any unauthorized access could not be guaranteed. At the same time, users become increasingly dependent on a developing system. To a large extent information is stored exclusively on electronic media and no longer on paper. Quite often work with the Computer Service cannot be scheduled, but requires immediate access. Thus the system is available around the clock. But systems do break down. Half a day's downtime every fortnight seems to be the maximum that users will tolerate.

The use of the system can be further illustrated by a few statistics. After two years, the volume of stored data amounts to the equivalent of 25000 pages of text. This volume has grown exponentially and continues to grow at the same rate. The average log-on time per user per day is around 100 minutes. The breakdown of function calls reads as follows: editing,

43%; printing, 17%; filing, 14%; mail 13%; other functions, 13%. The average number of files per user is around 150, although cases with less than 50 and more than 500 files do exist. Eighty per cent of the files contain less than the equivalent of 10 pages of text, so that on the whole small files are preferred.

But we should not be led astray by the mechanics of statistics. There is hardly an office, user or user group which seems to be average or representative. Work and working style and consequently the use of the Computer Service have varied much more than was anticipated.

Users who change offices during the course of a day may continue to process the same files from different terminals. In this way the system is used to overcome problems caused by varying working locations of users. Even more importantly, the Computer Service has proved to be an excellent support of cooperation and coordination within small working groups in which members are locally dispersed.

Both forms of communication, sharing files and exchanging files between electronic mailboxes, have been accepted. 'Sharing files' means that a group of people has the right to read and change the common files belonging to the group. There ist little communication between departments, however. Most of the communication takes place within small, cooperating 'closed user groups'. This means that a system architecture with local networks among working groups and with gateways to other networks seems to be the most appropriate approach.

Portable terminals are also used for this type of intra-office communication, but only a few executives use them and only on certain occasions. A typical application would be that during an extended absence from the office the portable terminal is used to receive messages from a manager's staff, entered at odd hours.

The communication feature also proves to be of particular benefit during training and for the subsequent on-the-job support. Users can be quickly contacted by circulars, and they in turn can ask questions via 'electronic mail'.

In a nutshell, the Computer Service is used to store and structure personal information as well as to record and schedule personal time and activities.

What would a better system look like? To serve users' purposes even better, the Computer Services should be expanded. We can identify several client needs: better tools for 'self-management'; forms and files, the structure of which can be defined by the user to cater for his individual tasks; flexible links between forms and files so that data can flow in either direction; a gateway to public communication services; gateways to existing in-house databases, in particular to support the process of planning; a good visual representation of an archive's structure and contents; and, in order to support group cooperation, to keep track of the contributions of individual group members to a joint effort and to make explicit the current state of work.

ACCEPTANCE FACTORS

Acceptance of the Computer Service as a resource depends first and foremost on the type of jobs to be done and the personal work structure. In other words the organization of the work is the crucial acceptance factor.

The application possibilities of the Computer Service were not fixed from the beginning, but were 'open', i. e. they allowed the users to restructure their work in a controlled fashion. An office system that forces users to do everything completely differently 'from the word go', and in a prescribed manner, would hardly have any chance of being accepted by our circle of users. The Computer Service supports evolutionary transition to the reorganization of work processes.

In our opinion the essential precondition for success was the fact that no attempt was made to offer users preprogrammed solutions to tackling work, but that the Computer Service gave them room and freedom to structure it themselves.

User-related factors were shown to have less influence. Contrary to widespread prejudice, it became apparent that the age of the users had no influence on their readiness to learn and their acceptance of new technology.

The group to which a user belongs plays a significant role. Colleagues can behave in a motivating but also in a demotivating manner. Our experience has been that the users communicate with each other, that they help one another and that they pass on ideas. A sense of belonging to a group emerges. This was encouraged from the beginning of the constructive research method.

Perhaps the best indication of acceptance can be seen in the fact that so far hardly a single user of the Computer Service has been willing to give up his/her workstation. Criticism of the functions and operation features was indeed expressed. But nobody want to do without the Computer Service - unless a more powerful system is made available.

Of course this result should be seen in the context of a total absence of 'pressure from above'. The application of the technology was not a rationalization program and the users were never assessed on their performance with the system. Transfers or even dismissals as a result of its application were never contemplated or discussed.

DEMANDS ON FUTURE SYSTEMS

The question is: what features and capabilities does the user attach particular importance to? This section is not about theoretical requirements, but about essentials that become apparent from experience in the application of modern office technology: availability, flexibility and data protection.

Availability means: the office system has to be available at any time and if possible right at the operator's usual workplace. System-related waiting periods, particularly during text entry, are unacceptable to users. Procedures which understandably take more time, such as search and copy procedures, are an exception to this requirement. The capacity of an office system should therefore be geared to peak load. Availability consequently means both a 'user's own workstation' and a 'continually running, stable system'.

Yet another feature which the design of office systems will have to take increasingly into accout is the flexibility of its application possibilities. Each user should be able to decide for himself how and whether he uses the technology for his own purposes. There is a great deal of individual freedom in the use of office systems. This motivates the user and leads to creative solutions. After all, it is only the users who can judge which functions are of benefit to them. This also means that an office system may allow continuous improvement and onward development - not just in the framework of a subsequent system version, but in ongoing operation. There will be no place for 'fixed-state' systems in the future.

Office systems interlink individual workplaces. This does not mean, however, that all work-related data, designs and documents should be accessible to anyone as a result of networking. For another feature valued by users is data protection. What one person does with 'his' part of the office system is taboo for other users. Although it is quite conceivable and necessary to allow for access privileges arranged according to user groups and for common documents to be maintained and updated centrally. But the office system cannot become an integral part of daily office work unless the users are convinced that their documents are protected from access by unknown parties.

The essential factor is that a certain amount of privacy should be accorded in the office of the future as a matter of course, just as it is at workplaces today. Office systems should under no circumstances be used for checking up on and monitoring the users.

THE ERGONOMICS OF HUMAN-MACHINE DIALOG

In the past ergonomics concerned itself mainly with physical aspects. Tools of work such as chairs, desks, keyboards, display screens, and on the other hand the work environment, had to be designed in a human way. The results of this work were the basis for today's design rules and standards.

But increased efforts are needed in a new subsection of ergonomics: software ergonomics. What is meant here is the designing of the user interface of an office system. Buzz words like 'easy-to-learn' or 'user-friendly' give an indication of what is to be aimed for. There is still a good deal of vagueness, however, about specific guidelines for design (Smith & Green 1980).

Experience shows that the key to user-friendliness lies in a carefully worked-out system interface with clear dialog prompting and understandable error messages. The user should be able to keep to rules that correspond to everyday logic. He cannot be expected to concern himself with the intricacies of system architecture.

The correct measure of help information is also to be found. A beginner evidently needs more help from the system than a skilled user. Furthermore, office systems should offer the possibility of cancelling, i. e. 'undoing', completed actions. The user then has the chance of acting 'on a trial basis'.

What is vital in the design of multifunctional office systems is to create a homogeneous standard user interface. The user generally attaches more importance to integration at the human-machine interface than to a wealth of functions.

That means, for instance, a consistent style of interaction no matter whether a user deals with text, menus or forms, and no matter what process is operating 'behind' a form. The system's 'office semantics' should mirror the objects, tools and procedures of the real office environment.

A system should be sufficiently transparent. A user should be able to ask for other participants, groups, services, functions, devices, processes, data, organizational rules, etc. Among many other elements relating to user convenience one more should be mentioned: to personalize a system, adapting it to a personal office routine. Again, there are many alternatives. One is to build highly parameterized systems where a user can adjust parameters rather like the stops of an organ. Thus the reaction or appearance of a system, data structure and state transition may be tailored to routine work.

INTRODUCTION AND TRAINING

All previous experience has repeatedly shown that the way in which an office system is introduced and the training of users have a decisive influence on acceptance. In the introductory phase the future user should be informed about the new technology from the very start and is to be involved in the decisions about its application. The introduction of an office system presupposes a high degree of willingness amongst users, organizers and system developers to cooperate with each other (Eason

1982, Otway & Peltu 1983, Pava 1983).

With new office technology complex systems are incorporated into complex organizations. This cannot be achieved 'in one fell swoop' but may be tackled gradually. The starting point for the application of office systems should therefore be an area that is easy to survey. The user community has to 'grow' from there.

It would be wrong to assume that innovation in the office can be achieved simply by installing state-of-the-art technology. Much more has to be done, including the creation of a suitable environment for the technology. The introduction of office systems may be incorporated in a program of organizational development. This means initiating a planned and continuous structuring process which gives equal consideration to the needs of people and tasks, and which works with the active participation of managers and staff.

Training does not simply mean practicing operating procedures. Usually it is possible to work with an office system after a few hours of practice. But then the real learning starts: What tasks can be tackled with the system? What changes are possible in the user's personal work organization? In which tasks is the new technology of no advantage?

From this moment it is no longer a question of which key to press when, but of the advantage each individual can gain for his work from the technical system. In this phase users need encouragement and support. The cost of looking after their needs is not inconsiderable. The person charged with this responsibility should first get to know the user's job and style of work in order to be able to make suggestions as to system utilization. This learning phase may take several weeks, often months.

Training courses with one large user group at a time are not effective with powerful multifunctional office systems. Individual instruction at the workplace, combined with a concise manual, may appear costly but provides considerable benefits. The pace of learning, for example, can be adapted to individual needs. The user practices on tasks that have to be performed in the office concerned, and it is possible to ascertain from the very start which of the many system functions are particularly important to the user.

This 'learning by doing' results in a situation where users differ greatly in their knowledge of the system. Functionally powerful office systems necessitate this kind of variation.

The more the functionality of office systems increases, the larger the system manuals become. This is a problem as users are generally unwilling to read a thick book. They would rather listen and try things out themselves. This is only successful, however, with 'tolerant' user interfaces. It is to be expected that office systems of the future will be so easy to use that the manual will simply serve the expert as a reference book. A contact person with in-depth knowledge, whom users can ask for advice at any time, is far more important than written material.

PROSPECTS

The question of user acceptance will be at the center of future research and development activities into office technology. To a large extent this research will be dependent on the cooperation of users, organizers and system developers. It will be necessary to find new forms of cooperation that differ substantially from the type of developer-user relationship generally found today.

When acceptance becomes a problem it is usually already too late. If the opportunity to shift from acceptance research to acceptance planning is grasped, however, both the developer of modern office systems and the user will benefit. On the one hand the risk of misguided developments can be avoided, and on the other, disappointments on the part of the user can be prevented.

The office of today is by no means perfect. Technical systems present themselves as a means of changing the office world. Technology should not be introduced for the sake of technology, however, but with the objective of making innovation possible. It is essential that all those affected contribute actively. The result must be to make office jobs more humane and more cost-effective.

REFERENCES

Allerbeck, M. & Helmreich, R. (1984). Akzeptanz planen - aber wie? *Office Management 32, Heft 11*, 1080-1082

Beckurts, K. H. & Reichwald. R. (Hrsg.).(1984). *Kooperation im Management mit integrierter Bürotechnik*. München: CW-Publikationen

Eason, K. D. (1982). The process of introducing information technology. *Behaviour and information technology 1*, 197-213

Helmreich, R. (1980). Was ist Akzeptanzforschung? *Elektronische Rechenanlagen 22, Heft 1*, 21-24b

Helmreich, R. (1984a). Human Aspects of office systems - User acceptance research results. *Interact '84, First IFIP Conference on Human-Computer-Interaction* (Proceedings)

Helmreich, R. (1984b). Geplante Akzeptanz - Aspekte bei der Gestaltung von Bürosystemen. *Siemens-Zeitschrift 58, Heft 5*, 8-10

Helmreich, R. & Wimmer, K. (1982). Field study with a computer-based office system. *Telecommunications Policy 6*, June, 136-142

Johansen, R. (1984). Teleconferencing and Beyond. New York: McGraw-Hill

Keen, P. (1981). Information Systems and Organisational Change, *Comm. ACM 24*, 24-33

Kreifelts, Th. (1982). *Anwenderanforderungen an ein Bürokommunikationssystem*. München: Oldenbourg

Otway, H. J. & Peltu, M. (Eds.). (1983). *New Office Technology - Human and Organisational Aspects*. Brussels: Ablex

Pava, C. (1983). *Managing New Office Technology - An Organisational Strategy*. New York: Free Press

Picot, A. & Reichwald, R. (1984). *Bürokommunikation - Leitsätze für den Anwender*. München: CW-Publikationen

Reichwald, R. (Hrsg.). (1982). *Neue Systeme der Bürotechnik*. Berlin: Schmidt

Smith, H. T. & Green, T. R. G. (Eds.). (1980). *Human interaction with Computers*. London: Academic Press

Uhlig, R. P., Faber, D. J. & Bair, J. H. (1979). *The Office of the Future*. Amsterdam: North Holland

Psychological Issues of
Human Computer Interaction in the Work Place
M. Frese, E. Ulich, W. Dzida (Editors)
© Elsevier Science Publishers B.V. (North-Holland), 1987

PLAYING AT INNOVATION IN THE COMPUTER REVOLUTION

Jerome A. Katz

School of Business and Adminstration, University of St. Louis,
3674 Lindell Blvd., St. Louis, MO63108

Approaches to unplanned innovation that emphasize playfulness are introduced and described. Three outcomes of play are detailed: creativity, mastery and affect, which are related to play research and game design theory. The three outcomes are used to analyze innovative behaviors among statistical computing users in primarily mainframe and mixed mainframe-microcomputing environments. Three contextual variables derived from the research are identified: ownership, access, and workload. Pathological forms of playful behaviors such as perfectionism and flightiness are then described, and research implications of play based approaches to the analysis of innovation are considered.

INTRODUCTION

If there is a mythology of innovation in computer science, its gods must be the designers of computer hardware and software, while the role of mortals is carried out by the millions who sit before their computer screens following its signs and auguries as our instructions.

What is missing are the intermediaries, those who take initiative to make the godlike mundane. In the business world, this role is played in white-collar ranks. Managers and professionals decide whether, when and often what to computerize, appealing to both those above and below for guidance. This role of innovator has recurrently been portrayed as a heroic figure. In the mythology above, the role is most often written as a promethean one, after he who stole fire from the Gods to give to the mortals. The names for such innovators have a promethean ring to them: change master (Kanter, 1983), intrapreneur (Pinchot, 1985), or product champion (Schon, 1963).

In many cases the metaphor is a useful one for teaching managers and professionals about the innovation process and the critical role played by the innovator, but it neglects another way in which innovations can come about.

If Prometheus represents the solid, sober, serious approach to innovation, the counterpoint must be Pan, the piping playful one, the teaser. Stories suggest that much of the inventiveness of mortals comes from attempts to best Pan. Why? Pan offers challenge, but when bested, Pan offers no retribution, only more challenges.

Often computerization proceeds because managerial and professional workers find using a computer to be fun. The remainder of this paper explores this idea of play as a basis for fostering innovation among white-collar employees. The nature of play and innovation will be briefly reviewed, and then an explanation of how the computer fosters the mixing of these two processes is given. Three outcomes from play research are postulated as important, and a variety of examples from the anecdotal and research literature on computerization is given to explain how these ideas apply.

PLAY AND COMPUTING

Play has traditionally been thought of as "a time and place apart from ordinary life in which the player is free from "serious" pursuits, where he may be absorbed intensely, and where he may nevertheless conduct his activities in an orderly, partially secret, yet rule bound way" (Sutton-Smith, 1971:85, describing Huizinga, 1949). Folklorist and play analyst Brian Sutton-Smith contends that ".. As we move upwards through the species, the period of play activity extends for an increasing period of the life span. It is arguable that in humans it never completely ceases to be an important response system" (Sutton-Smith, 1971:87).

But if the importance of play is readily recognized for children, it is treated as a necessary evil in the business world. Play, if it gets considered at all, gets institutionalized, foremost in the existence of the vacation, but also through company organized sports programs, socializing, and the like. And yet this approach misses the individual experience of play and innovation - a process that is mixed into the worklives of organizational members.

There is ample anecdotal (e.g. Carroll, 1982) and empirical (e.g. Carlson, Grace and Sutton, 1977; Curley and Pyburn, 1982:35) evidence that suggests how many people have found an element of playfulness in their experience of the computer. For example, Turkle reports on the playfulness of computer users, especially during their learning phase, and the continuing playfulness of hackers. But Turkle's observations are not the only ones indicative of a sense of playfulness in computer use.

A few studies have viewed the impact of computer technology on the writing process of professional writers (Bridwell, Johnson, and Brehe, 1984) and student writers (Bean, 1983; Collier, 1983). These various reports suggest that word processing users find the experience to be a satisfying one; that computer utility is greatest in revising documents rather than in the initial writing, and that word processing use leads to more and more detailed revisions.

A more thorough consideration of affective as well as cognitive elements in using the computer comes from the electronic mail research of Sproul and Kiesler (1986). They report that the electronic mail users exhibit extremely uninhibited behavior in their messaging. This takes a variety of forms: emotional punctuation (e.g. ?, !, and @#$%*ing) and word choices (e.g. flaming), communicating bad news or negative information, and flouting social conventions such as including nonwork material on a work related electronic mail system.

These findings were equally true for executives, professionals, and non-exempts. This was so much so that the authors reported that "Messages from superiors and managers looked no different from messages from subordinates and nonmanagers" (p.1509). This referred not only to the similar appearance of all electronic mail, but also to its forms of expression and content.

Taken together, there seems to be a recurring indication that adults using computers may report or engage in a variety of playful behaviors. The affect surrounding this use appears in both empirical research and anecdotal accounts.

Research in two areas of design has considered affective as well as masterly based components. These areas are job design, typified by the theory of Hackman and Oldham (1976), and the design of computer games, typified by the work of Malone (1980). Less well known, the latter is summarized below.

Malone (1980) developed a theory of intrinsically motivating instruction design that was specifically concerned with game design. His work leads to a number of other studies aimed at developing highly involving computer games (Mehrabian and Wixen, 1986; Morlock, Yando, and Nigolean, 1985; Myers, 1984) and educational programs (Chaffin, Maxwell and Thompson, 1982).

The outcome, an intrinsically motivating play activity, is composed of three major variables, each of which is composed of subscales. They are:

Challenge composed of variable difficulty level, multiple level goals, hidden information, randomness,

Fantasy composed of cognitive and emotional factors intrinsic and extrinsic fantasies, and

Curiosity composed of completeness, consistency, parsimony.

Components of challenge and fantasy are positively related to their major variable, while components of curiosity are inversely related. For example, while a variety of difficulty levels is associated with a challenging game, curiosity is aroused by the *in*completeness of the game.

Based on Malone's and Sutton-Smith's works, the remainder of this paper explores three purposes served by play for adults: creativity, mastery and affect.

The exploration will combine two types of data sources in order to explain and demonstrate each of the purposes. The data sources are literature on statistical computer applications, and observations of statistical computing at two sites.

The observations come from a pilot study of how professionals performed statistical analysis using low-barrier-to-entry (LBE) techniques, notably microcomputer based statistical and social surveying programs. The goal of the original research was to develop a set of rules-of-thumb for performing LBE social surveying. The two sites are called for convenience's sake School A, which had a EBCDIC based mainframe with a home-grown interactive statistical package (called here SAM) and School B, which used a smaller, ASCII-based computer with batch statistical programs.

Creativity

The literature on creativity gives the clearest indication of the ambivalent position of play in the organizational world. The norms are decried by creativity consultants and researchers in comments such as "Playfulness if for children only" (Adams, 1979:53) or serious people have a "fear of fun" (Olson, 1980:37). This contrasts with the research findings on the importance of play such as noted above in the summary of Sutton-Smith (1971:87).

The relationship of playfulness to creativity has been evidenced in a number of ways. From a developmental perspective, the works of Wallach and Kogan (1965) and Lieberman (1965) show a strong relationship between play and creativity. In group theory, Taylor (1975) spontaneity as a precursor of more serious innovative behaviors. While Hare (1982:161) sees the expression of spontaneity, particularly in self-oriented work, as a "warm-up" for more group oriented creative activity.

Building on these approaches, particularly in techniques such as frame-changing or frame-of-reference-breaking, experts in long range planning have long indicated that playful comments, humor, and play can offer insights and ideas for planners (Michaels, 1973).

Creativity is one of the hardest outcomes to recognize and assess insomuch as the observer must exercise a qualitative judgement regarding the extent of the creativity. A simpler, behaviorally anchored technique is to look at experimental or exploratory behaviors. This approach can be readily applied in the case of statistical microcomputing.

For example, as was predicted by Velleman (1980), it became evident that users of interactive statistical systems will experiment with a greater variety of statistical procedures than will users of batch systems. Velleman (1980: 23) suggests that:

> *The freedom to select analyses encourages the data analyst to tailor the details of the analysis to the specific need of a particular data set.*

Observation of users suggest that this experimentation is far greater among microcomputer users than among mainframe batch program users, and appears to be greater, based on early reports, for those who have a microcomputer at home and the office than for those with a computer at only one location. This suggests that experimentation is something of a happenstance, or spur of the moment effort.

This exploration is performed in a more tentative manner than the already-mastered "what-if" optimizations described below. Tentativeness is evidenced by greater reliance on advice, manuals and statistical texts, longer perusals of outputs, fewer within-procedure optimization runs, and greater use of graphical displays of the results.

The major form of exploration is labelled browsing. In browsing a computer user identifies programs used by other professions, e.g. an organizational theorist looking at a demographic analysis program. The browser then tries out the program with a dataset, usually a small one of known qualities, to discover what the program can do. What prompts choice among browsers can be a search for alternatives when facing a dead end in their own analyses, or trying to find an analytic method to test a specific theory, where the existing methods in the browser's home field are inadequate (e.g. using ecological analysis programs for studies of social ecology in organizational formation and death), or just to add variety during a period of slack or tedium. Once again, design issues affect this. Where computer program information is easily accessible, through a program library or a program listing, such browsing behavior is more likely.

The happenstance approach, tentativeness, and browsing suggest that experimentation, and possibly creativity, will be greater where there is little in the way of potentially threatening negative reactions of others. Given the above it is understandable why users will prefer to use the personal computer for statistical analysis over the mainframe where problem size and procedure availability permits.

What remains lacking at this stage is a comparison of the nature of the statistical thinking done by those using interactive *vs*. batch programs.

Mastery

Mastery refers to the growth in capability that can occur through play. This growth can be based on a striving to add abilities, or in a remedial capacity as when "the player develops confidence and competence to handle real-life situations toward which the original anxieties point (Sutton-Smith, 1973: 79-80).

Surprisingly, there is little work on the relationship of play among adults to mastery of living and working skills. Practitioners, such as Reuben (1980) stress the importance of understanding games, particularly athletic games for understanding how some organizations are run, but there is little evidence to suggest how adult games might prepare individuals for work day tasks.

In considering statistical program use mastery would be evidenced by two things: the use of appropriate statistical procedures, and the completeness of the analysis (e.g. full checks of data quality, assumption testing, outlier checks, cross-validation, etc.).

In 1969, at the dawn of the proliferation of mainframe statistical computing in universities, George Box gave the definitive statement regarding the relationship of computing mastery to statistical mastery. He observed:

There was a time when people who shouldn't do regression analysis or factor analysis didn't because it would have taken too much time to find out how to do the calculations and carry them out. Only the more determined spirits went ahead, and these were perhaps also willing to spend time to find out something about the assumptions and the pitfalls of the calculations they were making.

But now it is really too easy; you can go to the computer and with practically no knowledge of what you are doing, you can produce sense or nonsense at a truly astonishing rate (Box 1969, p.6).

Box's concern, which continues to the present (Kennedy, 1983; Velleman, 1980) explains only one side of the issue, with another concern voiced by Lefkowitz (1983) and Novick (1984), who states:

(I)t is all too often the case that arithmetic gets in the way of the professional's decision-making by breaking his concentration and train of thought. At times the sheer bulk of computations precludes the use of advanced techniques by the untrained researcher...(A) monitoring system is needed that does all the arithmetic, and even further, guarantees that all of the steps in the analysis are performed correctly and in their proper sequence (Novick, 1984: 33).

In response to Box's fears of wanton computation and Novick's fears of stifled creativity, most players seem to use different strategies at different times. Assumptions get checked either at the early database

building stage or when an interesting finding emerges and requires confirmation. Comparatively little checking of the appropriateness of tests
appears to be done, unless the program warns of a problem (e.g. a matrix
inversion failure due to its singularity). This is due in part to software
design, which tends to separate the procedures for checking data quality
(e.g. wild codes) and distributional characteristics (e.g normality) from the
major data analysis procedures such as regression, factor analysis and the
like, as well as the stylistic factors and time pressures of the players
themselves.

Additionally, only one mainframe program (CADA, see Novick,
1984) and only one microcomputer based statistical program (i.e. Epistat)
offer even elementary information on how to choose a statistical procedure given a particular type of outcome, such as a comparison of differences. This is particularly surprising given the availability of an extensive,
already constructed decision tree for statistical analysis (Andrews, et al.,
1981), and a number of elementary statistics textbooks which use similar
conventions for guiding statistical choice.

On the surface at least, interactive statistical program users have a
greater potential for achieving a complete analysis. Interactive program
users do at least spend more of their time working with their data rather
than awaiting results. Users of interactive statistical systems perform more
analyses than batch system users. This is partially due to the longer turn-
around time of batch systems, which poses a physical limit to the number
of computing runs, and in part due to the ease of reanalysis in interactive
programs.

Users of personal computer based statistical systems will spend more
time in analysis than will users of mainframe based statistical systems, and
little of this is due to the relative slowness of microcomputers' CPUs. It is
due largely to the greater appeal of working with the data interactively,
based on reports of users. In game design theory (e.g. Malone), the element that makes this work appealing is the desire for completeness as a
curative for curiosity.

As was found among spreadsheet users, using an interactive statistical program will produce a greater number of variant runs of an analysis.
Part of this, even in knowledgeable users, appears to be an attempt at
"what-if" forms of optimization, seeking a combination of data selection,
statistical, and presentation options that produces the most compelling
result.

A major factor in the quality of the completeness is the location of
the user's terminal. Working from a terminal in a computer center, apparent wild codes in the data cannot be checked, since ordinarily the raw
data will be kept elsewhere. Where the terminal in use is near the raw
data, these checks are more frequent, and corrections tend to be made
based on the original data materials and the permanent dataset, rather than
as a temporary recoding in the data. This produces a higher-quality archi-

val dataset and a clearer record of how the data and analyses changed with successive cleanings.

Affect

As Huizinga's definition of play above indicates, a person can be intensely absorbed in play. This intensity is an important part of what distinguishes play from other involvements. But the most important differentiation is the freedom from serious pursuits. In that freedom lies the opportunity for playfulness, for experimentation and for creativity that are the important hallmarks of play considered from the organizational perspective.

Play provides the player with energy for pioneering. Mastering a game is a learning experience, and like most learning fraught with delay, trial and frustration. The more complex the game, and adults eventually tend to like a moderate complexity, the longer this takes. At work, the demands of authorities or clients keep an individual working in the face of frustration, but what keeps an player playing? It may be an abundance of energy.

This may operate as does overlearning or other implosion based behavior modeling techniques. As the player develops the overabundance of involvement and energy, that energy is producing a behavioral potential sufficient to survive an extinction process which can occur during periods of mastery problems.

Another impact of this energy is its social element, as the player becomes a proselytizing computer zealot. This energy is communicated to others and is associated with computer play, further adding to the adoption of the innovation, and the development of a social support network for the zealot.

If affect in the promethean approach to innovation is described as satisfaction, then under the panish approach it should be described as fun. Given the seriousness of computer play even away from serious contexts, it would be unwise to expect to see fun modeled as laughter and smiles. It is more evident in a number of behavioral ways - through the expression of emotion to the computer itself or to others mediated through computer networks, through the way people spend their time, and through the ways people engage in practical jokes around the computer or with it.

As Sproul and Kiesler (1986) suggest, affect is strongly effected by the medium of its expression. For many users, it is easier to express strong emotions in computer communication than in face-to-face communication.

Paralleling the findings of Sproul and Kiesler (1986) in electronic mail situations, playing at statistical analysis on a computer is punctuated by moments of elation or lightheartedness and periods of intense concentration. Anger is freely expressed, directed both outward e.g. shouting curses, and inward, e.g. typing gibberish into the computer to force unwanted answers.

The reaction to failure is also more pronounced when involved on a play project than a work project. There are fewer inhibitions in expressing anger or frustration, and analysts are more inclined to put the play project away than when work projects are involved.

Continuing along this topic of affect and time use statistical analysts at play spread their personal statistical projects out over longer periods of time than they do when on a work project. They will mix non-analytic activities more during these play sessions, and in general show a more relaxed attitude toward the activity than they do when doing work analyses. Perhaps reflecting their valuation of the intrinsic quality of play and work projects, given free choice, e.g. when there is little time pressure, analysts will opt for their play projects over work projects.

One surprising method for analysts to make themselves feel good was to structure a "triumph of mastery of man over machine" as one player put it. Loosely translated, this involves playing practical jokes on the computer, forcing it to do useless work. This commonly involves producing as much output as possible using the fewest commands. A popular example is to request descriptive statistics or correlation matrices of all variables in a dataset.

Taken together, these indices of affect suggest that these players are deeply involved in the analytic tasks, and may even prefer play tasks to work ones. Evidence regarding how and when these people have fun with their computers, such as playing games, or completing a project, or uncovering a particularly interesting datum remains spotty, as individual mention these occurrences, but without a pattern as to their frequency of general categories emerging as yet.

CONTEXTUAL VARIABLES

In prospect, given the relative paucity of consideration of contextual variables in job design and game design theories, it was difficult to determine what contextual variables might become important. As the pilot study progressed, three variables seemed to play a major role in the play process. They are called ownership, access, and workload.

Ownership

Ownership is an oblique way of referring to the player's identification with the computer. Few mainframe users outside computer service units think of or refer to mainframe computers as "theirs." Mainframes are usually owned by the organizations, housed in an area the user doesn't think of as his or hers, and are collectively used.

Microcomputers are often distributed with a one-person-one-processor goal in mind. This leaves computer users with the impression that they control, or more naively, own, the personal computer in their possession. This sense of ownership appears to give a type of permission to make more extensive use of the computer than does collective ownership of a mainframe. This follows the conventional reasoning of the diffusion of responsibility literature (Latane, Williams, and Harkins, 1979).

Access

Ownership and the web of computer policies in which possession is embedded often raises issues of access. As one statistician stated:

Thus far the statistics community has tended to take the general view that a computer is for computing, regardless of its size or physical location. If it is placed on a table next to one's desk, so much the better (Kennedy, 1983: 65).

The possession of a personal computer means that the person can gain access to computer power at the time and place of their choosing. This type of access facilitates analysis done in a manner most consistent with the work habits of the player. As access increases, usage appears to increase, and the increase is greatest for small scale or short single purpose analyses, which are exactly the types of analyses most likely to be driven by exploratory or intuitive, alias creative, goals.

Workload

Ownership and access can be strongly effected by the work demands on the player. Large datasets require a mainframe approach, while small datasets can be usefully analyzed on microcomputers. Workload also has a strong, but exceedingly transient effect on play. Its relationship to play appears to be imperfectly curvilinear. In periods of slack workload, play increases, and many "back burner" projects get activated. As workload increases, play decreases, but under conditions of high workload, it appears that many users increase their amount of play slightly, as a means of providing a brief recreational break. Usually play in these periods is of the video games rather than programming variety.

PATHOLOGIES OF PLAYFULNESS

In keeping with the individual level approach to play and organizational life, it is worth considering how extreme forms of play can produce counterproductive or counter-innovative behaviors. Two extremes seem likely. One is perfectionism, which would be based on unreasonably high desires for mastery. The other is flightiness, based on an affect so strong that it precludes concentration. The extreme outcome of creativity might be a composite of the two pathologies.

The tendency for computer users to use the computer to optimize work and play outcomes has been recounted in a number of different ways above. Practice for achieving mastery hinges on the player. But when left unchecked, this desire for optimization becomes a drive for perfectionism. Often this takes the form of unkept promises for software or analyses. The player continues to rework the material. With reworking comes greater insight, and a belief that (1) all the needed information and changes will be near at hand, and (2) if the material had been released earlier it would have been inadequate.

In the pathology of perfectionism, the player has stopped having fun, and engages instead in a ritual rather than a game. The ritual provides comfort, which is a pale form of affect in comparison to playfulness or fun, but the ritual does not permit a clean point of closure. This provides the player with some motivation, as any incomplete game might in Malone's theory, but also poses an element of discomfort, as the player becomes as locked-in in play as in of work. The pursuit of mastery, and the realization that it remains just out of reach can start by having a motivating effect, but with the replacement of fun by comfort, the failures of mastery take on a more self-deprecating and negative tone.

Flightiness on the other hand, comes from an overabundance of energy and information. If perfectionism refers to the dogged pursuit of one item, flightiness reflects the approach of the dilettante, taking superficial account of a variety of items.

The computer permits the superficial perusal in ways never before dreamed. Entire libraries can be surveyed in seconds. Every incident of a topic, even a word, of interest can be found in the text of magazine, journals and newspapers instantly. Thousand of people with similar interests can be found and their biographies viewed immediately on the major networks.

And yet all the individual needs to do is ask the computer for the information, it doesn't even have to be viewed as it arrives, since the computer is capable of storing the information away for review at the player's leisure.

Part of the power of the computer is the way it opens the individual to vast stores of information, experience, and social exchange. It can be intimidating at first, and often individuals find their success in using the computer depends on their ability to recode some information as noise to be dismissed. Those who fail to develop or exercise this judgement suffer from flightiness, an inability to concentrate on the task at hand, whether it be play or work.

Like perfectionism, while in flight, the player has replaced fun producing behaviors with rituals. This person remains locked in the early player stage in terms of mastery, although this is often masked by the wealth of information regarding the potentials for computer use that is the hallmark of flightiness.

In considering these pathologies, it is worthwhile to remember that pathology in general can be applied to "all of the people some of the time, some of the people all of the time". Pathological behaviors are more likely to be caused by extreme pressures from a boss, project or family member as by some deep characterological flaw.

In either type of pathology the problem from the organization's perspective is that there is considerable effort but not performance. Unfortunately, computer problems of the types described here might be describable, but not necessarily altered. It is helpful to realize that in the above observations, the incidence of pathology was very rare overall, and most likely to occur in the early stages of the innovation. Social networking, involvement in organizational computer programs and institutional pressures seemed to coincide with more even-handed approaches to computer innovation.

IMPLICATIONS OF PLAY FOR RESEARCHERS

Research considering panish issues in innovation requires using an unconventional frame. Different variables are studied, e.g. fun rather than satisfaction. Panish innovation may violate organizational procedures, with the classic catch-22 being the purchase of a computer through petty cash because its use cannot be justified for a conventional purchase order, and that justification requires the user to spend time using the computer. Because play in organizations is a *sub rosa* activity, researchers must be indirect in their data gathering or hold a high level of trust among respondents.

Panish innovation holds important data for organizational and innovation researchers. The panish innovators may in many cases lay the groundwork for subsequent promethean innovation efforts. This groundwork may include the legitimization of computer-based innovation, the identification of innovators for later promethean efforts, as well as the content of subsequent innovations. In order to study promethean innovations, it may be necessary to occasionally study panish efforts, just as it is sometimes necessary to study an organization's founder to understand the organization later in time.

In other cases, panish efforts may reflect a computer subculture paralleling the conventional computer culture, and contributing vitality, experimentation, ideas or even opposition to the predominant promethean culture. This subcultural approach is evident in Turkle's discussion of hackers, but can also apply to organizational power users who develop their skill through panish efforts.

Although this paper has focussed on white-collar play on computers, play can be more widespread in the workforce. In practice, computers become a double-edged sword in lower ranks, as some workers (notably assembly line and telephone response workers) find the pacing of their work determined and monitored by computer, while others (notably secretaries in non-pooled settings) find the computer increasing their skills and saving time on the most boring of tasks. For the former group, asserting mastery over the computer by testing its limits reflects some element of play, albeit not necessarily well-intentioned. For the latter group, other observation not reported above suggest that some secretaries see the computer in much the same panish way as do white-collar employees. Play approaches may offer ways to consider the relation of blue- and pink-collar groups to computers.

Finally, with the growing interest in charismatic aspects of organizational motivation and commitment, it is important to realize that play, and particularly ways to combine work and play, represent a major vehicle for increasing an individual's involvement in and commitment to the organization (e.g. Berlew, 1974). For the people observed above, the opportunity to play with their personal computers became a reason to become more involved in their work. As their mastery grew in advance of others, their involvement in the organization also grew through advice giving, demonstrating, teaching, and challenging others. Computer play is not the only form of play in organizations, but it is an easy one to track down - one looks for new personal computers or people with lots of computing "toys". It is a form of play that is not seasonal; that takes place in the locale of the office; and that has the potential for group play through networking as well as individual play.

CONCLUSION: PLAYING AT ORGANIZATIONAL INNOVATION

This paper started with the idea that innovation, particularly regarding the process of computerization, could occur through the effort of managers and professionals having fun as well as through the more conventional method of scanning, planning, and implementing. These innovations occur at the individual level, but with their diffusion by computer zealots, take on an organizational impetus of their own.

There are famous examples of where a chief executive decides that computers would be useful, and in implementing the top executive's wishes, an organization innovates (Rockart and Treacy, 1982). These represent clear cases of where the design of an innovation includes how it will be institutionalized from the innovation's inception.

In other cases, like those described here, the innovation may start out among individuals with less power. In these cases, the organization's efforts to institutionalize the innovation come later in the decision process, e.g. *de facto* standards for hardware and software may already exist, and institutionalization may be more difficult to manage. Perhaps even more importantly in those *post hoc* attempts to institutionalize individually made innovations there comes a fundamental cultural or climate change in the manifest seriousness of the innovation process.

Essential to the definition of play is the idea of its distinctiveness from the serious forms of work. In its early stages, "playing with the computer" may literally embody the element of play, an element distinguished in part by its lack of seriousness. With the advent of organizational efforts to incorporate microcomputers, the potential for play declines as the organizations expectations for work from personal computer users changes. What was once fortuitous and exceptional is now expected and treated as commonplace. In short, institutionalization may not just be the death of innovation, it might also be the death of fun.

Maintaining innovation as an enduring revolution is a topic considered by change theorists (Hackman, 1984; Kanter, 1983), and is beyond the scope of this paper, but it is important to recognize that computer inspired playfulness in organizations may be a transient or episodic thing. It can be a vital force for innovation, but like other forms of organizational change cannot be depended upon to hold the interests or motivations of people for long. Even Pan can becoming boring.

ACKNOWLEDGMENT

This research was sponsored through Project Threshold, a joint project of the University of Pennsylvania and IBM. The preparation of this report was sponsored by a grant from IBM through the Management of Iformation Systems Program of the Wharton School.

REFERENCES

Adams, J.L. (1979). *Conceptual blockbusting.* New York: W.W. Norton & Company.

Andrews, F.M., Klem, L., Davidson, T.N., O'Malley, P.M., & Rodgers, W. L. (1981). *A guide for selecting statistical techniques for analyzing social science data.* Ann Arbor: University of Michigan, Institute for Social Research.

Bean, J. (1983). Computerized word-processing as an aid to revision. *College Composition and Communication, 34,* 146- 148.

Berlew, D.E (1974). Leadership and organizational excitement. *California Management Review, 17 (2),* 21-30.

Box, G.E.P. (1969). The challenge of statistical computation. In R.C.
        Milton & J.A. Nelder (Eds.), *Statistical computation*. New York:
        Academic Press.

Bridwell, L., Johnson, P., & Brehe, S. (1984). Composing and computers:
        Case studies of experienced writers. In A. Matsuhashi (Ed.),
        Writing in real time: Modeling production processes. New York:
        Longman.

Carlson, E.D., Grace,B.F., & Sutton, J.A. (1977). Case studies of end user
        requirements for interactive problem- solving systems. *Manage-
        ment Information Systems Quarterly, 51-63.*

Carroll, J.M. (1982). The adventure of getting to know a computer.
        Computer, 15 (11), 49-58.

Chaffin, J.D., Maxwell, B. and Thompson, B. (1982). Arcade curriculum -
        the application of video game formats to educational software.
        Exceptional Children, 49 (5), 308-311.

Collier, R. (1983). The word processor and revision strategies. *College
        Composition and Communication, 34,* 149- 155.

Curley, K.F. & Pyburn, P.J. (1982). "Intellectual" technologies: The key to
        improving white-collar productivity. *Sloan Management Review,
        Fall,* 31-39.

Hackman, J.R. (1984). The transition that hasn't happened. In J.R.
        Kimberly and R.E. Quinn (Eds.) *Managing organizational
        transitions.* Homewood, IL: Irwin.

Hackman, J.R. and Oldham, G.R. (1976). Motivation through the design
        of work: test of a theory. *Organizational Behavior and Human
        Performance, 16,* 250-279.

Hare,A.P. (1982). *Creativity in small groups.* Beverly Hills: Sage.

Huizinga, J. (1949) *Homo ludens: The play element in culture.* London:
        Routledge and Kegan, Paul.

Kanter, R.M. (1983). *The change masters.* New York: Simon & Shuster.

Kennedy, W.J. (1983). A curriculum in statistical computing? *American
        Statistical Association Proceedings,* 65-66.

Latane, B., Williams, K. & Harkins, S. (1979). Many hands make light the
        work: Causes and consequences of social loafing. *Journal of
        Personality and Social Psychology, 37* (6), 822-832.

Leavitt, H.J. (1965). Applied organizational change in industry. In *Hand-
        book of Organizations.* Chicago: Rand McNally.

Lefkowitz, J.M. (1983). Teaching the use of statistics packages. *American
        Statistical Association Proceedings,* 60- 62.

Lieberman, J.N. (1965). Playfulness and divergent thinking: An investiga-
        tion of their relationship at the kindergarten level. *Journal of
        Genetic Psychology, 107,* 219-224.

Malone, T.W. (1980). What makes things fun to learn? A study of in-
    trinsically motivating computer games. *Dissertation Abstracts
    International, 41,* 1955 B. (University Microfilms No. 8024707,
    93)
Mehrabian, A. & Wixen, W.J. (1986). Preferences for individual video
    games as a function of their emotional effects on players. *Journal
    of Applied Social Psychology, 16* (1), 3-15.
Michaels, D.N. (1973). *On learning to plan - and planning to learn.* San
    Francisco: Jossey-Bass.
Morlock, H., Yando, T. and Nigolean, K. (1985). Motivation of video
    game players. *Psychological Reports, 57* (1), 247-250.
Myers, D. (1984). The patterns of player-game relationships - a study of
    computer game players. *Simulation and Games, 15* (2), 159-185.
Novick, M.R. (1984). Human factors in computer-assisted data analysis.
    American Statistical Association Proceedings, 33- 36.
Olson, R.W. (1980). *The art of creative thinking: A practical guide.* New
    Rok: Barnes and Noble/ Harper and Row.
Pinchot, G. III (1985). *Intrapreneuring.* New York: Harper and Row.
Reuben, H.L. (1980). *Competing.* New York: Pinnacle.
Rockart, J.F. and Treacy, M.E. (1982). The CEO goes on-line. *Harvard
    Business Review, January-February,* 82-87.
Schon, D. (1963). Champions for radical new inventions. *Harvard Business
    Review, 41* (2), 77-86.
Sproul, L. and Kiesler, S. (1986). Reducing social context cues: Electronic
    mail in organizational communication. *Management Science, 32*
    (11), 1492-1512.
Sutton-Smith, B. (1971). Play, games, and controls. In J.P. Scott and S.F.
    Scott (Eds.). *Social control and social change.* Chicago: University
    of Chicago.
Taylor, I.A. (1975). An emerging view of creative actions. In I.A. Taylor
    and J.W. Getzels (Eds.) *Perspective in Creativity.* Chicago: Aldine.
Turkle, S. (1984). *The second self: Computers and the human spirit.* New
    York: Simon and Schuster.
Velleman, P.F. (1980). Do statistical packages help or hinder data analysis?
    American Statistical Association Proceedings, 21-26.
Wallach, M.A. and Kogan, N. (1965). *Modes of thinking in young children:
    A study of the creativity-intelligence distinction.* New York: Holt,
    Rinehart and Winston.

THE FIT
BETWEEN THE WORK PLACE
AND THE HUMAN

Psychological Issues of
Human Computer Interaction in the Work Place
M. Frese, E. Ulich, W. Dzida (Editors)
Elsevier Science Publishers B.V. (North-Holland), 1987

COMPUTERIZATION VERSUS COMPUTER AIDED MENTAL WORK

Winfried Hacker

Technische Universität Dresden, Mommsenestr. 13
DDR-8027 Dresden, German Democratic Republic

The design of human-computer interaction is best
treated as a dependent component of the more comprehensive design of computer aided work. The hierarchical structure of activities results in a hierarchy of
objects in task design. The design of the comprehensive
task which can be oriented by the concept of sequentially and hierarchically complete activities determines and
restricts the design of subtasks and task details. Identical
designs, for example on the level of dialogue structures,
may have opposite effects on the human depending upon
higher order design solutions (e.g., of task complexity).
A set of objective task characteristics of a design instrument permits both desired mental requirements and social implications.

THE SUBJECT MATTER: TASKS OR INTERFACES?

Design of human-computer interaction means information centered
task design. Before one is able to design details of this interaction, for
example the dialogue structure, some basic decisions have to be made.
How does one allocate the functions between humans and computers (including interface problems) and how does one design the organizational
division of tasks among the workers? Both questions pertain to key problems of task design and require a diagnosis and an evaluation of task
demands.

Unfortunately, computerization often does not spontaneously generate human-centered job contents (Hacker & Schönfelder, 1986, Rudolph,
1986). Evaluating a representative sample of computerized white-collar
jobs by means of a supplement of the Task Diagnostic Survey (Rudolph,
Schönfelder & Hacker, 1987), we found that here are no cogent relationships between computerization of wide spread data and text processing
tasks and the enhancement of the quality of working life. This is so, even
though the potential efficiency of human-computer interaction depends on
the health and personality promoting design of those task contents that

remain with the human. Given a bad design, the new tasks may even be more monotonous and may provoke more mental health risks after the introduction of computers than before (e.g., Greif & Holling, 1986). Moreover, the potential economic efficiency of human-computer systems are not realized, as well. This is particularly so when human routine tasks are computerized within the tradition of a Taylorist division of labor. Relatively complex human processing operations are replaced with narrowminded and simple input operations in such a case.

Differences in the task content of computer aided mental work are not only caused by software, of course. A bad design of the work place that is due to a technocentric allocation of functions between human and computer and a Taylorist division of labor between several persons cannot be repaired even by the best software.

In order to design computer aided mental work, the following is required:
- an adequate conceptualization of working activities and
- an adequate development of goals and evaluation characteristics of how working activities should be designed.

The concept of goal directed working activities leads to some fundamentals of work and software design. The task and goal orientation for the user (concept-driven user) includes:
- establishment of plans for reaching a goal,
- the hierarchical structure of working activities,
- the flexibility in the use of plans which is dependent on the task and the working conditions, and
- individual modifications within a given set of degrees of freedom (cf. Hacker, 1986a).

Computer aided work should be designed in terms of this concept based on desired characteristics of the working persons' activities. Thus, the basic question of design is: What should be reserved for th human, and what should be computerized? The anthropocentric allocation of functions between human and computer will lead to a such a division of labor between different people that all of the tasks involve a high degree of stimulating task content.

Concerning mental work, this concept of goal-directed activity is to be differentiated further. The rough term "mental work" is not suitable for the description of task requirements. Mental work cannot be reduced to thinking or solving problems. It will rather involve the following as well:
- processes of merely transferring information, i.e. perception and rehearsal without thinking at all,
- information processing, i.e. classification and reasoning according to a set of given rules,
- thinking determined by algorithms, and
- information generating processes, i.e. finding and solving problems in a creative way.

Consequently for a clear characterization of requirements for mental work, the processes required in each case have to be analyzed. The introduction of information systems may yield extremely different sets of requirements leading to very different effects on workers' wellbeing and performance.

The concept of *"user-friendliness" of software* is a more limited approach. Interfaces between the human and the tool are to be matched to the human. However, the danger arises that the approach of user-friendliness leads to the conventional adaptation of the machine surface to the human, but nothing more because once a certain interface is given, the questions of allocation of functions between the human and the computer and the division of labor are not important issues any more. Although the adaptation of the interface is necessary, the more important issues of how work impairs or promotes personality are easily forgotten. Therefore, task design has to go beyond ergonomic design of workplaces and software ergonomics and include the design of the content of computer-aided work. This is the only way that the central contradiction in this area can be solved: Human-computer interaction should be simple (i.e. not additionally demanding, DIN 66234/8) but the task should be stimulating and result in intrinsic motivation. A solution is possible only on the superior level of the overall task characteristics. This level includes both the quality of software and the content of work. Consequently, design goals and evaluating measures are demanded for the total tasks and not only for interfaces.

DESIGN GOALS AND EVALUATING CHARACTERISTICS FOR COMPUTER AIDED MENTAL WORK

The goals for design and the methods by which the design is evaluated must be valid for computer aided work; merely trying to achieve userfriendly software is not sufficient. For example, an error-resistant, self-explanatory and reliable dialogue does not make an overall monotonous task more stimulating. Therefore conventional and general design criteria of a good work place, should be applied for computer-aided mental work as well. When designing tasks, three golas have to be met: (1) improvement of efficiency, (2) optimization of psychophysiological demands, and (3) health and personality enhancement. To meet these goals, it is possible to use the well-known ergonomic criteria for evaluating design solutions. These criteria have to be adapted to the question of designing computerized *cognitive* tasks instead of manual tasks (which they were originally developed for). The criteria can be hierarchically ordered, as discussed in detail in the following:

The first level is *feasibility*. This level is often underestimated in the area of mental work. Cognitive feasibility, is jeopardized by overload of human information processing capacities. There are three types of deficiencies that lead to cognitive overload: First, people will be overloaded if mentally efficient information on a required action is *lacking*. Not all information that is physically there in a given setting is also represented mentally. Two examples: About 1800 pure tones can be discerned, but only 4 to 5 can be precisely identified. Feedbacks, which are delayed by more than 100 to 200 msec or which are not available in time to take effect on the next operation will disturb the regulation of action. Second, people will be overloaded if an information is mentally efficient, but *cannot be used* in regulating the action. For instance, the span of short-term memory in serial tasks does not exceed 3 to 4 chunks. Third, people will be overloaded if the information itself leads to its wrong utilization. Coding that is incompatible with normal habits of interpretation, e.g. blue for hot steam and red for cooling water, would be an example for information that prompts wrong responses. The second and third forms of overload can be expected in working with information systems.

The second level refers to the *level of harmlessness*. This is important as investigations reveal that about half of VDU data input operators show eye complaints and complaints in the shoulder-arm region due to inadequate workplace design. Thus, long-term health risks may be implicated. The tendency to show high health complaints and illness rates is more pronounced in those jobs with a high division of labor and high partialization of mental work. The degree of completeness (as opposite of partialization) is a measure of this phenomenon; we will come back to this issue.

The third level refers to *health impairments*; in contrast to the level before, established occupational diseases are not implicated here, but the less clearly defined complaints, like psychophysiological complaints, unacceptable degrees of fatigue or the experience of monotony, satiation and stress. They are equally associated with inadequate design of contents and execution conditions of computer aided mental work. Restricting the degrees of freedom for independent decisions or reducing the completeness of actions by giving several subtasks with differing demands lead to higher degrees of fatigue, monotony, and satiation.

The fourth level concerns *personality enhancement*. Important aspects are whether a worker can develop skills and can learn in his or her job. This is closely related to intrinsic motivation for work.

ON THE HIERARCHY OF DESIGN MEASURES

Tasks and activities are structured hierarchically. The overall activity can be subdivided into individual activities. These in turn consist of subactivities or actions; these again concist of routine operations. The existence of several levels of regulation of an activity also results in the demand to develop a hierarchy in the design of activities. When looking at the design of computer aided mental tasks, the hierarchy of design levels as shown in Figure 1 is obtained.

Figure 1: Hierarchy of design objects

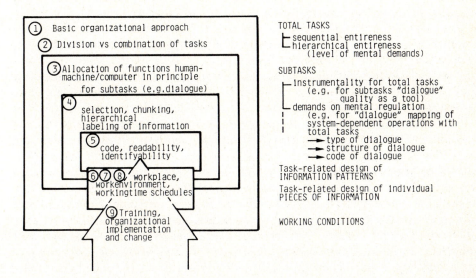

The *total* task with its physical and mental spectrum of requirements is determined by basic organizational concepts (e.g., by the degree of centralization of decisions or by the number of management levels) and by the division and combination of labor between the workers (cf. Nullmeier & Rödiger in this book). Guidelines and evaluation measures for the design of the total task are founded on the principle of *complete activities*, i.e. an activity that embraces all levels of regulation, the intellectual and the sensorimotor level as well as organizational aspects (this is explained in detail in the next section).

Subtasks are to be analyzed in terms of their instrumentality and their demands made on central processing capacity. The individual *subtasks* are determined by the allocation of functions between human and hardware as well as software. *Instrumentality* means that the subtasks should help to solve the total task. Human computer interaction consists of subtasks that should help in the solution of the total task.

On of these subtasks is the human-computer dialogue which is instrumental fo the total task (cf. Spinas in this book). Raum (1986 a), for

example, showed that both inexperienced workers and experts prefer simplified and transparent dialogues. These dialogues must, however, allow
for individual modifications of the actual task treatment. The reason for
this preference lies in the better chance to cope with the actual main task.
This coping is dependent on individual preferences and the specifics of
the individual's interactions with the task. Since this is so, only he chance
to modify the actual task treatment allows the individual to adapt the
situation to his or her limits of the central processing capacity (cf. Frese
in this book). However, one precondition for this is that there is a sufficiently broad main task. This implies that a dialogue can be computer-
guided and without any degrees of freedom as long as the main task permits sufficient degrees of freedom. It is not the subtask "dialogue" but
rather the entire activity that determines the effect of the work place on
the human.

The second issue - the *demands on mental regulation* - refers to the
question which cognitive processes and representation are implicated in the
specific task regulation. Task related design of *patterns of information* is
related to the design of subtasks. Patterning the information has to be
done to assure task related groupings, a good structure of the information,
meaningful labels and finally has to be oriented to different kinds of user
groups. Two examples: (1) Clustering information helps to save time in
information input tasks. This is even more so when the information is
complex. (2) Time requirements can be reduced by providing insight into
the structure of the information. This can be done by presenting a mental
model of the task structure. However, this is only true if the representation is coded iconically *and* conceptually -- a purely conceptual one does
not work well (Hacker & Meinel, 1978).

These examples confirm hierarchical principles. The use of even
universal principles like the Gestalt laws or the principle of double coding
as in the experiment described above is related to the task. Information
design will be useless without considering task characteristics .

The design of patterns of information can be subdivided into *individual pieces of information*. Thereby special attention is to be devoted to
enhancing storage as well as to securing legibility of information.

Finally, the *organizational and time conditions of subtask executions*
have to be designed as part of the total task. Here it is important to give
guarantees to keep one's workplace and to consider the work environment,
and the work time regimes. The processes of introduction of the new
technology and of training are aspects of these conditions as well.

This hierarchy of design levels has two consequences:
(1) The different levels of task design vary in their *range of effects*.
Design on superior levels has more comprehensive effect on workers' efficiency and well-being than design of subordinate ones. For example, the
optimization of single commands or data formats will not lead to an enrichment of the content of work.

(2) Design solutions of superior levels *determine* the effects of design solutions of subordinate ones. Therefore, equal design measures will have different effects depending upon the design solutions on superior levels. The determining effect of the overall task is decisive. For example, the task compatibility of the linguistic form of an instruction depends on the task's complexity. In a low task complexity situation, people like to get grammatically more demanding descriptions of relationships. Conversely in a high task complexity situation, grammatically simple descriptions of the sequence of operations are preferred (Scholz, 1986).

Thus, the design of superior task characteristics determines the possible design scope of the individual task characteristics. Therefore, there is not one optimum "user-friendly" dialogue form, grouping of information or command structure *per se* but rather only solutions for *classes of tasks and users*!

What has to be done in the case of unknown users and tasks? In this case, the presentation of the most appropriate forms of dialogue, information patterns, etc. cannot be achieved. The principle of selectable information offers a way out of this dilemma (Raum 1986 b): Different selectable variants of dialogue types, help functions, forms of data configuration, codings, or commands are presented. The users can then utilize the choices and use those options that are commensurate with their individual prerequisites and with their tasks.

This principle of selectable information is based on the most important principle of up-to-date job design, namely the principle of offering autonomy which is related to the concept of complete actitivities.

DESIRABLE OBJECTIVE ACTIVITY CHARACTERISTICS: COMPLETE ACTIVITIES.

Technological systems should be developed so as to enhance human tasks instead of generating functions that remain in the hands of the human in a more or less arbitrary way. Therefore, a well-defined set of objective task characteristics that are desirable from this point of view is required. These characteristics have to be technolologically possible but they should also be based on predictions of how these tasks will affect the human on a short and long term basis. The predictions should be concerned with performance, perception and evaluation of job contents, physical and mental well-being as well as the chances of further learning at work.

For the description of these desirable task characteristics in information systems it is not sufficient to be concerned only with the lowest level of activity, i.e. the motor and mental operations as keystrokes and "mental motions" as in the conceptualization of Card, Moran & Newell (1983). We discussed at the outset of this article: Even at work with the tool "computer", the human attempts to pursue goals and realize plans. Goal oriented activities, however, cannot be reduced to a sum of actions, nor actions to a sum of operations. The Taylor model of job design has failed, it is not worth reviving (Volpert, 1985).

Furthermore, efficient actions are more than just quick and faultless reactions. Efficient actions have no negative effects but rather enhancing ones: The acting person is not overloaded, bored or frightened and does not become de-skilled. Rather he has the chance to be stimulated, motivated and to learn. There is little to gain if a millisecond low-level approach reduces cognitive complexity of tasks but leads at the same time to major losses (calculatable in minutes) due to the side-effects of monotony or de-skilling of users (Greif & Holling, 1986).

It is useful to describe and design tasks in information systems in terms of the concept of a complete activity (cf. Figure 2).

Figure 2: Sequential and hierarchical aspects of a complete activity

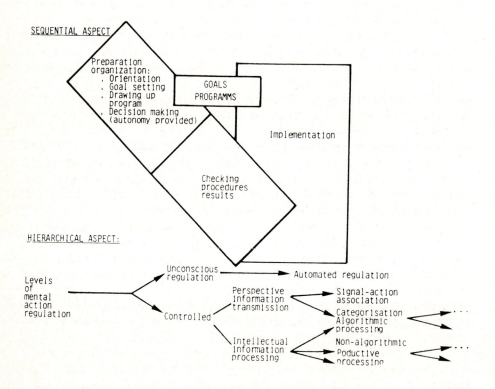

A complete activity is complete in terms of the sequential and hierarchical aspects. The sequential aspect includes:
- preparation functions (determination of goals, development and selection of procedures),
- organizational functions (coordinating tasks with other people),
- inspection and control through which workers get feedback,
- implementation in terms of executing the procedures developed before.

The *hierarchical* aspects of complete activity include different levels of regulation. The worker alternates between them. Consequently, tasks should allow the worker to use both mental routine operations and thinking processes of different types.

The precise mixture of demands that leads to using these different levels of the hierarchy is yet to be found. It appears that humans should be liberated from those mental processes that lead to overload whereas others that are stimulating should remain. The following experimental findings are pertinent here:

(1) With an increase of working memory load, the quantity and quality of performance deteriorates and fatigue increases. In contrast, increasing the complexity of intellectual tasks does not yield such a deterioration, at least as long as memory load remains constant (Hacker, 1986c).

(2) If external memory aids are given, deterioration of performance and well-being does not occur. An increase of fatigue and growing task complexity leads to a more frequent use of external memory aids (Schönpflug, 1985, Hacker, 1986b).

(3) Different mental processing operations exert different effects on performance and well-being. Processing operations do not mean simple transformation of data (essentially, a routine task), but in contrast higher order cognitive facilities are used. For example, the quantity and quality of routine performance deteriorates linearly with a decrease of the necessary processing operations and the increase of mere information input. In contrast mental tasks with sufficient processing requirements do not lead to a high load and result in better performance (Hacker, 1986 c).

What are the reasons for incomplete activities? Sequentially and hierarchically incomplete activities (i.e. partialized activities) can be caused by insufficient job design (Volpert, 1983). One possible reason for this occurrence is the inappropriate allocation of functions between humans and computers and by a Taylorist division of labor. For instance, data processing operations are frequently done by a computer, while low demand monotonous data input operations which require only perception and rehearsal but no thinking are done by humans. Similarly, Humans have to carry out operations that are preplanned and organized in every detail by the machine or by somebody else and are controlled by other people. Hence the worker who is actually executing a specific task is "released" from thinking, planning, and deciding.

Opportunities for setting goals and making decisions, for developing individual working methods, and for getting sufficient feedback are lacking in incomplete activities. In particular, one of the following aspects may lead to incomplete activities:

(1) Lack of sufficient activity: Chances for sufficient and active interference into the technical process are too small, for example, when a person has to essentially only monitor a process passively.

(2) Lack of chances to determine goals and make decisions and thus to take responsibility: Under such conditions the chances of autonomous and thus motivating goal setting and deciding on individual work procedures are lacking. Goal setting and decisions of this sort is dependent on the degrees of freedom that a job offers. Programming languages and dialogue types also differ in how much they offer these degrees of freedom. It could be shown that there is a negative correlation between autonomy on the one hand and anxiety and blood pressure on the other hand. Procedural autonomy should enable one to decide on the sequence of subtasks to avoid anxiety. Temporal autonomy helps to avoid critical values of blood pressure (Hacker, Iwanowa & Richter, 1983).

(3) Absence of thinking requirements in work: Activities can be incomplete in terms of lacking or insufficient thinking requirements. These requirements should be of a non-algorithmic and, occasionally, even creative type.

(4) Lack of cooperation: Cooperation means more than exchange of thoughts and communication. Incomplete activity does not allow the giving and receiving of social support and cooperation that leads to enhancement of personality.

(5) Lack of learning requirements: Insufficient chances to utilize and maintain as well as develop one's qualifications is a hallmark of incomplete activities. There should be at least occasional chances to learn new things. Learning should not only include abilities and attitudes, i.e. not only knowledge and routines. They should be transferable to varying tasks both within and outside of the functions agreed upon by the employment contract.

In short, it may be said that incomplete activities which come about as a result of inappropriate work design, impairs intrinsic motivation and learning potential of work. The higher the degree of incompleteness of the activities, the lower the well-being, mental health, satisfaction, intrinsic motivation, and learning potential. An example for the empirical relationships is given in Figure 3. Thus, the approach of complete activities provides guidelines for designing desired characteristics of working activities with useful economic and social implications.

Figure 3: Relationsship between learning potential and task perception

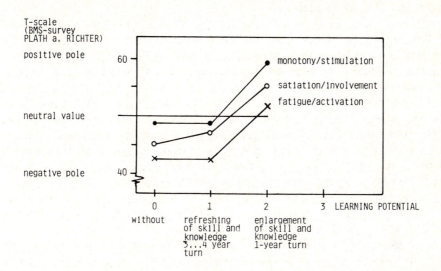

T-scale
(BMS-survey
PLATH a. RICHTER)

positive pole

60

monotony/stimulation

satiation/involvement

fatigue/activation

neutral value

negative pole

40

0   1   2   3   LEARNING POTENTIAL

without   refreshing   enlargement
          of skill and   of skill and
          knowledge   knowledge
          3...4 year   1-year turn
          turn

TECHNOLOGICALLY DESIGNABLE CHARACTERISTICS OF MENTAL ACTIVITIES

We have argued that software design is a part of task design. Therefore, designers of user software as task designers need the following:
- participation of designers even in the problem analysis phase since eraly stages of task definition determine the possible characteristics of software;
- adequate conceptions concerning what users want in terms of their work, for example, complete activities because they render personal and social advantages;
- instruments for the analysis and design of tasks.

We shall discuss only the last item here. Task designers need instruments of task analysis and design that concentrate on technologically designable task characteristics. The goal is to give the worker a possibility for complete activities. However, it is not possible to *directly* design mental processes; for example, one cannot design thinking patterns. But it is possible to design a job, so that it may enhance thinking processes. Those aspects of the design, I call technologically designable characteristics.

Hence, we are looking for a limited set of the most important objective task characteristics (technologically designable characteristics). Examples are:

- frequency of repetitions of uniformly repeated mental operations;
- degrees of freedom concerning time and content, decision and planning requirements (autonomy) and thus
- type of dialogue as well as
- sequential completeness (which was discussed in Figure 2).

These characteristics are clustered, i.e. they correlate highly with each other. For example the type of dialogue correlates with the degrees of freedom concerning content of work with r=.78 (p<.01).

Figure 4:   *Intellectual demans as a function of the type of human-computer interaction (Rudolph TUD 1986)*

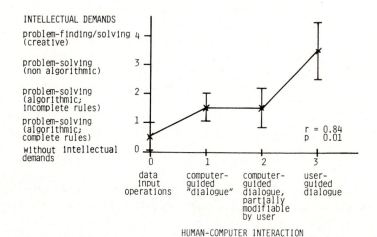

It is decisive for design purposes that these technologically designable characteristics (for example the dialogue type) correlate highly with thinking requirements as well (r=.84, p<.01, cf. Figure 4). Being forced to repeat frequently some uniform subactivities (as in the data input operations) correlates with thinking requirements .82 (p<.01).

Another example of the correlation between objective task characteristics and mental demands is shown in Figure 5. Mental requirements are plotted as a function of autonomy of the activity to be determined by the task designer, i.e. as a function of the type and extent of chances for setting goals and making decisions.

Figure 5: Mental requirements as a function of procedural anatomy

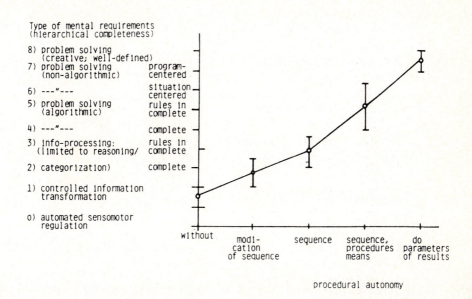

DESIGN OF FUTURE WORKING TASKS WITH DESIRED CHARACTERISTICS

It is urgently needed to concentrate on the design of tasks that will appear in the future and cannot yet be found in the industrial reality now. Currently, the majority of job design measures is just done to correct insufficiencies in jobs which already exist. Such corrections take longer and cost more. Moreover, the danger arises that undesired solutions of job design will be at a deadlock.

The important question of the design of future working tasks will be: Are there any patterns of task characteristics which result in desired social and economic effects? We know already something about *single* characteristics. For example it is well confirmed that sequential and hierarchical completeness of activities and sufficient degrees of freedom are in close correlation with performance efficiency, word satisfaction, well-being and low illness rates. For job design, however, such correlations on single task characteristics are not sufficient.

Patterns of task characteristics can be detected by discriminant analyses. The following example comes from an investigation by Rudolph et al. (1987). About 60 activities of 300 employees were researched. It is evident that fatigue, monotony, and satiation as well as complaint and illness rates can be predicted by justifyable error rates from sets of 3 to 9 task characteristics (cf. Table 1).

Predicted (re-classified) task outcome	error rate $\left[\begin{smallmatrix} 0/0 \end{smallmatrix}\right]$	technologically designable task characteristics	
		number	examples
Experienced fatigue/ activation	13	5	- temporal degrees of freedom - sequential completeness
" monotony/ stimulation	18	3	- variability of tasks - cooperation requirements
" satiation engagement	7	5	- sequential completeness - communication chances - required information on work organization
" work motivation	7	5	- sequential completeness
" complaints (concerning wellbeing)	14	9	- temporal degrees of freedom
rate of sickness: duration	18	8	- degrees of freedom concerning contents - feedback - predictibility of requirements
" " : freuency	20	6	- knowledge required - responsibilities

Table 1: *Prediction of some effects of whitecollar tasks from designable task characteristics (discriminant analyses)*

One example: At an error rate of 20%, perceived monotony can be predicted with three activity characteristics: number of different subtasks, repetition of uniform orders, and temporal degrees of freedom. The rise of monotony emerges if the workers do not have to process more than 2 to 3 subtasks with different subtasks, if uniform orders are to repeated over the day and if temporal degrees of freedom are not high during the workday.

The generality of these results still has to be established. But these results suggest that the design process will lead to positive social and economic results if the following conditions are met: It gives an equal share to technological as well as to social objectives; it is organized in an iterative and participative manner (cf. Figure 6); and it offers chances to develop designs of computer aided mental tasks. Design of human-computer interaction should be implemented as a component of this type of design of computer aided work tasks of the future. This may help to overcome the short-lived Tayloristic concepts of design in order to develop

Figure 6: Approaches of system design (Kemp, Clegg and Wall, 1984)

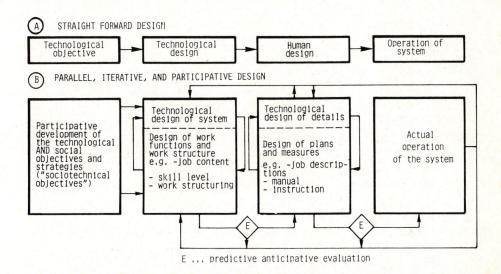

E ... predictive anticipative evaluation

software and jobs that are conducive to reduce potential harms and increase motivational and learning potentials of tasks.

REFERENCES

Card, S. K., Moran, T. P., & Newell, A. (1983). *The psychology of human-computer interaction.* Hillsdale, N.J.: Erlbaum.

DIN 66 234. Normenausschuß Informationsverarbeitungssysteme (NI) (1984 als Entwurf verabschiedet). *Bildschirmarbeitsplätze. Grundsätze der Dialoggestaltung.* Berlin: Deutsches Institut für Normung e. V.; Beuth-Verlag.

Greif, S., & Holling, H. (1986). Neue Technologien. In D. Frey & S. Greif (Eds.), *Sozialpsychologie* (2. Auflage). München, Wien: Urban & Schwarzenberg.

Hacker, W. (1986 a). *Arbeitspsychologie.* Bern: Huber.

Hacker, W. (1986 b). Memory for its own sake? Coping with optional memory demands. In F. Klix & H. Hagendorf (Eds.), *Human memory and cognitive capabilities* (pp. 1057 - 1070). Amsterdam: Elsevier.

Hacker, W. (1986 c). What should be computerized? Cgnitive demands of mental routine tasks and mental load. In F. Klix & H. Wandke

(Eds.), *Man-computer interaction research I* (pp. 445 - 461).
Amsterdam: Elsevier.

Hacker, W., Iwanowa, A., & Richter, P. (1983).
*Tätigkeitsbewertungssystem (TBS). Verfahren zur objektiven
Tätigkeitsanalyse.* Berlin: Psychodiagnostisches Zentrum an der
Humboldt-Universität.

Hacker, W., & Meinel, M. (1978). Kognitive Komponenten beim Erlernen
interner Repräsentationen: Sind behaltensökonomische Repräsen-
tationen stets regulativ zweckmäßig? In G. Clauß, J. Guthke, &
G. Lehwald (Hg.), *Psychologie und Psychodiagnostik lernaktiven
Verhaltens* (Tagungsbericht, pp. 54 - 61). Berlin: Gesellschaft für
Psychologie der DDR.

Hacker, W., & Schönfelder, E. (1986). Job organization and allocation of
functions between man and computer: Analysis and assesment. In
F. Klix & H. Wandke (Eds.), *Man-computer interaction research I*
(pp. 403 - 419). Amsterdam: Elsevier.

Moran, T. P. (1983). Getting into a System: External-internal task mapping
analysis. *CHI'83 Proceedings*, 45 - 49.

Raum, H. (1986 a). Aufgabenbezogene Dialoggestaltung bei Bildschirm-
arbeit. In H. Raum & W. Hacker (Hg.), *Optimierung geistiger
Arbeitstätigkeiten* (Referate des Dresdener Symposiums zur
Arbeits- und Ingenieurpsychologie 1986, pp. Band 1; 52 - 57).
Dresden: Eigenverlag Technische Universität Dresden.

Raum, H. (1986 b). Alternative information presentation as a contribution
to user related dialogue design. In F. Klix & H. Wandke (Eds.),
Man-computer interaction research I (pp. 339 - 348). Amsterdam:
Elsevier.

Rudolph, E. (1986). Neue Erfahrungen zur Analyse, Bewertung und Gestaltung rechnergewstützter geistiger Arbeit. *Sozialistische
Arbeitswissenschaft, 6.*

Rudolph, E., Schönfelder, E., & Hacker, W. (1987). *Verfahren zur
objectiven Analyse, Bewertung und Gestaltung geistiger Arbeitstätigkeiten mit und ohne Rechnerunterstützung (TBS-GA).* Berlin:
Psychodiagnostisches Zentrum an der Humboldt- Universität.
Hogreffe-Vertrieb, Göttingen.

Schönpflug, W. (1985). *The trade off between internal and external
information storage.* (Paper submitted for publication). .

Scholz, G. (1986). *Zur sprachlichen Darstellung von Aufgabentext.* Infor-
mationen der TU Dresden 1986.. Dresden: Eigenverlag der Tech-
nischen Universität Dresden.

Volpert, W. (1983). *Handlungsstrukturanalyse als Beitrag zur Qualifikationsforschung.* Köln: Pahl-Rugenstein.

Volpert, W. (1985). *Zauberlehrlinge: Die gefährliche Liebe zum Computer.*
Weinheim: Beltz.

Psychological Issues of
Human Computer Interaction in the Work Place
M. Frese, E. Ulich, W. Dzida (Editors)
© Elsevier Science Publishers B.V. (North-Holland), 1987

THE CHANCES OF INDIVIDUALIZATION IN HUMAN-COMPUTER INTERACTION AND ITS CONSEQUENCES

David Ackermann and Eberhard Ulich

Work and Organizational Psychology Unit
Swiss Federal Institute of Technology (ETH)
Nelkenstr. 11, CH-8092 Zürich

This paper presents – after a theoretical summary – the results of investigations based on the principles of differential and dynamic work design. The experiments display that dialog forms meeting the requirements of these principles cause no discernible reduction in efficiency or increase in strain. On the contrary there are some hints that the individualization of dialogs leads to improved efficiency. Finally we demonstrate the principle's application in the developping process of software with user participation.

INTRODUCTION

This paper is based on the assumption that the scope for setting up organizational structures as well as the scope for work structuring has increased substantially with the recent technological developments. Hence the use of computer-aided work systems requires fundamental decisions to be taken concerning the formulation of company strategy and work design philosophy.

Earlier concepts (e.g. Lipmann 1932) as well as recent results of research (e.g. Triebe, 1980, 1981; Zülch & Starringer, 1985; Grob, 1985) confirm the assumption that the concept of an existing "one best way" for every work activity, which has only to be discovered and taught to people, is a portentous error of the traditional work design theory. On the contrary the principle of differential work design calls for a "simultaneous offer of different work structures among which the worker can select" (ULICH, 1978, 1983). The principle of differential work design shall guarantee an optimal development of personality in the interaction with work activity based on interindividual differences. In order to meet these requirements and take into account processes of personality development, the principle of differential work design needs to be supplemented by the principle of dynamic work design. Accordingly, there has to be the pos-

sibility to enlarge existing and to create new work structures or to select
from different systems (Ulich, 1978, 1983). Therefore it is not sufficient
to fullfill the requirements due to possible interindividual differences by
differential work design. Moreover, it is necessary to take into account
intraindividual differences over time. Possible sources of such differences
can be (see Ulich, Frei and Baitsch, 1980)

- increasing reduction of the degrees of freedom caused by the habituation to certain styles of work in the sense of the development of a
  "subjective one best way"
- increasing formation of decision routines with repeating demands
- changement of the level of aspiration e.g. due to new work experiences
  and the resulting impact on self-concept and reaction to the environment
- qualitative changes in the satisfaction with work, for example substitution of a form of resignative satisfaction by a more progressive
  form of (dis)satisfaction (see Bruggemann, 1974, Bruggemann, Groskurth and Ulich, 1975)

This raises the question "how work as one of the most important
learning treatments can be designed, so that work supports the development of the workers qualifications and not only the application of them."
(Triebe and Ulich 1977, 270).

In this connection the demand for flexibility and user definability of
interactive dialog systems is very important (Ulich, 1986, 1987). "If from
the user's point of view 'software' is defined as all the parts of a computer
system which can be modified by the user and 'hardware' as all those
parts which once there, cannot be modified any more, then present day
computer systems consist almost exclusively of hardware" (Fischer, 1985,
p. 37). If one accepts this definition of software then the criterion of
"flexibility / user definability" should be considered as one of the essential
criteria of user-oriented dialog-design.

Four experimental studies carried out in our research group concerning ways of making computer-aided work activities more flexible and
adaptable as well as the consequences arising are described below. All are
pilot studies requiring further examination and amplification.

ON THE USE AND EFFECTS OF FLEXIBILITY

The first experiment concerns the question of the efficiency of
flexible dialog forms and how they will be used. Aschwanden and
Zimmermann (1984) worked with two groups of subjects with 15 members
each who were presented with a task concerning the processing of orders
with two different dialog versions. A characteristic of dialog version 1 was

the high degree of rigidity whereas dialog version 2 was noticeably more flexible (see Table 1). In the planning stage of this study , measures were taken which would minimize the difficulties of applying the experience gained in the experiment to a normal work situation. These involved creating experimental conditions which were as realistic as possible. To satisfy the criterion 'representative activity' a typical of a business situation task was chosen, i. e. the preparation of a tender for an order of office material. Experienced personnel from the telephone information service of the Swiss Postal Office operated the computers in order to get as close as possible to a 'representative subject'. Finally, to satisfy the criterion 'representative environment', the experiment was carried out in the training center of the post office known to all participants. Each subject had to prepare 6 tenders. On the average the experimental processing time lasted three hours. Before and after the experiment, the subjective state was measured using Nitsch's "EigenZustandsskala" (scale to evaluate the subjective self-condition) (1974).

The main task - the drawing up of a tender - was identical for both groups. A certain degree of freedom for the way the work was carried out was allowed independently of the dialog version used. The subjects working with the flexible dialog version had an additional scope for choosing the modes of data-input (see Table 1).

Table 1: Differences between the two dialog versions used (Aschwanden and Zimmermann, 1984)

	DIALOG VERSION 1	DIALOG VERSION 2
DISPLAY 1	Preset	User-definable
DISPLAY 2	Procedure: fixed, line format, field by field Automatic calculating	Procedure: user-selectable Calculator key
ALL DIS- PLAYS AND LISTS	Memory line function Corrections: - Backspace - 1 Cursor key, field by field - 'Go' function display 2	No memory line function Corrections: - 4 Cursor keys, field by field - 4 Cursor keys, character by character - Insert - Delete
TOTAL NUMBER OF FUNCTION KEYS	9 keys each with 1 function	17 keys each with 1 func- tion +2 keys each with 2 func- tions +1 key with 3 functions

Based on the results, the authors conclude that "The strain on the user of having to keep information in mind should be reduced as far as possible by providing an external memory in which memoranda can be stored" (Aschwanden and Zimmermann, 1984, 41). Furthermore, the results of the experimental study can be summarized as follows:

(1) The additional freedom provided by the flexible dialog version was actually used.
(2) An increase in the degree of freedom used did not lead to any discernible reduction in efficiency or increase in strain.
(3) Easing the burden on the retention memory in favour of processing performance stimulated innovative behaviour.

A PILOT STUDY ON THE QUESTION OF INDIVIDUALIZATION

Based on the hypothesis of "semantic information transfer" of Krause (1982), Ackermann (1983) formulated the hypothesis that difficulties in human-computer interaction during task solving processes are caused by the discrepancy between individual mental representation and cognitive styles on the one hand and the given operations of the scope of action prescribed by the software on the other hand. Therefore, cognitive and action regulation processes are the most important aspects in this research.

To investigate fundamental aspects of the principle of differential work design, such as the basic question of efficiency of user-definable versus fixed dialog forms, the computer game PRIMP-1 (Programmable Robot for the Investigation of Mental Processes) was developed. The task of this game is to steer a robot through a maze in which there are three rooms containing wine bottles. The bottles have to be sorted according to their contents - full, half-full and empty - and put onto shelves. The robot can be controlled by basic commands. The six basic commands can be combined into hierarchical command units, so-called 'macros', allowing the formation of iterations and selections according to the player's intentions and reflections. These macros represent the action-schemes and the structuring of the scope of action by the user. Figure 1 shows the screen and the basic commands of the game.

Experimental design

In a first test series, 6 students of the ETH Zürich were given the task of developing the most efficient set of commands with as few steps as possible and in the shortest possible time to perform the task. "The number of games which had to be played before the command set was complete was unlimited and log-files could be used for analyzing the game" (Ackermann, 1986a, p. 3). Finally each subject had to play the

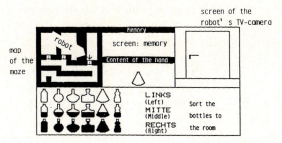

Figure 1: *Part of the manual of the game: screen layout and command set*

game five more times using all the command sets of the other subjects. In this way all the subjects worked with one set of self-defined commands and 5 preset command sets. Detailed interviews were also conducted with the subjects. In addition the questionnaire HAKEMP devised by Kuhl (1983) for determining action-oriented and situation-oriented subjects was applied.

Results

The students redefined the task according to their own demands, goals and image of a potential user. The constructed command sets reflect their own model of the needed scope of action. The general objective designing the command programs was to prevent errors of the designer and errors of possible users. The other tendency was to find an optimal strategy to sort the bottles.

Command programs / Type of Command	AROBBY	B-BEFEHLE	D.BEF	ECMD2	GLOBI	HCOMMANDS
left		LEFT	L	L		
turn round		TURN ROUND	TURN ROUND			
right		RIGHT	R	R		
go ahead		GSTOP				
(Combinations)		RUN		GL/GR/VL/VR		
move left				XT		
recognizing Corners		WLEFT	RR (F)			
checking for Walls						
move right						
recognizing Corners		WRIGHT				
checking for Walls						
search empty Rack	DEPOSIT R		SLD +	PUT +	SKR R	PLACE L
search full Rack	SEARCH R			NEXT	SVR R	BOTTLE L
search Door	EXIT R		AUSGANG	TOR	ST R	EXIT L
bottle in Memory	GETBOTTLE R		GET	GET		
(+ with deposit/take)						
(L left/R right)						
from Room(x) to Room(y)		x.y (x.y E A,B,C)	Rxy (x.y E A,B,C)	xGOy	Rxy	
to Room(y)	RL/RM/RR					LEFT/RIGHT
from start to Room(y)		START (nur R)	RSX	BEGIN (only R)	ROx	START (only R)
from Room(y) to Start	STARTRACK	GOSTART	RXS	GB (only R)		
Bottle in Memory autom.				GETL/GETM/GETR		BRING

Figure 2: Synopsis of the command sets

Figure 2 presents a synopsis of the solutions. Some solutions seem to be quite similiar, for example "a" and "h", but they show large differences in the implementation of the commands and the basic intentions. The designer of "a" looked for a simple solution. Therefore the player has to indicate only the goal-room and the robot will run along the walls trying to find the indicated room itself. The designer of "h" tried to structure the whole task in simple and intelligible units. The selection of the appropriate command to steer the robot from one room to another was reduced on the decision "LEFT" and "RIGHT" in front of the doors.

The designer of "e" intended to automatize the tedious aspects of steering the robot as well as possible. Evaluating his solution, he realized that the game appeared monotonous to him. Therefore, he extended the scope of action by commands to optimize the robot's path in the maze. This offered the possibility to change between two scopes of action with different "granularity". In contrary, "b" was designed deliberately to offer a large scope of action on the cost of a longer learning process.

The quantitative analysis of the command sets (Figure 3) shows a large variety of programming styles: Designer "H" used the command "go" only once, whereas programmer "E" used it 79 times. However, the quality of the command sets is comparable as shown in Figure 4. The only difference in the manuals (Figure 3) is that programmer "E" offers more sub-commands to the user than programmer "H".

Command set	MANUAL Total commands	Main commands	Help commands	CONSTRUCTION ANALYSIS OF THE COMMAND SETS Total commands	Used as subprogram	deposit	turn	go	remember	take	open	compare	if	until	not	door	rack	wall	free	empty	equal	Mean length	Standard deviation	Used basic commands
a	11	6	5	24	30	2	4	2		1	3	1		8	9	2	4	4		6	2		3.69	2.56	13
b	20	19	1	19	46		6	11		5				6	4	6	2		1	6			5.22	2.86	9
d	31	24	7	31	107	1	8	9	1	18	4			4	4	2	2	1		1	1		4.07	4.99	13
e	19	8	11	33	112	4	4	79	1	17	2			4	10	8	2	2		5	2	1	10.07	20.31	14
g	28	19	9	28	77		6	24		18				2	6	2	1	2		3	2		6.6	7.9	10
h	11	7	4	24	76	1	1	1		1	2	1		19	5		8		7	4	5	4	1	4.28	4.87	14

Figure 3: Quantitative analysis of the command sets

In the second part of the experiment, the subjects had to work with the command sets of their colleagues. Figure 4 shows

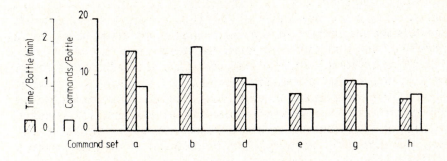

Figure 4: Quality of the command sets (mean of all played games with these command sets)

the quality of the command sets in respect to "needed time per bottle" and "used commands per bottle" evaluated as mean ratio of all played games. The results presented in Figure 5 show that the subjects had difficulties in using command sets whose structures were different from the command sets developed by themselves. The difficulties are demonstrated by increased error rates, reduced time-efficiency, as well as by increased number of commands needed (Ackermann, 1986b). In 10 out of 18 possible scores working with user or self-defined-commands took first place in this ranking and in three more cases second place (see Figure 5).

		Subject (Player)				
Parameter	A	B	D	E	F	G
Time / Bottle	1.	2.	4.	1.	2.	1.
Commands/ Bottle	1.	6.	3.	1.	2.	1.
Errors/ Bottle	4.	3.	1.	1.	1.	1.

Rank orders of the individual developed commandsets in 6 trials (individual commandset + the best trial of each other)

Figure 5: Rank orders of the individual command sets in 6 trials com pared with the best trial of each other

Subjects who were situation-oriented formulated significantly more short, single commands which were not combined into command units (macros). Action-oriented subjects made more use of the scope of action than state-oriented ones (Ackermann, 1986a).

The results show that the possibility to adapt action-schemes to own goals and redefinitions of the task according to the individual mental representation of the task will improve efficiency in man-computer dialog. Therefore, this give additional weight to the concept of differential work design (Ulich, 1978, 1983). Data from two other test series which will be presented now seem to confirm the above experience.

A PILOT STUDY ON THE INDIVIDUALIZATION OF AN INPUT MEDIA

There is clearly a descernible trend toward 'simple mice' based on the assumption that "the user is worried by too many function keys" and on the premise that "if you only have one key to press, you can't press the wrong one". Nievergelt took the opposite view; he proposed a 5-finger mouse which should contribute to optimization of dialog monitoring and control. This tool was developed by Nippon Telegraph and Telephone Company (Ohno, Fukaya & Nievergelt, 1985).

Based on the fact that the thumb and forefinger have the greatest mobility and are therefore particularly suitable for fine adjustments, "the first and second keys are designated for analog-input and the remaining three can only be used for digital input" (Ackermann & Nievergelt, 1985, p. 377). On the underneath side is a ball as in other mouse designs for cursor control and movement. The concept of NTT that this mouse should be constructed as a 'personal mouse' for individual requirements, it complies closely with the concept of differential work design.

The experiments were conducted using the computer game PRIMP-1 described above. The assignment of the basic commands (GO, TURN, DEPOSIT, TAKE, OPEN) to the five function keys of the mouse was either fixed or could be chosen by the user. The user-selected assignment could be changed during the game. The ball for moving the robot could be used in all four directions as long as it was not disabled. As a basis for

Table 2: Experimental conditions for examining different types of input tools (Ackermann & Nievergelt, 1985)

Subject	Trial 1	Trial 2
Inexperienced	Mouse with preset key order without ball	Mouse with preset key order with ball
Inexperienced	Keyboard	Mouse with preset key order with ball
Inexperienced	Mouse with user-defined key order without ball	Mouse with user-defined key order with ball
Experts	Mouse with user-defined key order with ball	Mouse with user-defined key order without ball

comparison it was intended to carry out the same task using a normal keyboard. An overview of the various conditions of the exeriment is given in Table 2. It can be seen from this table that each subject had to carry out the task of sorting the bottles under two different experimental conditions. The time interval between the trials was 15 minutes.

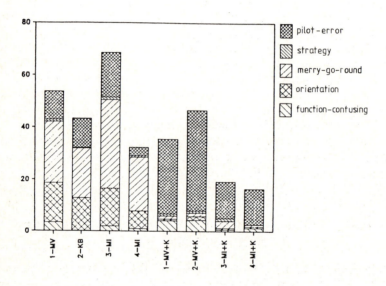

Figure 6: Statistic of different kinds of errors

The results show (Figure 6) that the keyboard group performed the worst with regard to the time per task and the number of commands per unit of time. With regard to the number of commands per task and the number of errors per task this group was placed in the third and second from the last respectively. The possibility of using the moving element i.e. the ball of the mouse led to an improvement in performance in all cases and all parameters. With regard to the parameters of efficiency and error statstics in most cases the user-defined order turned out to be the best. Subjects who where able to define their own key order did not mix up the keys as often as those with preset key order (Figure 7). (Mann-Whitney U-Test, p < .05). We hypothesize, that this result is due to an improved mental representation of key-functions and intended strategy.

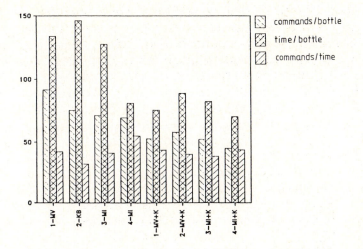

Figure 7: "Commands per bottle", "Time per bottle" and "commands per minute" for the different experimental conditions.
The differences are statistically significant (Mann-Withney U-Test $p \leq 0.05$)

WORK PSYCHOLOGY AND THE CHALLENGE OF SOFTWARE DEVELOPMENT

Is it possible to apply the principles of differential and dynamic work design to the software developing process? To answer this question we made the following case study. In order to improve the evacuation planning for the Swiss civil defense organisation of the city of Zurich, Luethi (1982) developed a mathematical solution based on the transshipment algorithm described by Ahrens & Finke (1980). The implementation was running on a main-frame computer and was only accessible to a few specialists. But the Swiss civil defense organisation is formed by militiamen not acquainted with mainframes. This raised the question how this evacuation planning system could be redesigned for the use by militiamen on ordinary personal computers. The system to be developed was primarily intended to serve for instruction purposes. We realized that the system to be developed had to be easy to learn and to offer different ways of problem solving to prevent difficulties and delays in the problem solving process. Furthermore the system had to support decision making in every stage of the evacuation planning process.

The principle of differential and dynamic work design mentioned above were used as the guideline for dialog design. Our hypothesis was that difficulties in the human-computer interaction during task solving processes are caused by the discrepancy between individual mental representation and cognitive styles on the one hand and the given scope of action prescribed by the software on the other hand. Therefore we divided the developing process of the program into three phases: First a careful task analysis to understand correctly the existing scope of action and suggest possible forms and interaction structures, especially its semantical structure (Ackermann, 1987), second an evaluation of possible dialog forms by "paper-and-pencil"-simulations and third experimental evaluations of parts of the dialog with user participation during the process of implementation. To meet these intentions a flexible software concept in MODULA-2 was developed (Boesze, 1986).

The developing of EPILOG
(Evacuation Planning In DiaLog)

Step 1: Task analysis. Because only a few specialists were able to manage the evacuation planning process, we had only a few clues to possible solutions. Therefore we decided to develop the system mainly on the basis of the cycle of problem-solving proposed by Daenzer (1978):

- fixing or correcting the goal
- looking for possible solutions
- evaluation and selection

Step 2: Modelling possible forms of the scope of action. We decided to use a town map of Zürich of the civil defense organization as a basis of the planning process since we knew that every militiaman was acquainted with it. We made comic-strips of possible layouts of the screen and the menu-structures for partial simulations of the evacuation planning process.

Step 3: Implementation and evaluation. The different software modules were designed according to the experiences of step 2. Afterward the selected solution was implemented and the running parts tested by specialists and militiamen of the civil defense organisation with and without computer experience. The system was redesigned according to the subject's reactions, errors and suggestions. Two different menu-structures had to be implemented as well as different kinds of information display selectable by the subjects to fullfill requirements due to individual differences.

Step 4: Evaluation of the Desicion Support System "Epilog". The resulting system was tested again with other militiamen to investigate the appropriateness of the menu structures and the desicion process.

During the implementation and evaluation process the subjects made a lot of important suggestions about command structures and information displays they needed for an optimal evacuation plan. A great deal of individual differences were considered in dialog design. One subject stated in the beginning that she detested computers but afterwards she asked if she might come again voluntarily. This example shows that the possibility to participate in the developing process leads to a good acceptance of the final product and a good support of the desicion making process in evacuation planning. The results prove that it is possible to develop software according to the user's needs and the task's requirements. The demand for flexibility of dialogs has also consequences for software design, especially for the software architecture or structure.

CONCLUSION

This experimental development of software shows that it is possible to "tailor dialogs for and by the individual to his or her own individual demands, abilities or cognitive styles in order to improve efficiency and to give optimal chances of task orientation and achievment motivation" (Ackermann, 1986b, p. 295) according to the principle of differential work design. The changes of the user's qualification will be investigated in further experimental series to test the above mentioned question "how work... can be designed so that work suports the development of the workers qualifications and not only the application of them" (Triebe and Ulich, 1977).

REFERENCES

Ackermann, D. (1983). *Robi Otter oder die Suche nach dem operativen Abbildsystem.* Interner Bericht über die Studienarbeiten SS 1983. Zürich, Lehrstuhl für Arbeits- und Organisationspsychologie.

Ackermann, D. (1986a). Untersuchungen zum individualisierten Computerdialog: Einfluss des Operativen Abbildsystems auf Handlungs- und Gestaltungsspielraum und die Arbeitseffizienz. In: Dirlich G., Freksa, Ch., Schwatlo, U., & Wimmer, K. (Eds.) (1986a). *Kognitive Aspekte der Mensch-Computer- Interaktion.* Ergebnisse eines Workshops vom 12./13. April 1984 in München. Berlin: Springer Informatik-Fachberichte Nr. 120, p. 96 - 110.

Ackermann, D. (1986b). A pilot study on the Effects of Individualization in Man-Computer-Interaction. In: Mancini, G., Johannsen, G. & Martenson, L. (Eds.) (1986b). *Analysis, Design and Evaluation of Man-Machine-Systems*. Proceedings of the 2nd IFAC/IFIP/ IFORS/IEA Conference, Varese, Italy, 10.- 12. September 1985. Oxford/New York: Pergamon Press, p. 293 - 297.

Ackermann, D. (1987). *Handlungsspielraum, Mentale Repräsentation und Handlungsregulation am Beispiel der Mensch-Computer-Inter-aktion. Untersuchungen zum Prinzip der differentiellen und dynamischen Arbeitsgestaltung*. Unpublished doctoral dissertation, University of Bern, Department of Psychology.

Ackermann, D. & Nievergelt, J. (1985). Die Fünf-Finger-Maus: Eine Fallstudie zur Synthese von Hardware, Software und Psychologie. In: H.-J. Bullinger (Ed.) (1985) *Software-Ergonomie '85 Mensch-Computer-Interaktion*, p. 376 - 385. Stuttgart: B. G. Teubner .

Ahrens, J. H. & Finke, G., (1980): Primal transportation and transshipment algorithms. *Zeitschrift für Operations Research, 24*, 1 - 32.

Aschwanden, C. & Zimmermann, M. (1984). *Flexibilität in der Arbeit am Bildschirm*. Psychologische Lizentiatsarbeit. University of Zürich.

Boesze, J. Z. (1986). *EPILOG: Evakuationsplanung im Dialog*. Unveröffentlichte Diplomarbeit im Fach Informatik. Swiss Federal Institute of Technology (ETH), Zürich, März 1986.

Bruggemann, A. (1974). Zur Unterscheidung verschiedener Formen von "Arbeitszufriedenheit". *Arbeit und Leistung, 28*, 281 - 284.

Bruggemann, A., Groskurth, P. & Ulich, E. (1975). Arbeitszufriedenheit. *Schriften zur Arbeitspsychologie* (Ed. E. Ulich) Bd. 17. Bern: Huber.

Daenzer, W. F.(Ed) (1978). *Systems engineering*. Köln: Hanstein, 1978.

Fischer, G. (1983). Entwurfsrichtlinien für die Software-Ergonomie aus der Sicht der Mensch-Maschine Kommunikation. In: Balzert, H. (Eds.): *Software-Ergonomie*. Stuttgart: Teubner, 30 - 48.

Grob, R. (1985). *Flexibilität in der Fertigung*. Berlin: Springer.

Krause, B. (1982). Semantic information processing in cognitive processes. *Zeitschrift für Psychologie, 190(1)*, 37-45.

Kuhl J.: Action- vs state-orientation as a mediator between motivation and action. In: Hacker, W., Volpert, W. & Cranach, M. von (Eds) (1983). *Cognitive and motivational aspects of action*. Amsterdam: North-Holland Publishing Company.

Lipmann, O. (1932). *Lehrbuch der Arbeitswissenschaft*. Jena: G. Fischer.

Lüthi, H.-J. (1982). Computerunterstützte Planung im Zivilschutz. Zuweisungsplanung mit CASA. *Output, 12*, p. 19 - 22.

Nitsch, J. R. (1974). Die hierarchische Struktur des Eigenzustandes - ein Approximationsversuch mit Hilfe der Binärstrukturanalyse (BISTRAN). *Diagnostica, 20*, 142 - 164.

Ohno, K., Fukaya, K.-I. & Nievergelt, J. (1985). A five key mouse with built-in dialog control. *SIGCHI-Bulletin, 17(1)*, 29 - 34.

Triebe, J. K. & Ulich, E. (1977). Eignungsdiagnostische Zukunftsperspektiven: Möglichkeiten einer Neuorientierung. In: Triebe, J. K. & Ulich, E. (Eds.): *Beiträge zur Eignungsdiagnostik. Schriften zur Arbeitspsychologie* (Ed. E. Ulich) Bern: Huber, p. 241 - 273.

Triebe, J. K. (1980). Untersuchungen zum Lernprozess während des Erwerbs der Grundqualifikation (Montage eines kompletten Motors). *Arbeits- und sozialpsychologische Untersuchungen von Arbeitsstrukturen im Bereich der Aggregatefertigung der Volkswagenwerk AG, Band 3*. Bonn: Bundesministerium für Forschung und Technologie (HA 80-019).

Triebe, J. K. (1981). *Aspekte beruflichen Handelns und Lernens. Feld- und Längsschnittuntersuchung zu ausgewählten Merkmalen der Struktur und Genese von Handlungsstrategien bei einer Montagetätigkeit.* Unpublished doctoral dissertation, University of Bern, Department of Psychology.

Ulich, E. (1978). Ueber das Prinzip der differentiellen Arbeitsgestaltung. *Industrielle Organisation*. 566 - 568.

Ulich, E., Frei, F., & Baitsch, Ch. (1980). Zum Begriff der persönlichkeitsförderlichen Arbeitsgestaltung. *Zeitschrift für Arbeitswissenschaft. 34*, 210-213.

Ulich, E. (1983). Differentielle Arbeitsgestaltung - ein Diskussionsbeitrag. *Zeitschrift für Arbeitswissenschaft, 37(9)*, 12 - 16.

Ulich, E. (1986). Aspekte der Benutzerfreundlichkeit. In: Remmle W. & Sommer, M. (Eds.): *Arbeitsplätze morgen*. Berichte des German Chapter of the ACM, Band 27. Stuttgart: Teubner, p. 102 - 122.

Ulich, E. (1987). Some aspects of user-oriented dialog-design. In: Fuchs-Kittow, K., Docherty, P., Kohn, P. and Matthiassen, L. (Eds): *System design for human development and productivity. Participation and beyond.* In Press.

Zülch, G., & Starringer, M. (1984). Differentielle Arbeitsgestaltung in der Fertigung für elektronische Flachbaugruppen. *Zeitschrift für Arbeitswissenschaft, 38*, 211-216.

Psychological Issues of
Human Computer Interaction in the Work Place
M. Frese, E. Ulich, W. Dzida (Editors)
  Elsevier Science Publishers B.V. (North-Holland), 1987

VDU-WORK AND USER-FRIENDLY HUMAN-COMPUTER-INTERACTION: ANALYSIS OF DIALOGUE STRUCTURES

Philipp Spinas

Work and Organisational Psychology Unit, Swiss Federal Institute of
Technology (ETH), 8092 Zürich, Switzerland

Based on concepts of cognitive and industrial psychology
we designed a field study in order to obtain more data
about experiences and requirements of computer users in
office work. The goal of the study was the comparison
of different forms of VDU-work and human-computer-
interaction. Employees of four companies were asked to
judge the quality of the used dialogue system relative to
several psychological aspects by means of interviews and
questionnaires. The inquiry is completed by an observation of the user behaviour during a terminal session. The
results confirmed the importance of a varied job content
and user control over the computer system.

INTRODUCTION

If we consider the use of new technologies as an *option* in the way
described by Ulich (1980), then many more possibilities become available
for the creation of humanly adequate - and at the same time economically
feasible - working conditions in connection with the design of the different interfaces between man, task and computer (Spinas, Troy & Ulich,
1983). Resulting from one-sided *technical* orientation, these possibilities
have frequently been - and still are today - little recognized and used. But
if we take *man* and his *task* (or problem) as the starting point of the interface design, then new alternatives become available. The computer can
be understood as an aid in the sense of a convivial tool (Illich, 1973),
which man has at his disposal for the fulfilling of a task. From this point
of view, an important goal should be to facilitate the use of the tool while
- at the same time - providing a variety of application possibilities within
the frame of an appropriate scope of action. 'User friendliness' in this
sense means an adaptation of the software to the perception, memory,
thinking and action of man. Of central importance are the user's mental
representations of the work process and available tools, because any
planning and subsequent carrying out of work activity are based upon it

(Hacker,1978). Previous experience would appear to support the assumption that insufficient transparency and influenceability of the dialogue structures represent a main problem of computer use. Nievergelt (1982) formulated this very aptly with four questions that he suggests a user should be able to answer: "Where am I? What can I do here? How did I get here? Where can I go and how can I get there?" The user is frequently confronted with "sequentially appearing fragments from an 'inner world' consisting of the information structure represented in a system which is otherwise hidden from him" (Fähnrich & Ziegler, 1983), and this fact can greatly inhibit the construction of an adequate mental representation. In addition to being confronted with a more or less inflexibly prescribed series of dialogue steps, the user has little opportunity to develop own plans of action and is instead expected to simply react with relatively passive patterns of behavior in response to given signals.

Our study was designed to investigate the criteria which dialogue software would have to satisfy in order to meet the needs of the user. In addition, it was our goal to increase our knowledge of cognitive-psychological aspects of the complex problems of human-computer-interaction.

DESIGN OF THE STUDY, METHODS AND SAMPLE

On the basis of previous investigations (Spinas, 1983), departments of four different companies were chosen to serve as our research field. Our criteria in the selection were (1) similarity of work activity and (2) dissimilarity of dialogue structure. Along with general analyses of representative work places and observation of work activities (in diagramming dialogue sequences), interviews were conducted with supervisors (of the departments involved) and with those responsible for the computer department. The employees' evaluation of the work at the VDU-terminal and of the quality of the dialogue system used - in terms of various psychological criteria - were gathered by means of individual interviews and questionnaires (N=88). The analysis of the dialogue structures was based upon such materials as user manuals, flow charts and block diagrams.

Our sample consisted of qualified office clerks who had used computers one to five hours daily over a period of three years (average). The age of those questioned averaged 34 years and the proportion of female employees, at 44%, was somewhat less than that of the men.

APPLICATIONS AND EMPLOYEE EVALUATION OF COMPUTER USE

In the four departments selected for investigation, computer systems served mainly to support the following activities:

- Company 1 (Insurance): registration and processing of claims; correspondence
- Company 2 (Insurance): compilation of insurance policy offers; correspondence
- Company 3 (Trade): registration and processing of orders; correspondence
- Company 4 (Insurance): registration and processing of claims; correspondence

Figure 1 provides a breakdown of the different categories of computer activity in each of the four companies in relation to the total daily time spent working at the VDU-terminal. The employees themselves provided the raw data whose accuracy was confirmed by our own observations and information provided by management. Of particular interest is the relatively high percentage of data entry time in Companies 1 and 2 in contrast to Companies 3 and 4, where a more balanced relationship exists between the different categories.

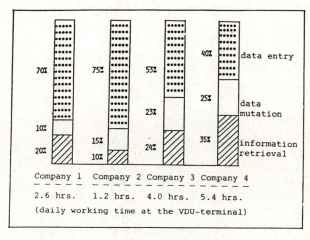

Figure 1: Percentage breakdown of VDU-activity

There were striking differences between the companies in the planning and integration of their computer systems. For example, the employees in Company 3 were informed much earlier (approx. 6 month) and more thoroughly about the impending changes, were better trained for computer work and, above all, participated more in the developmental process (92% of those questioned considered their wishes with regard to the planning of the system to have been taken into consideration) than those in the other companies.

Figure 2 shows how the employees evaluate the support provided by the computer system (all differences - except those between companies 3 and 4 - are significant; Mann-Whitney U-Test, $p < 0.05$). The completely positive evaluation found in Companies 3 and 4 is impressive. The benefit consists mainly of a simplification and taking over of routine, administrative work steps ("less paper-work") and the extensive possibilities of information retrieval, which amounts to enormous support in connection with customer counseling - especially, for example, in the providing of data about articles (e.g., inventory, delivery dates, replacement parts, etc.). Company 1's employees also considered the instant accessibility of up-to-date information to be a help; but this advantage was offset by the "unpleasant extra work" (increase in number of administrative work-steps)

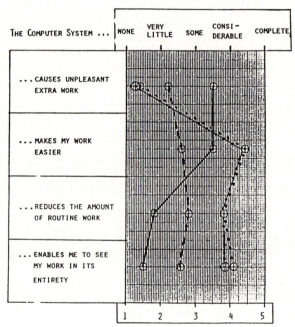

*Figure 2: User Evaluation of the Benefits of the Computer-System
(Comparison of Median Values)*

```
Company 1 (N=20):  ———————
   "    2 (N=21):  ▬ ▬ ▬ ▬
   "    3 (N=25):  ● ● ● ●
   "    4 (N=22):  ●—●—●—
```

required for the registration of damages and the fact that the original hopes of being relieved of routine work were disappointed. Company 2 takes a middle position in this regard. Its computer system – particularly in the processing of big jobs – provides assistance by taking over certain routine tasks without adding complications to the other work. Distinct differences are also evident in the extent to which the computer system demonstrates to the user the value of his activity and its connections to the preceeding and subsequent work steps.

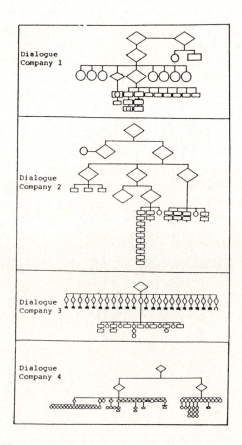

Figure 3: Comparison of the four Dialogue Structures (simplified)

◇ = Menu   ◯ = Information Mask

☐ = Data Entry Mask

DESCRIPTION OF THE DIALOGUE STRUCTURES

The exchange of information between user and computer takes place in all four companies by means of a VDU-terminal and a keyboard. In figure 3, the *structure* of the dialogues (static aspect) is illustrated. The four dialogues are all based on the same basic techniques - menu, data entry mask and information mask -, which are also known as so-called "passive" dialogue forms. However the particular overall structure in each of the four companies is different.

In Company 1, the hierarchical order of the individual elements is arranged according to criteria of the (mainly mechanical) logic of procedure *and* in part also according to the type of insurance. As can be seen, this 'mixed strategy' results in a muddled (and thus difficult to retain) overall structure; it also necessitates the user to take "detours" for certain steps. A similar strategy determined the dialogue design of Company 2. Since there are only two types of insurance, a consistent menutree structure, a linear positioning of the data entry masks with pre-determined sequence and the increased automatization of entire work processes, the overall structure of the dialogue proves to be more simple, more uniform, and thus also more terse. The dialogues in the Companies 3 and 4 were also designed from a 'mixed strategy', but one which clearly differentiates between various parts of the overall structure. The work areas are offered at the first level (main menu), and they can be differentiated at the second level. Then relatively homogenous (i.e., self-enclosed), plausibly defined processing units (information masks and data entry masks) follow. The consistency of these structures greatly contributes to their 'terse form' (for reasons of clarity, in figure 3/dialogue 3 only one processing unit is shown as an example at the third level).

The supply of dialogue *functions* in Companies 1 and 2 is limited to those absolutely essential for completion of the task, in contrast to the situation in the Companies 3 and 4, where additional helpful functions (for example, interruption, sorting, statistics, etc.) are available. Similarly, the search attributes available in the dialogues 3 and 4 - through the various possibilities of combination, their broad possibilities of application (customers, objects, orders), and the minimal demands of entry - allow the goal to be reached more quickly than in either of the other dialogues.

With regard to the *vocabulary*, it is worth mentioning that in dialogue 1, the most - and also the most out-of-the-ordinary - codes and abbreviations are used, and in dialogue 2, there are some language inconsistencies, i.e., the programmers did not always adhere to the company's customary use of language. To minimize data entry operations, dialogue 4 uses a great number (300-500) of codes and abbreviations.

THE DIALOGUE STRUCTURES AS EVALUATED BY THE USERS

The judgement and evaluation of the dialogue structures by their users is illustrated in figure 4, which graphically portrays the mean values of the scales (which were generated by factor- and item-analyses of 53 questions).

As expected, dialogue 3 was, without exception, given a more positive rating by its users than either of the other dialogues (t-test, p <.05). The differences in the dimensions 'Flexibility' and 'Feedback' are the most pronounced. The objective differences between the dialogue structures in terms of opportunities for personal styles of behaviour are clearly reflected in the user evaluations. The more or less strongly predetermined dialogue path was evaluated negatively by the users in Company 1 and even more so by those in Company 2. As expressed in their interview

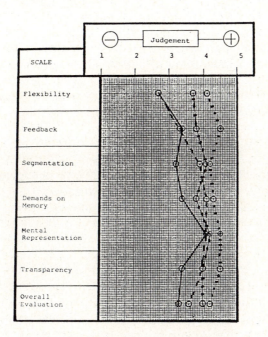

Figure 4: Evaluation of the Dialogue by the User

Dialogue Company 1 (N=20): ————
     "   "   2 (N=21): — — — —
     "   "   3 (N=25): • • • •
     "   "   4 (N=22): —•—•—•—

statements, they feel pressed into a mold that doesn't fit their individual needs and ways of approaching the task, thereby degrading them to the role of a servant of the computer ("feeding" data).

Above all, the more negative evaluation of 'Feedback' in dialogues 1 and 2 can be attributed to the fact that the cause of an error is explained too little or not at all. Thereby learning processes, which are essential for the modification and refinement of mental models, are rendered more difficult or even made impossible.

It is interesting to note that the differences with regard to the possibility of forming adequate mental representations are not as great as expected. Daily use of the computer system apparently has lead to the formation of a structural- and process-model of the dialogue. More pronounced are the differences in evaluation of transparency, which refers more to the outer form of the dialogue structures than to the possibilities for their mental representation; here effects of practice only with regard to demands made on memory, it can be seen that especially the users of dialogues 1 and 4 are forced to retain too many details in memory whose meaning is difficult to differentiate, because they do not easily initiate associations to existing memory contents.

Concerning the segmentation of the dialogue into many small operations (equal to many subgoals), dialogue 1 is judged the worst by its users which can be explained by the way the registration of claims has to be done: the user is forced to work sequentially in a time-consuming manner, step by step.

In the overall evaluation, dialogues 1 and 2 do not differ very much. Maybe the minimum transparency and average flexibility of dialogue 1 just offset the almost completely absent flexibility and average transparency of dialogue 2 (as far as the ratings are concerned). Dialogues 3 and 4 clearly are evaluated better; the main reasons for this result are discussed in the next section.

EXTENDED DISCUSSION OF SELECTED ASPECTS: 'USEFULNESS', FLEXIBILITY AND SEGMENTATION/TRANSPARENCY

In the following section, mainly three important characteristics of the dialogue structures will be discussed more in detail. These characteristics are shown in figure 5.

The number of choice possibilities per menu gives a hint at the variety of applications. Accordingly, dialogue 3 provides the greatest number of application areas. This seems to be an important determinant of user satisfaction, because it indicates the range of assistance available for the user to complete his tasks. With caution it can be interpreted as a measure of 'usefulness' of the dialogue system.

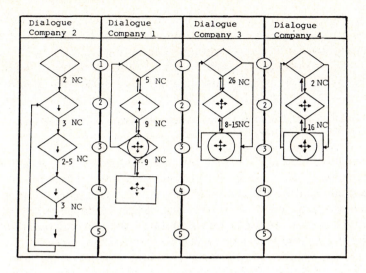

Figure 5: Selected Characteristics of the four Dialogue Structures

◯ =Hierarchy Level
NC =Number of Choices per Menu
↓ =Possibilities of Movement (Flexibility)

The arrows in figure 5 show that the dialogues 3 and 4 offer the user the most degrees of freedom for his activity. He can almost always move 'forward', 'backward' or 'sideways' at every level; in addition, by jumping over the second menu level, he is able to proceed directly from the main menu to the desired mask. In this regard, as mentioned previously, dialogue 2 stands in striking contrast to dialogues 3 and 4, and dialogue 1 takes a middle position. In all four dialogues, the dialogue path taken is determined by menu choice and function keys; for the experienced user, the entry of mask numbers is also possible in dialogue 3. This path flexibility is illustrated in the sense of a 'navigation-map' in figure 6, which also gives an impression of the complexity of the dialogue system.

The extraordinary significance of dialogue flexibility is seen in the high correlation with the scale 'Overall Evaluation' (rs=.70); the greater the user's flexibility rating of a dialogue, the more positively will be the overall rating.

Based on concepts of differential work design (Ulich, 1978), Ackermann (1985; see also Ackermann, this volume) investigated experimentally
the effect of flexibility in human-computer-interaction on user behaviour.
In a specially designed computer game, subjects had to solve a problem
using both individually developed and prescribed command sets. The re-

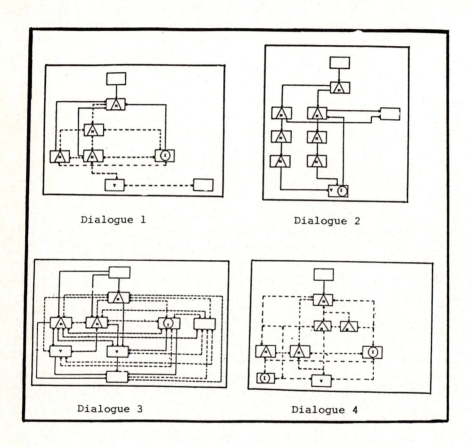

Figure 6: Flexibility by possible Paths (simplified)

sults show that the individualization possibilities improved efficiency and offered more chances for task orientation and achievement motivation. Obviously, dialogue flexibility is necessary to take account of *inter*-individual differences in user behaviour and of *intra*individual differences in action regulation, which are mainly due to learning processes. Rigid dialogue structures force the user into a scheme of given (sub-) goals and prescribed sequence of operations, whereas flexible dialogues allow the user to develop his own problem solving and action strategies. According to results of various studies, flexibility and individualization possibilities improve efficiency and/or performance as well as user satisfaction and motivation (see for example Ackermann, 1985; Aschwanden & Zimmermann, 1984; Broadbent & Broadbent, 1978; Frese, this volume; Gilfoil, 1982). All these studies cited here confirm the concept of differential and dynamic work design formulated by Ulich (1978) in order to improve conditions for an optimum development of personality in working life.

Looking again at figure 5 it is evident that dialogues 2 and 1 have the strongest *segmentation*. The dialogue structure is divided into five respectively four hierarchy levels, most of them containing several small operations. This fragmentation of a whole into many small parts can reduce dialogue transparency (see figure 7) and greatly increase the difficulty of forming adequate mental representations in the sense of a cognitive map (Downs & Stea 1973; Moar & Charleton 1982), for - in the terminology of Gestalt psychology - the parts tend to dominate the whole. There is a risk of an overload of the short-term memory capacity.

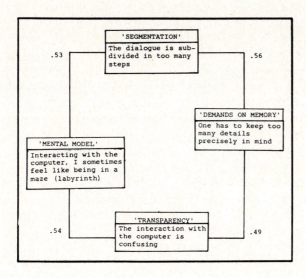

Figure 7: Correlations between Items of Dialogue Judgement (r_s)

Possible consequences are:
- little transparency ("seeing the forest for the trees", Lewis & Mack 1982, 388)
- orientation problems
- regulation of action guided by perception (reacting to signals) instead of plans and anticipation

Sometimes users who got completely lost reported that they did not even remember what their aim originally had been. For us it was interesting to see that the findings of our field research were confirmed by various experiments investigating the role of depth and breadth of menus and tree structures in computer interfaces.

Miller (1981) stated that the structure of the menu hierarchy has a profound effect upon goal acquisition performance in a menu based system. "The data support the conclusion such that a menu hierarchy of two levels was the fastest, produced the fewest errors, showed the least variability, and was the easiest to learn" (Miller 1981, 300). Kiger's experiment dealt with preference issues as well as performance. He concludes: "The data seem to indicate both performance and preference advantages for broad, shallow trees. As a general principle, the depth of a tree structure should be minimized by providing broad menus of up to eight or nine items each" (Kiger 1984, 208; see also Allen 1983, Snowberry et. al. 1983). Returning to our study figure 5 shows that the users of the dialogues 3 and 4 have quick and comfortable access to the desired information and processing functions, for the menu system has only two hierarchical levels but a great number of choice possibilities. On the other hand dialogue 2 has five levels but few choices per menu; once the working level has been reached, (the 5th level), it takes a series of 10 single steps to complete a task. This sequence is predetermined and unalterable, therefore the user is forced to work sequentially: to reach the first actual work mask, he has to struggle through four menus step-by-step in a laborious and time-consuming manner! As already mentioned, the registration of claims in dialogue 1 has to be done in a similar way.

Summarized in a few words one could say that rigid menu systems which are strongly hierarchically designed and subdivided in many small dialogue steps force a user to work sequentially, increase the difficulty to form adequate mental representations of the tool, cause orientation and memory load problems and finally make it impossible to develop own strategies of problem solving and action regulation. Seen in a longterm perspective, systems of this kind - unfortunately boosted for being 'easy to use' and 'userfriendly' by the marketing of the producers - even endanger an optimum development of personality by stunting some basic human abilities (they are not used and trained anymore) and deforming others (see Rose & Jansen 1981, Volpert 1983).

DEMANDS OF THE USERS

Summarized briefly, a 'user friendly' dialogue system, according to our subjects, should exhibit the following characteristics:
- broad application field
- user control
- restricted use of codes, abbreviations, etc., in favor of understandable terms and signs
- uniformity
- explanatory error messages
- short response times (about one second) and guarantees against system breakdown

In addition, the desire was expressed for better testing of programs (*before* their release for use) and for more participation opportunities in the process of software development. In response to our direct question concerning the preference between a simple, system-guided dialogue and a more complex one offering more degrees of freedom, we received an impressively clear answer (see figure 8): 84% of those questioned chose the dialogue variant offering the user possibilities for the development of individual action strategies, although a greater amount of knowledge

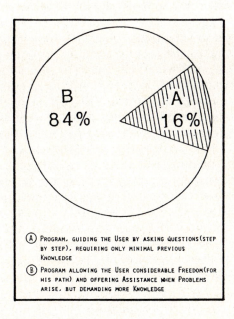

Figure 8: Preference of different Man-Computer-Interaction (N=88)

acquisition is required to master the tool! This can be understood as a sharp rejection of all those conceptions in which 'user friendliness' amounts to fool-proof, system-guided dialogues, boosted   for their advantages of being easily learned and operated.

CONCLUDING REMARKS

In our opinion, the results of this study confirm the necessity of modifying traditional concepts of user friendliness, which try to reduce the complexity of a dialogue system by restricting the variety of applications and/or the degrees of freedom in completing a task. Such a system - usually realized as a deep hierarchy of menus, followed by a series of data entry masks and a strongly system-guided dialogue - in fact is easy to learn and convenient for beginners during their first weeeks of computer use. But learning processes change the demands and attitudes of the user very fast, therefore the 'beginner-system' is going to frustrate the user, because it can't satisfy his growing needs anymore. Another concept of user friendliness is proposed: A dialogue system can be called user friendly, if the user perceives a satisfying relationship between the expense for system handling and a broad potential of possible uses within the frame of an appropriate scope of action. According to our data, the cognitive control - whose components can be described as possibilities of orientation (transparency, predictability) and of exerting influence - which the user has got over the computer is of decisive importance (see also Gilfoil 1982). The user must be able to form an adequate mental representation of the content (informations, tools) and organizational form (dialogue-paths, arrangement of informations) of the system in order to use it efficiently and recognize its support. Moreover, we consider the idea of providing individualization possibilities (see Ulich 1978, 1983, 1985) - for example through user-definable keyboard functions - to make a lot of sense.

Also it should be obvious that the future user of a system should be included in the development process right from the beginning so as to minimize the likelihood of subsequent corrections (concept of participative system development; see Ulich 1981). Together with an intensive training that concentrates not only on operational techniques, but also on teaching functional connections, the dialogue system would be of genuine assistance for the employee in the carrying out of his task.

REFERENCES

Ackermann, D. (1985). A pilot Study of the Effects of Individualization in Man-Computer-Interaction. *Proceedings of the 2nd IFAC/IFIP/*

IFORS/IEA Conference on Analysis, Design and Evaluation of Man-Machine-Systems. London: Pergamon.

Allen, R.B. (1983). Cognitive Factors in the Use of Menus and Trees: An Experiment. *IEEE Journal on selected areas in communications, 2,* 333-336.

Aschwanden, C. & M. Zimmermann (1984). *Flexibilität in der Arbeit am Bildschirm*. Psychologische Lizentiatsarbeit. Zürich: Universität/ ETH.

Broadbent, D.E. & M.H.P. Broadbent (1978). The Allocation of Descriptor Terms by Individuals in a Simulated Retrieval System. *Ergonomics, 21,* 343-354.

Downs, R.M. & D. Stea (1973). *Image and Environment*. Chicago: Aldine.

Fähnrich, K.P. & J. Ziegler (1983). Die Benutzerschnittstelle des Arbeitsplatzrechners Xerox X8010. *Office Management, 31,* 12.

Gilfoil, D.M. (1982). Warming up to computers: a study of cognitive and affective interaction over time. *Proceedings 'Human Factors in Computer Systems'*, Gaithersburg, 245-250.

Hacker, W. (1978). Allgemeine Arbeits- und Ingenieurpsychologie. *Schriften zur Arbeitspsychologie Vol.20*; Bern: Huber.

Illich, I. (1973). *Tools for Conviviality*. New York: Harper and Row.

Kiger, J.I. (1984). The depth/breadth trade-off in the design of menu driven user interfaces. *Int. J. Man-Machine Studies 20,* 201-213.

Lewis, C. & R. Mack (1982). Learning to use a Text Processing System. *Proceedings 'Human Factors in Computer Systems'*, Gaithersburg, 387-392.

Miller, D.P. (1981). The depth/breadth tradeoff in hierarchical computer menus. *Proceedings of the Human Factors Society*, 296-300.

Moar, J. & L.R. Charleton (1982). Memory for routes. *Quarterly Journal of Experimental Psychology, 34A,* 381-394.

Nievergelt, J. (1982). Errors in dialog design and how to avoid them. *Proceedings Intern. Zurich Seminar on Digital Communications, IEEE,* 199-205.

Rose, H. & H. Jansen (1981). Behinderung statt Entwicklung der Arbeitnehmerpersönlichkeit durch Computertechnologien? *Zeitschrift für Arbeitswissenschaft, 35,* 247-253.

Snowberry, K., Parkinson, S.R. & N. Sisson (1983). Computer display menus. *Ergonomics, 26,* 699-712.

Spinas, P. (1984). Bildschirmeinsatz und psycho-soziale Folgen für die Beschäftigten. In: *Arbeit in moderner Technik. Referate der 26. Fachtagung der Sektion 'Arbeits- und Betriebspsychologie' im BDP,* 503-516.

Spinas, P., Troy, N., & E. Ulich (1983). *Leitfaden zur Einführung und Gestaltung von Arbeit mit Bildschirmsystemen*. Zürich: Industrielle Organisation.

Ulich, E. (1978). Ueber das Prinzip der differentiellen Arbeitsgestaltung. *Industrielle Organisation, 47*, 566-568.

Ulich, E. (1980). Psychologische Aspekte der Arbeit mit elektronischen Datenverarbeitungssystemen. *Schweizerische Technische Zeitschrift, 75*, 66-68.

Ulich, E. (1981). Humanisierung - Wirtschaftlichkeit? *Sysdata, 12*, 13-15.

Ulich, E. (1983). Differentielle Arbeitsgestaltung - ein Diskussionsbeitrag. *Zeitschrift für Arbeitswissenschaft, 37*, 12-15.

Ulich, E. (1985). Arbeitspsychologische Konzepte für computerunterstützte Büroarbeit. In: Oesterreichische Gesellschaft für betriebliche Ausbildung (Ed.): *Spectrum, 14*, 1-30.

Volpert, W. (1983). Denkmaschinen und Maschinendenken: Computer programmieren Menschen. *Psychosozial, 18*, 10-29.

Psychological Issues of
Human Computer Interaction in the Work Place
M. Frese, E. Ulich, W. Dzida (Editors)
Elsevier Science Publishers B.V. (North-Holland), 1987

PSYCHOPHYSIOLOGICAL INVESTIGATION OF STRESS INDUCED BY TEMPORAL FACTORS IN HUMAN-COMPUTER INTERACTION

Wolfram Boucsein

Department of Physiological Psychology, University of Wuppertal
Max-Horkheimer-Str. 20, 5600 Wuppertal, F. R. Germany

As human-computer interaction approaches dialog structures at an increasing number of work places, temporal factors like system response times which cause marked delays in this interaction increasingly take on stress-inducing properties. In a methodological section, this paper points out the need for multivariate psychophysiological research at simulated work places as a complement to field studies. In an empirical part, a short report of three investigations carried out by the author's group is presented, concerning psychophysiological stress reactions and performance decrement induced by different system response times. Future research in this field should combine laboratory and field studies and include concepts of task-analysis to separate different temporal aspects of human-computer interaction; these could be varied systematically to test their influence on performance and stress.

INTRODUCTION

With computers coming into widespread use at work places in offices and industry, a lot of research work on classic ergonomic aspects of visual display terminals (VDTs) as tools has been generated. Rules have been developed for physical properties of e.g. the display, the keyboard, the work place as a whole, and its surroundings (e.g. Grandjean & Vigilani 1980). Hence, a rapid development of VDT-work places from simple input-, coding-, and control-tasks to more dialog-structured tasks shifted research interest to so-called software-ergonomy (e.g. Dzida, Herda & Itzfeld 1978). With regard to temporal aspects of human-computer interaction (HCI), interest focussed at first on work pauses and developing appropriate rules. However, when the computer's role in HCI becomes more that of a dialog partner than a mere tool, temporal factors concerning single steps of that interaction have to be taken into consideration.

A model combining and extending the temporal aspects of HCI given by Williges and Williges (1982) and Shneiderman (1984) is shown in figure 1. Using terms from learning theory, we divide user's behavior in alternating "operant" and "respondent" parts depending on who initiates this part of interaction, man or computer. These operant and respondent sections may alternate as shown in figure 1, or sequences of operant parts may result when the computer's response is a "prompt"(> in figure 1), or sequences of respondent sections may result when work is formed by a series of re-action tasks.

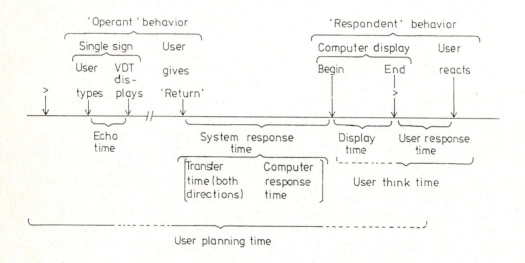

Figure 1: Temporal factors in human-computer interaction.

Prior to each respondent or operant section there is a delay of the computer's response to a user's input which may be caused by different features - both hardware and software - of the computer system and hence is labelled system response time (SRT). A further division of SRT into transfer time and computer response time made by Thadhani (1981) is usually not really perceptible to the user, and therefore is put into brackets in figure 1. Display time is measured from the beginning to the end of a computer's output on the VDT depending on display rate and amount of information displayed, e.g. the mask's dimension. It may in part be utilized as user think time (Shneiderman 1984), which overlaps the user response time (Williges & Williges 1982) that ends with the user's reaction.

Even closer to micro-sections of HCI is echo time, a delay between the keystroke and the appearance of the corresponding character on the screen. User planning time as well as user think time, both introduced by Shneiderman (1984), are not very clear-cut temporal factors in HCI, as is shown in figure 1 via dotted lines.

Almost no attempts have been made to investigate the influence of a variety of temporal aspects of HCI. Williges and Williges (1982) varied SRT, display time, echo time, an additional keyboard entry time factor, and number of characters to be held in the input buffer, in a very limited repeated measurement design with 4 subjects. They found that delays caused by SRTs and echo time delays were the most important timing parameters in operator performance. The majority of studies on temporal factors in HCI focussed on SRTs, since computer response times became a serious problem with the introduction of time-sharing systems as can be seen in older summaries (Carbonell, Elkind & Nickerson 1968, Miller 1968, Martin 1973). With computers becoming faster, temporal delays caused by features of the system tend to fall into a negligible range. This may be true for parameters like echo time within the VDT, but even with increasing speed of central processors, SRTs are not unusual in time sharing systems, in which every user has access to big data banks thus temporarily blocking other users. Additionally, with the introduction of faster computer systems, there is a tendency to increase the number of VDTs, and/or to introduce time consuming complex programming languages and comfortable routines, thus prolonging SRTs. As Thadhani (1981) pointed out, a cost-shift has taken place during the last ten years, since system costs rapidly decreased while user costs now outweigh the combined hardware and data processing center costs. Apart from economic aspects which led to elaborated calculation procedures for cost-reductions through SRT-shortening (Smith 1983), several authors pointed to the stress-inducing properties of SRTs at computer aided work places (Martin 1973, Youmans 1983, Boucsein, Greif & Wittekamp 1984, Shneiderman 1984, 1987), but very few attempts have been made to quantify stress reactions with respect to methodological standards given by experimental stress research. Therefore, the first aim of the present paper is to outline the application of psychophysiological paradigms for studying stress at simulated and real work places. Secondly, a short report is given of an investigation of stress induced by temporal factors in HCI by a variation of SRTs at simulated VDT work places.

METHODOLOGICAL ISSUES

The Study of Human-Computer Interaction at Simulated Work Places as a Method in Stress Research

Since VDTs are being used at more and more work places, an increasing number of office and industrial tasks can be simulated in laboratories because these VDT-dialogs can be emulated by laboratory computers in a realistic manner. This opens possibilities for stress research in several respects:

1. Introduction of experimentally controlled factors for stress-induction. An analysis of factors that may be sources of stress at work places demands a systematic variation of isolated stress-inducing variables. To perform this within a real-life setting is normally prevented by methodological problems as well as by economic boundaries. So an additional analysis of work places in the laboratory where those investigations can be made under highly controlled conditions is necessary. VDT work places as compared to others require only a restricted amount of movement from the worker which is hence easily controlled. In this regard, Sondheimer and Relles (1982) pointed to a need for the extensive use of controlled laboratory investigations of interactive computer system's influence on human factors to develop adequate field settings.

2. Enlarging the theoretical background with respect to various concepts of general psychology. Highly controlled experimental settings in the laboratory allow an exact testing of predictions from psychological theories. An attempt in this direction is made by key-stroke models [1] (e.g. Card, Moran & Newell 1983) which, however, have severe limitations in explaining more complex cognitive processes. Controlled experiments at simulated work places make it possible to include additional concepts of e.g. time estimation, development of work strategies, anticipation of threat, or controllability and predictability which cannot be transferred easily into complex work situations but must be adapted to specific task structures and context conditions.

3. Use of multivariate psychophysiological recording to measure stress reactions at work places. Field conditions normally restrict the amount and/or kind of variables that can be recorded at work. As pointed out in the next section, investigations following standards given by psychophysiological stress research should be multivariate, including variables from different functional systems. This can be performed in the laboratory at simulated work places, and variables that prove to be good stress indicators may later be used in field studies.

Strategies for Psychophysiological Measurement at Real and Simulated Work Places

The use of physiological measures within medical research in the field of occupation and industry is well established (Astrand & Rodahl 1977; Rohmert & Rutenfranz 1983). Psychologists in this area also make use of physiological variables as indicators of mental or emotional strain. As compared to other objective measures like flicker-fusion frequency which demands an interruption of the task, physiological measures have the advantage of continuous recording with minimal impact during work. However, investigations at real work places are often restricted to a few variables that are easy to record like heart rate. Meanwhile, multivariate methodology is well established in psychophysiology (Fahrenberg 1987), and theoretical framework has much improved in this field including concepts of activation, orienting reaction and habituation, homeostasis and autonomic balance, stimulus- and reaction-specifity, as well as psychophysiological theories of emotion, stress, and individual differences (Gale & Edwards 1983). Particularly, the unidimensional concept of activation has been replaced by multidimensional concepts, a development which canalized the search for empirically determined separate physiological indicators for different kinds of strain, e. g. physical, mental or emotional.

Several methodological issues are raised by the use of psychophysiological recording. Firstly, covariations between physiological measures themselves and with other indicators, e.g. behavioral and subjective measures, are generally low. Secondly, large individual differences dependent on personality and situational characteristics as well as on their interaction must be taken into account. Thirdly, dependencies on initial values are frequently discussed, leading to the use of analysis of covariance (ANCOVA) or related designs.

In addition to taking these problems into account, in the field of occupational and industrial psychophysiology there must be a careful control of measurement artifacts when physiological recordings are made in real as well as in simulated work places because movements during tasks are often accompanied by changes in physiological variables, which are in the same range as the phenomena under investigation. On the other hand, multivariate research is alleviated, since the fussy polygraphic recording and hand-survey used in earlier days have been replaced by computer-aided techniques for simultaneous recording, data reduction, and evaluation of various physiological measures (Martin & Venables 1980).

Psychophysiological concepts do not only include physiological measurements but also biochemical, behavioral (e.g. performance), and subjective variables, according to a complementary multilevel view (e.g. Fahrenberg, Foerster, Schneider, Müller & Myrtek 1986). This requires a wide range of measures taken at the same time which is only realizable in the laboratory at simulated work places. Designs with related laboratory

and field studies should be used, carrying across the most important indicators into real life situations.

Hypotheses can be developed and tested concerning differential
validity of functional systems like the central nervous system indicating
vigilance changes (Luczak 1975), the cardiovascular system reflecting
mental as well as physical strain (Mulder, Mulder & Veldman 1985), or
the electrodermal system which mainly reflects more emotional changes
during work (Kuhmann, Boucsein, Schaefer & Alexander 1987).

EMPIRICAL PART

In this part, a short report is given of a project on
psychophysiological stress reactions and performance decrement induced
by different SRTs carried out by the author's group [2].

Theoretical Background: System Response Times as a Stress-Inducing Factor in Human-Computer Interaction

Research on SRT-duration dates back about 20 years. On the basis
of communication theory Miller (1968) recommended an upper limit of 2
sec for intratask-SRTs and 15 sec for intertask-SRTs. If these were not
possible, they could be prolonged to allow the user himself to behave like
a time-sharing system, executing other tasks during SRTs. This type of
working behavior has been labelled "job swapping" by Nickerson, Elkind
and Carbonell (1968). SRTs not exceeding 2 sec were also adopted by
Martin (1973) based on an analogy to human conversation; Youmans
(1983) reported a change from satisfactory to unsatisfactory work when
mean SRTs increased from 1.8 to 2.5 sec. Other field studies with trained
subjects found performance decrement most pronounced when SRTs increased in the range from 0.5 to 1.5 sec (Holling 1987).

While prolonged SRTs will interrupt the task, extremely short SRTs
may induce an agitated work-style, leading to a reduction in accuracy and
an increase in error. To find optimal values for SRTs, it is necessary to
take task- as well as user-characteristics into account, and to distinguish
between inter- and intratask-SRTs (Carbonell et al. 1968, Shneiderman
1979).

In addition to the mean duration of SRTs, their variability is
considered to be another important factor of influence on the user's
behavior, leading to uncertainty concerning the temporal course of events
in HCI, and thus reducing effectiveness in using the system (Carbonell et
al. 1968). While Martin (1973) generally proposed a maximum of 50 %
standard deviation from mean SRT, Gallaway (1981) limited deviation to
5% for SRTs up to 2 sec and to 10% for SRTs between 2 and 4 sec.

Sackman (1970) concluded that the acceptance of mean duration and variability of SRTs depends much on task complexity, reporting that users become very impatient if intertask-SRTs for simple tasks exceed 10 sec and/or become irregular, whereas if the user assumes the computer is busy with a great amount of data, SRTs up to 10 min will be tolerated. The user's acceptance may thus depend on his model of the computer, tolerating assumed necessary computing times for the tasks themselves but no arbitrary delays (Shneiderman 1984).

Apart from the possible influence of SRTs on the acceptance of computers as tools or even as dialog partners via cognitive processes in HCI, additional effects of SRTs can be inferred from an analogy to time-dependent working situations in industrial manufacturing: a quick worker's involuntary working pauses caused by slowing down the assembly-lines do not represent recovery times, as had been suggested, but increase subjective stress (Graf 1970). Similarly, prolonged SRTs, which on the one hand reduce working speed and thus the amount of work in HCI, will, on the other hand, lead to an increased stress response to the work situation since they act as involuntary working pauses (Peters 1977).

Therefore, in addition to the already known effects of different SRTs on performance (Shneiderman 1984, 1987, Holling 1987), stress-inducing properties of SRTs have to be investigated. From a standpoint of psychological stress theory, mean duration as well as variability of SRTs may influence stress reactions in several respects (Boucsein et al. 1984):

1. Mean duration of system response times. Under the view of models which mainly regard working behavior as directed to an entire goal of work, prolonged mean SRTs will lead to a general delay of the state "end of work" and thus to an anticipation of aversive consequences (Greif 1983), e.g., overtime work or salary reduction.

2. Variability of system response times. Increased variability of SRTs will be the main cause of stress when the focus is on single task-units within a series: a continuous working-course that is interrupted by intervals of unpredictable length will produce uncertainty which is known to be a factor in developing psychological stress (Monat, Averill & Lazarus 1972).

When we started our project, there had been only one controlled laboratory study on SRTs that used psychophysiological stress indicators: Weiss, Boggs, Lehto, Shodja, and Martin (1982) recorded blood pressure and heart rate during a time-shared process control at simulated work places introducing SRTs of 2, 6, and 10 sec with variances of either 0 or 0.33 sec as within subjects factors. They found large individual differences that interacted with SRT-factors but no significant main effects for SRTs. However, those authors used an incomplete design which did not allow 2 sec SRTs to be fully included in the analyses, and they did not record initial values which are of great importance for psychophysiological evaluation.

The aim of our project was to evaluate stress-inducing effects of mean length as well as variability of SRTs that were independently and systematically varied in a well-defined HCI. To permit an optimal control of task- and environmental variables, a time-sharing VDT-work place was simulated by using a series of simple error-detection and -correction tasks with varying intertask-SRTs. An additional advantage of the laboratory investigation was the opportunity to measure not only subjective stress effects but to monitor continuously several physiological variables with a minimum of artifacts that may have occurred from uncontrollable sources in the field. Three laboratory studies with unexperienced subjects at simulated VDT-work places were performed, and their results are reported below.

Psychophysiological Stress Reactions to Changes in Mean Duration and Variability of System Response Times

The first two studies investigated effects of SRTs varied systematically with respect to their mean duration and variability on performance and stress reactions as independent experimental factors.

In the first study (Schaefer, Kuhmann, Boucsein & Alexander 1986) performed with 20 students (4 men, 16 women), the effect of different SRT-conditions on the psychophysiological, the subjective, and the performance level were tested. SRT-conditions were experimentally controlled with mean duration (2 sec vs. 8 sec) and variability of SRTs (constant vs. 80 % variability) as factors in a 2 x 2 design with independent groups. In each of 5 trial blocks subjects had to perform 50 tasks as following: a single line of 80 characters (60 capital letters, 20 spaces) appeared on the VDT, the target for the correction procedure was defined as identical letters surrounding a space, and subjects had to respond by pressing one key for target lines and another one for non-target lines. Heart rate and electrodermal activity were measured during trial blocks as well as in resting periods of 5 min following each trial block, where also blood pressure was recorded, and measurements of subjective stress responses with an adjective check list and a list of bodily symptoms were taken. To obtain initial values for ANCOVA, all measures were also taken before the first trial block.

Apart from a significant effect of task series for most variables indicating an overall adaptation in physiological and subjective parameters, differential effects of a systematic variation of SRTs were found in electrodermal and cardiovascular variables: while longer SRTs led to an increased (but not significant) number of spontaneous skin conductance reactions, blood pressure was elevated when SRTs were short, possibly reflecting the greater work density. Heart rate was influenced solely by the time course under all experimental conditions. In addition, the group with short and constant SRTs showed more errors in task-performance and an increase in self-rated bodily symptoms.

Unfortunately, there was a significant continuous increase of working speed and error rate especially within the first 3 trial blocks, indicating a large practice gain which may have obscured the effects of our experimental conditions. Another critical point of this study was the use of equal numbers of 50 tasks per trial-block leading to differences in working time dependent on SRT-duration (from 12 min with the 2 sec SRTs to 20 min with the 8 sec SRTs), so that influences of SRT-duration could not be clearly separated from those of different working times.

Therefore, a second study (Kuhmann et al. 1987) was performed with 68 students (46 men, 22 women) using a design similar to that of the first study, except that increments of SRTs in the variability conditions were steps of 50 %, since in an unpublished experiment of our group concerning the psychophysical threshold between adjacent SRTs those increments could be differentiated confidently. Furthermore a 20 min training trial (T0) was introduced as a first working block with constant SRTs of 1 sec, and identical working times of 20 min were used in the subsequent trial blocks T1 to T5 for all groups. Subjects were told to work as quickly and as accurately as possible. They were also told the number of tasks they had to perform during the whole experiment, which was 1248 for the conditions with 2 sec SRT and 624 for the 8 sec-conditions. To give an incentive for accuracy, subjects were told that faulty tasks would have to be repeated, increasing the session's length, though this was not really carried out.

In contrast to the first experiment, tasks were presented with a non-blinking cursor at the left margin of the line, and individual lines were reduced in length to 40 characters with 10 spaces distributed in a random order, to reduce practice gain during the experimental conditions, as well as aversiveness of the task, both of which had been found in the first study. The subject's task was to detect a target and to mark it with the cursor which was moved from one blank position to the next by pressing the right- and left-arrow cursor keys of the keyboard for movements to the right or left. The up-arrow key was used for marking the target when the cursor was positioned. For non-target lines subjects had to move the cursor to the right margin position before pressing the up-arrow key. The same physiological and subjective measures were taken as in the first experiment, except that blood pressure was measured twice during the last 5 min of each trial block; these were averaged.

The results obtained could be regarded as a general confirmation of our first study. In both studies a decrease in performance over trials was seen together with an increase in subjective complaints. In all physiological variables recorded, adaptation to the experimental situation took place as discussed for heart rate by Luczak, Philipp, and Rohmert (1980). With

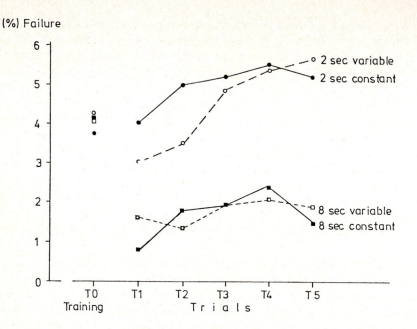

Figure 2: Mean error rate (%) in trial blocks T1 to T5, adjusted by
ANCOVA with training trial (T0) as covariate.

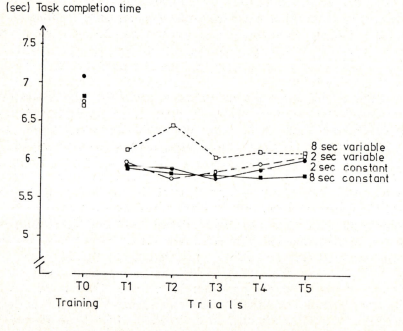

Figure 3: Mean task completion time in trial blocks T1 to T5, adjusted by
ANCOVA with training trial (T0) as covariate.

regard to the experimental factors (duration and variability of SRTs), statistically significant effects were seen for the duration factor only. Additionally, a few significant interactions occured with time course.

Under short SRTs higher error rates (Figure 2) appeared together with a greater number of cursor movements per task (without figure), but no such effects were found in the task completion times (Figure 3).

A similar tendency had been obtained in the first study, where subjects under constant SRTs of 2 sec produced more errors than the other groups, also without showing differences in working speed. Additionally, subjects reported more headaches and eye symptoms under 2 sec SRTs. The differences in error rates were clearly induced by the different SRT-conditions, since during the training trial with identical SRTs of 1 sec for all subjects, the groups did not differ from each other either in error rates, in task completion times, or in the number of cursor movements per task.

With regard to the performance measures, there seemed to be a clear advantage of longer SRTs at a first glance, since error rates were markedly reduced with long as compared to short SRT conditions. One explanation might be given by differences in the speed-accuracy trade-off between these conditions (Wickelgren 1977): since subjects tend to adapt their working speed to the response speed of the system, short SRTs should lead to a faster working speed and hence increase the probability of errors (Shneiderman 1984). There were, however, no differences between groups in working speed, as measured by the average task completion time. Therefore, a simple speed-accuracy trade-off explanation does not hold. Instead, the greater number of cursor movements per task paralleled the higher error rate in short SRT-conditions, which pointed to the use of different working strategies under short and long SRT-conditions (Kuhmann et al. 1987).

A further differentiation between short and long SRTs was seen on the physiological level: besides a common adaptation effect for the cardiovascular variables heart rate and blood pressure, higher systolic blood pressure levels were maintained over trials under short SRTs (Figure 4), while the corresponding effect in diastolic blood pressure did not reach significance. No differences in heart rate were obtained. This is in accordance with the results of the first study as well as with those of Weiss et al. (1982) who did not find heart rate differences between SRT-conditions ranging from 2 to 10 sec. Heart rate and blood pressure are known to be sensitive to different levels of work load and controlled processing demands in mental tasks (e.g. Mulder et al. 1985, Kuhmann et al. 1985). In SRT-studies, short SRTs represent a higher physical work load in that the subjects are presented with more tasks in the same time than in long SRT-conditions. Mental work load, in contrast, is primarily induced by different levels of task difficulty, which were identical over SRT-conditions in our two studies because the tasks themselves were not

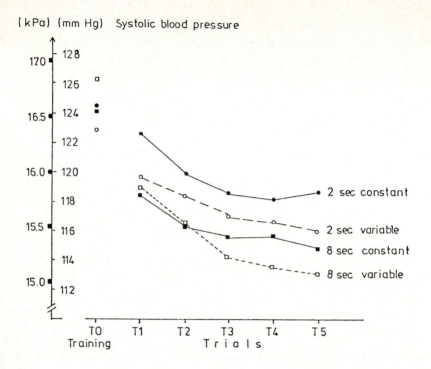

Figure 4: Mean systolic blood pressure in trial blocks T1 to T5, adjusted by ANCOVA with training (T0) as covariate.

different. The higher physical work load at similar levels of mental load resulting in differences in blood pressure between groups but not in differences in heart rate thus suggests different sensitivity of heart rate and blood pressure changes to physical work load at equal levels of altogether moderate mental load.

In contrast to the differences in blood pressure, there was a striking result for the higher level of electrodermal activity under long as compared to short SRT-conditions; this had been evident but not significant in the first study: a greater number of spontaneous skin conductance reactions (Figure 5) as well as a stronger increase of skin conductance level during the experiment with 8 sec SRTs. Since the groups with 2 sec SRTs performed about twice as many tasks as the 8 sec SRT groups in the same time, it can be inferred that greater electrodermal activity within the latter groups is not an effect of activation induced by the task performance itself. This is because in this case the electrodermal activity would have been much greater in conditions with short SRTs. Hence, in-

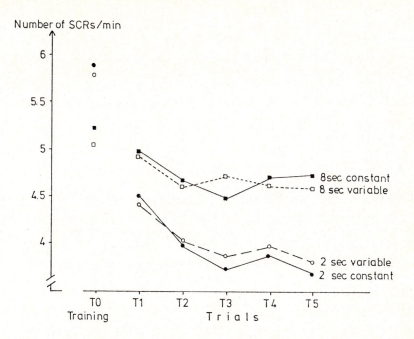

Figure 5: Mean number of skin conductance reactions (SCRs) per minute in trial blocks T1 to T5, adjusted by ANCOVA with training trial (T0) as covariate.

creased electrodermal activity must be mainly attributed to the involuntary working pauses induced by SRTs. As the subjects believed that they had to perform a particular number of tasks, long working pauses which could not be influenced by them will have caused emotional excitement and hence a reduced adaptation to the experimental situation. This could be shown in higher levels of skin conductance under the 8 sec SRTs, and in the number of spontaneous skin conductance reactions which decreased over trials in the 2 sec SRT-groups but remained nearly constant under 8 sec SRTs (cf. figure 5). This result points to the role of electrodermal activity as a specific indicator of emotional stress (Faber 1983, Boucsein 1987), which is likely to be cognitively mediated (Cox 1978): the subjects have more time to think about consequences of their working conditions when SRTs are longer, leading not only to better performance with respect to accuracy but also to emotional stress reactions, which is in accordance with the results of Graf (1970) and Peters (1977). Since this opposite effect of SRT duration on electrodermal activity and blood pressure had been also obtained in the first study, there is strong evidence for the differential validity of electrodermal and cardiovascular variables as indicators of emotional and physical stress, at least under conditions comparable to those of our experiments.

One further result that has been found in both studies was the lack of significant effects of SRT variability and of interactions between the duration and the variability factor. Thus, variability effects appear to be missing with either identical numbers of tasks and different working times as in the first study, or with identical working times and different numbers of tasks per trial block as in the second study. The implication here is that this lack of the expected variability effects must be due to something other than differences in the number of tasks or total working times.

Variability of SRTs is considered to be a factor inducing temporal uncertainty which is known to be a potent stressor (Monat et al. 1972). It may be possible that subjects cope with this stress-inducing factor by forming a mean expectation value of SRT duration to enable predictions of the temporal course of events, thus subjectively modifying the experimental condition of SRT variability. An alternative explanation might be that constant SRTs of 8 sec may not be represented subjectively as constant intervals but induce temporal uncertainty in the same way as variable 8 sec SRTs do, while subjects are able to differentiate between constant and variable SRTs when a mean duration of 2 sec is chosen. This raises the question of sensoric thresholds for SRT-differences and their dependency on mean duration of SRTs. Related results from psychophysics of time estimation are not really applicable, since in this field time estimation procedures normally are the only task that subjects have to focus on. In the case of VDT work, attention is mainly directed to the job itself, and detection of SRT differences is incidental.

Therefore, for the third experiment, a method was introduced which allowed difference thresholds to be obtained indirectly via reaction times to the absence of an expected event. Simulated system break-downs were introduced at random, to which subjects had to respond with a restart procedure, that took a distinct amount of time exceeding normal SRTs.

48 students (39 men, 9 women) took part in the experiment. Each subject performed 3 practice- and 5 trial-blocks (T1 to T5) of 20 min duration each. They were divided into 4 groups with 2, 4, 6 or 8 sec SRTs. During the first training, 1 sec SRTs were used for all groups, in the 2nd training subjects received the SRT duration assigned to their group, and the 3rd training made subjects familiar with the break-down prodecure. Perceived variability was evaluated indirectly via the reaction times on system break-downs.

These reaction times were calculated by subtracting SRT from the total time between disappearance of the last task and pressing the restart-key. Since there were no practice gains during trial blocks 2 to 5, reaction times of those blocks were evaluated together. To obtain values for psychophysical thresholds, standard deviations of reaction times were plotted against SRTs. The curve was extrapolated to a SRT of 0 sec by fitting a 2nd degree polynomial. This ordinate value represents sources of variance of reaction times due to other factors than time estimation (e.g. decision processes, motoric execution times, etc.). Standard deviations of reaction times under the 4 SRT-conditions were corrected by this ordinate value, and then transformed into relative sensitivity (equivalent to Weber's constant) by dividing the corrected standard deviations by the appropriate SRT-duration. As can be inferred from figure 6, there is a non-linear increase of Weber's constant with SRT duration, with a disproportionately greater value at SRTs of 8 sec, being twice as big as with 2 sec SRTs. This result, obtained on the basis of psychophysical evaluation procedures, clearly indicates that constant SRTs of 8 sec have an internal representation which is poorly selective in comparison to constant SRTs of 2 sec. The implication here is that constant SRTs of 8 sec do not induce predictability as short and constant SRTs do. This explains in part the fact that we could not obtain effects of SRT variability in our first two

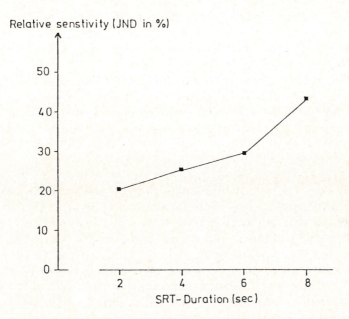

Figure 6: Relative sensitivity - in just noticeable differences (JND) in percent - to SRT variability at various mean SRTs, averaged across trial blocks T2 to T5.

experiments: constant and variable 8 sec SRT conditions must be regarded as psychologically equivalent with regard to temporal uncertainty, thus leading to no differences in stress reactions. Another possible explanation for our results from the first two experiments is that the greater stress-inducing property of 8 sec SRTs is not only due to increased time but also to a greater uncertainty which parallels prolonged mean SRTs, with a sharp increase between 6 and 8 sec SRTs.

We have to conclude that a plain separation of mean duration from variability of SRTs as experimental factors in a 2 x 2 design as used in our first two experiments is not appropriate for an unconfounded investigation of the stress-inducing properties of those two factors. Future research must give more regard to the internal representation of temporal factors of HCI in the subjetcs which can indirectly be inferred from determination of psychophysical thresholds as performed in our third experiment.

CONCLUSIONS

Temporal factors in HCI as SRTs were shown to have distinct stress-inducing properties, but there is no simple relation between SRT-parameters and the amount of stress. Under conditions of performing simple error-detection and -correction tasks with moderate time pressure as in our studies, the longest SRTs used (8 sec) as compared to the shortest ones (2 sec) led to a marked reduction of errors without extending time for individual tasks. This points to a greater thoroughness or carefulness during task completion which had been due to the use of SRT as a preparatory phase. Though tasks were rather simple, it is likely that subjects used the 8 sec SRTs as "user planning times" (cf. figure 1). However, as our psychophysiological stress recording showed, slow-paced work as induced by the longer SRTs led to an increased amount of emotional strain, indicated by an increased electrodermal activity and more bodily symptoms. On the other hand, the shortest SRTs used led to an agitated work-style with an increased error rate and cardiovascular strain as indicated by blood pressure. Our results point to the possibility of using different psychophysiological systems as indicators for mental as compared to physical strain. The results of our third experiment suggest an optimal mean SRT of 6 sec (or somewhat less) for the kind of tasks used here, since subjects were not able to maintain exact internal representations of 8 sec SRTs being constant. This may have led to a loss of predictability and thus to another factor that induced emotional stress in addition to an increased length of SRT.

The findings here are that too short as well as too long SRTs have stress-inducing properties resulting from different sources, and that a simple shortening of SRTs will not automatically lead to lower stress levels, nor even to better performance. This is principally in accordance with the U-shaped relationship between SRT duration and errors found by Barber and Lucas (1983) which, however, had its optimum around 12 sec. The difference in optimal SRT is easily explained by the more complex tasks used by those authors. This gives rise to the point that no general rules can be stated either for SRTs or probably for any other temporal factors playing a role in HCI; at the very least, task dependent SRTs have to be determined. This cannot be performed, as Shneiderman (1979) did, using the non-empirically based recommendations from Miller (1968). Recommendations must be preceded by thorough, controlled laboratory and field studies based on task-analyses, using not only performance- and subjective measures but also psychophysiological indicators of different systems which indicate different kinds of strain during HCI at the VDT-work place.

FOOTNOTES

1) A critical review of the key-stroke models and their methodological basis is given by Greif and Gediga in this book.
2) Together with Professor Siegfried Greif at Osnabrück University, supported by the German Research Society, Grant Bo 554/2-1.

REFERENCES

Astrand, P. O., & Rohdahl, K. (1977). *Textbook of work physiology*. New York: McGraw Hill.

Barber, R. E., & Lucas, H. C. (1983). System response time, operator productivity and job satisfaction. *Communications of the ACM, 26*, 11, 972-986.

Boucsein, W. (1987). *Elektrodermale Aktivität: Grundlagen, Methoden und Anwendungen*. Berlin: Springer (in press).

Boucsein, W., Greif, S., & Wittekamp, J. (1984). Systemresponsezeiten als Belastungsfaktor bei Bildschirm-Dialogtätigkeiten. *Zeitschrift für Arbeitswissenschaft, 38* (10 NF), 113-122.

Carbonell, J. R., Elkind, J. I., & Nickerson, R. S. (1968). On the psychological importance of time in a time sharing system. *Human Factors, 10*, 135-142.

Card, S. K., Moran, T. P., & Newell, A. (1983). *The psychology of human-computer interaction*. Hillsdale, N. J.: Erlbaum.

Cox, T. (1978). *Stress*. London: MacMillan Press.

Dzida, W., Herda, S., & Itzfeldt, W. D. (1978). User-perceived quality of interactive systems. *IEEE Transactions on Software Engineering, Se-4*, 270-274.

Faber, S. (1983). Zur Auswertemethodik und Interpretation von Hautleitfähigkeitsmessungen bei arbeitswissenschaftlicher Beanspruchungsermittlung. *Zeitschrift für Arbeitswissenschaft, 37* (9 NF), 85-91.

Fahrenberg, J. (1987). Psychophysiological processes. In J. R. Nesselroade
& R. B. Cattell (Eds.), *Handbook of multivariate experimental
psychology (2nd ed.)*. New York: Plenum (in press).
Fahrenberg, J., Foerster, F. Schneider, H.-J., Müller, W., & Myrtek, M.
(1986). Predictability of individual differences in activation pro-
cesses in a field setting based on laboratory measures. *Psycho-
physiology*, *23*, 323-333.
Gale, A. & Edwards, J. A. (Eds.). (1983). *Physiological correlates of
human behavior (Vols. 1-3)*. London: Academic Press.
Gallaway, G. R. (1981). Response times to user activities in interactive
man-machine computer systems. *Proceedings of the Human
Factors Society - 25th Annual Meeting* October 1981, 754-758.
Graf, O. (1970). Arbeitszeit und Arbeitspausen. In A. Mayer, & B. Herwig
(Eds.), *Handbuch der Psychologie (Band 9)*. Göttingen: Hogrefe.
Grandjean, E., & Vigilani, E. (Eds.) (1980). *Ergonomic aspects of visual
display terminals*. London: Taylor and Francis.
Greif, S. (1983). Streß und Gesundheit. Ein Bericht über Forschungen zur
Belastung am Arbeitsplatz. *Zeitschrift für Sozialisationsforschung
und Erziehungssoziologie*, *3*, 41-58.
Holling, H. (1987). *Wahrscheinlichkeitsmodelle und empirische Analysen
zur Beanspruchung durch Systemresponsezeiten*. (in press).
Janke, W., & Debus, G. (1978). *Die Eigenschaftswörterliste (EWL)*.
Göttingen: Hogrefe.
Kuhmann, W., Boucsein, W., Schaefer, F., & Alexander, J. (1987). Experi-
mental investigation of pychophysiological stress-reactions induced by different system response times in human-computer
interaction. *Ergonomics*, *24*, (in press).
Kuhmann, W., Lachnit, H., & Vaitl, D. (1985). The quantification of
experimental load: Methodological and empirical issues. In A.
Steptoe, H. Rüddel, & H. Neus (Eds.), *Clinical and methodological issues in cardiovascular psychophysiology*. Berlin: Springer.
Luczak, H. (1975). Untersuchungen informatorischer Belastung und Beanspruchung des Menschen. *Fortschritt-Berichte der VDI-Zeit-
schriften, Reihe 10*, Nr. 2.
Luczak, H., Philipp, U., & Rohmert, W. (1980). Decomposition of heart-
rate variability under the ergonomic aspects of stressor analysis.
In R. I. Kitney, & O. Rompelman (Eds.), *The study of heart-rate
variability*. Oxford: Clarendon Press.
Martin, I., & Venables, P. H. (Eds.) (1980). *Techniques in Psychophysiology*. Chichester: Wiley.
Martin, J. (1973). *Design of man-computer dialogue*. Englewood Cliffs,
N.J.: Prentice Hall.
Miller, R. B. (1968). Response time in man-computer conversational
transactions. *Proceedings of the Spring Joint Computer Conference, 33*, 267-277.

Monat, A., Averill, J. R., & Lazarus, R. S. (1972). Anticipatory stress and coping reactions under various conditions of uncertainty. *Journal of Personality and Social Psychology, 24*, 237-253.

Mulder, G., Mulder, L. J. M., & Veldman, J. B. P. (1985). Mental tasks as stressors. In A. Steptoe, H. Rüddel, & H. Neus (Eds.), *Clinical and methodological issues in cardiovascular psychophysiology* . Berlin: Springer.

Nickerson, R. S., Elkind, J.I., & Carbonell, J. R. (1968). Human factors and the design of time sharing computer systems. *Human Factors, 10*, 127-134.

Peters, T. (1977). *Arbeitsmedizinische Forderungen an die Bildschirm-textverarbeitung.* 5th European Congress for Text Processing, Intertext.

Rohmert, W., & Rutenfranz, J. (Eds.) (1983). *Praktische Arbeits-physiologie.* Stuttgart: Thieme.

Sackman, H. (1970). Experimental analysis of man-computer problem solving. *Human Factors, 12*, 187-201.

Schaefer, F., Kuhmann, W., Boucsein, W., & Alexander, J. (1986). Beanspruchung durch Bildschirmtätigkeit bei experimentell variierten Systemresponsezeiten. *Zeitschrift für Arbeits-wissenschaft, 40* (12 NF), 31-38.

Shneiderman, B. (1979). Human factors experiments in designing inter-active systems. *Computer, 12*, 9-19.

Shneiderman, B. (1984). Response time and display rate in human per-formance with computers. *Computing Surveys, 16*, 265-285.

Shneiderman, B. (1987). *Designing the user interface. Strategies for effective human-computer interaction.* Reading: Addison-Wesley.

Smith, D. (1983). Faster is better: A business case for subsecond response time. *Computerworld, 18*, 1-11.

Sondheimer, N. K., & Relles, N. (1982). Human factors and user assistance in interactive computing systems: An introduction. *IEEE Transactions on Systems, Man and Cybernetics, 12*, 102-107.

Thadhani, A. J. (1981). Interactive user productivity. *IBM Systems Journal, 20*, 407-423.

Weiss, S. M., Boggs, G., Lehto, M., Shodja, S., & Martin, D. J. (1982). *Computer system response time and psychophysiological stress.* II. Proceedings of the Human Factors Society, 26th Annual Meeting (pp. 698-702). Santa Monica, California.

Wickelgren, W. A. (1977). Speed-accuracy tradeoff and information pro-cessing dynamics. *Acta Psychologica, 41*, 67-85.

Williges, R. C., & Williges, B. H. (1982). Modelling the human operator in computer-based data entry. *Human Factors, 24*, 285-299.

Youmans, D. M. (1983). *The effect of system response time on users of interactive computer systems.* IBM United Kingdom Laboratories, Hursly Park, England.

COGNITIVE OPTIMIZATION
OF HUMAN-COMPUTER INTERACTION
IN THE WORK PLACE

Psychological Issues of
Human Computer Interaction in the Work Place
M. Frese, E. Ulich, W. Dzida (Editors)
© Elsevier Science Publishers B.V. (North-Holland), 1987

ERGONOMIC FEATURES OF INTERACTIVE SYSTEMS - THE INTERDEPENDENCY OF SOFTWARE AND HARDWARE

Ahmet Çakir

ERGONOMIC Institute
for Social and Occupational Sciences Research Co., Ltd.,
Soldauer Platz 3, D-1000 Berlin 19,
Federal Republic of Germany

The capabilities of computer systems to comply with the real needs of their users are limited by the features of physical devices, usually called "hardware". These needs can be specified as task adequate *refinement of data*, availability of user defined amount of information and processing and presenting the data within the time limits given either by the specific task and/or by human physiology. The quality and usability of methods and procedures of entering, processing, presenting and storing of data and information is severely limited by the features of devices available on the marketplace. The term "software ergonomics" is misleading because it lacks a usable definition and attracts the attention of designers toward programming, while successful working systems can only be created by considering these limitations while designing programs.

INTRODUCTION

Definitions

The term "software ergonomics" has become popular since its creation not very long ago. There is considerable confusion about the definition and scope of "ergonomics". In addition the term "software" in the conventional meaning of the phrase is quite useless for the understanding of "software ergonomics". What is the benefit of a combination of two terms when both of them lack a usable definition?

The historically and presently used definitions of hard- and software state that hardware is the "physical equipment used in data processing whereas computer programs, procedures, rules and associated documentation" are software (IBM dictionary of word and data processing). If this definition is accepted some important questions arise, e.g. how is a programmable keyboard or a non-volatile memory with a loaded program to be assigned - to "hardware" or to "software"? Can a computer program be assessed in relation to its ergonomic quality without the knowledge of the hardware on which it is implemented?

It is doubtful that the conventional definition of these two terms will ever help us to understand the goals that hide behind the ideas on "software ergonomics". The relevant aspect to distinguish between "hard" and "soft" from the user's point of view is his or her ability of personal control on the activities to be performed; where "personal control" should be understood as "having an impact on the conditions and on one's activities in correspondence with some *higher order goal*" (Frese, in this book). Most computer systems are consisting of hardware only as programs, procedures, rules and associated documentation are not object to user's control from this point of view. Really *soft* is only what is object to variation in correspondence with higher order goals of the user.

Hardware ergonomics includes not only the features of the physical devices but also all features of programs, procedures and rules on which the user's control cannot be established. Thus hardware ergonomics is an ongoing process of fitting the features of physical devices and/or programs and/or procedures ... to the needs of the user by a given task and not merely a definition of "ergonomic" features of physical devices only.

Software ergonomics can be defined as

fitting the properties of a dialogue-based working system to the cognitive and intellectual attributes of man working in an organizational environment (Cakir, 1986).

This definition incorporates the entire behaviour of the system including the hardware which covers all ergonomic aspects of the physical devices as far as these can be regarded or evaluated separately. The rational behind the definition can be easily understood observing some new developments on the market: By the end of April 1987 one of the leading software houses of the FRG will stop selling data base management systems with the argument that the standardization of operating systems by the biggest manufacturer of hardware is going to eliminate the boundaries between hardware, operating system and data bases thus leading to a monolithic structure (Handelsblatt, 03.12.1986).

Our definition of software ergonomics clearly shows the strong interdependence of hard- and software ergonomics but it also helps to understand why this term can be totally misleading. Thus we understand all of the aspects of the human-machine-interaction by using the phrase "software ergonomics". In addition, the scientific view should not focus on human-computer-interaction only as it is only a limited part of the human interaction with tools. A systematic approach in ergonomics must cover any interaction with the environment and should not be restricted to isolated parts of it. Many unwritten rules of human behaviour which also apply to the use of computers are a product of our cultural background that has developed long before computers have been invented. The interaction with a machine tool for example is ruled by the same basic principles although the kind of information to be handled is quite different. Therefore the term human-machine-interaction opposed to human-human-interaction seems to be appropriate as there are some differences in the basic principles which rule each of them.

From humans and machines

Since the time of Newton and Descartes the scientific approach of analyzing human beings and their behaviour has been very similar to the methods of analysis of mechanical systems. Even in our days the term "information" is widely used in the sense of Wiener and Shannon. One should keep in mind, that Wiener was a mathematician who did not emphasize that there are major differences between machines and animals (Cybernetics: or Control and Communication in the Animal and the Machine). His theory must be seen in connection with the automatic control of guns where he gained practical experience in two world wars (Bell, 1986).

Shannon, whose work can be considered to have *the* major impact on "information theory" developed his ideas while improving the performance of public exchange networks. The "communication" in such networks could be completely automated in the meantime, thus showing how predictable and predefined their operations are.

One of the worst results of this approach was and still is the way in which automation is realized: The human factor is treated as a "bottle neck" of automated systems, as a factor of inconsistency to be overcome by perfect automation. During the course of the 20th century the target of automation has been *replacing the skills of highly skilled workers*, either to replace them fully or partly by less skilled persons. The human skill of evaluating objective data subjectively has been regarded as a factor of uncertainty, thus organizations have been formed to be predictable and manoeuvrable by replacing the "human factor" by rules, fixed and virtually objective. The result and the success of this can be easily understood by the meaning of the phrase "work-to-rule". Any organization in the world can be paralyzed if people start "working to rule", this means to work precisely according to the rules the company provides.

On the other hand the human society possesses thousands of perfectly automated systems to our benefit, like the international telephone network which connects more than 500 million stations and approximately 25 % of all human beings fully automatically. Employing humans for predictable and predetermined work is inhumane. Such predictable tasks are best suited for machines. One of the ergonomic specialists has stated "only one man and a dog are needed to operate the international public exchange system: the man feeds the dog and the dog is employed to keep the man from doing anything else".

Today thousands of computers are employed for automated data exchange and the entire human society would collapse if they cease work. These systems are machines by definition. Beyond this area many organizations, ruled by inflexible methods and practices, do exist acting like machines towards anyone who wants to interact with them. Such "machines" will write you a letter confirming that "your personal income for the year 1987 amounts $ ***,***,000.00 and the taxes to be paid amount to $ ***,000.00 payable by ...". And unless you pay the sum of $ 0.00 you will receive another letter reminding you to pay $ 0.00 plus a fee for late payment.

Ergonomics of human-machine-interaction partly deals with the problems created by machine like organizations or organizational units. But the main approach reaches far beyond this, it can best be described as improving the abilities of data processing systems towards an informational technology where technology should be understood in the Greek meaning of tekhnologia = systematic treatment derived from techne = art, skill. Information itself is not an objective dimension alone but incorporates both the objective contents of data (e.g. *price*) and the subjective evaluation (e.g. *value*). A system of "information technology" can be operable and efficient without any technical devices whereas it is impossible to run it without the impact of humans.

Thus the human factor in information technology is not a bottleneck or a source for inconsistency or error, but the vital part of a system which is formed by humans and machines. Humans are most effective in cooperating with the "organizational context" which goes beyond the man-machine domain. The "organizational context" is one of the main issues of software ergonomics as defined in this paper.

PRINCIPLES OF DIALOGUE DESIGN AND IMPLICATIONS FOR DEVICES

Principles of DIN 66 234 Part 8
... and their implications for physical devices

Although any systematic approach may be successful and acceptable to reach improvements in this area, the German draft standard DIN 66 234 part 8 with five "principles of dialogue design" is discussed in this section mainly because it contains a *set of guidelines* from which one can see the goals and also the restrictions which makes it possible to detect what is missing.

This standard, commonly discussed as a standard for software ergonomics, has clear hardware implications. This means the conformance with this standard may require physical devices with certain features. Similar implications are required for the compliance with other parts of DIN 66 234.

Some of the following examples may serve as a demonstration of the interdependence between hardware and software ergonomics. The implications have been formulated after interpreting the principles of dialogue design in a government project.

Principle of dialog design	Implication for physical devices
o Suitability for the task (Aufgabenangemessenheit)	- CPU characteristics - quality of input devices - choice of input devices - quality of output devices - choice of output devices - speed and capacity of storage devices - data security (tempest) - backup processing at least with a streamer tape
o Self-descriptiveness (Selbstbeschreibungs- fähigkeit	- capacity of storage devices (help files) - screen capacity (additional lines for additional information) - additional keys
o Controllability (Steuerbarkeit)	- multi-tasking - failure-restart facilities - UNDO-function keys - number of function keys
o Correspondence to user expectations (Erwartungskonformität)	- standard keyboard layout - standard response times - quality of screens and printers
o Error tolerance (Fehlerrobustheit)	- variety of implications

In this project a considerable number of decisions on the characteristics of physical devices have been changed after recognizing the implications of these principles of dialog design. This project has been the most unlikely case in industrial environments. In "real" environments a number of limitations rule the choice of the physical devices and thus the maximum achievable quality of "software ergonomics".

LIMITATIONS OF HUMAN-MACHINE-INTERACTION BY
PHYSICAL DEVICES

Human-Machine-Interaction (HMI) is restricted by the relevant features of physical devices. Restrictions imposed by physical devices can be easily understood by looking at a design process for a computer system or just at a bookshelf.

In designing a new system the designer takes into consideration e.g. the price, quality and other relevant features of input/output devices or e.g. the clock frequency of the processor.

A successful system cannot be created without detailed knowledge of the technical properties of physical devices to be used. Systems developed contrary to this rule may face some disastrous problems like the German interactive videotex which could attract only 10 % of the predicted number of users.

Scanning a bookshelf one notices the different formats of books, and the different print qualities chosen to present the information in the very same manner the author wishes or believes to be adequate. This is the result of approximately 5,000 years experience in the ergonomics of books. Contrary to this, most workplaces are equipped with one single screen forcing the user to keep all those pages in his mind which may be needed at the same time but are only accessible one after the other. The meta-communication for the access can also be so demanding that one forgets the last page when the next page is displayed. For example reading the weekend issue of a daily newspaper in the interactive videotex system means to work through 10,000 screens accessible by a tree structure.

"Task adequate dialog design" for the constructor of a valve in a power engine may be interpreted today as finding a way of structuring a CAD system which generates drawings in adequate time periods after entering a considerable amount of data and which is able to display 2D- or 2 1/2 D-graphics in limited resolution and a just acceptable flickering image. Task adequate, for someone who wants to construct a valve, is a system which can generate all information needed for the product, display a true 3D image, give a dynamic simulation with different parameters or static graphics, including tables and generate the entire information for the production after the constructor gives his or her approval to the set of parameters. Of course, this is a problem of programs. But given the fact, they were available, only a limited number of computers at this time have the ability of processing the amount of data needed in this case and within the time scale adequate from the user's viewpoint.

Thus the main problem of human-machine-interaction is to make available a clearly (user) defined structure of data, with a task adequate refinement and within the time limits, given either by the physiology of humans and or by the requirements of the task. These are problems of physical devices and will remain so for a long time.

If one intends to apply the ergonomic principle, "What you see is what you get" to a system to be designed for writing and editing a book with text, color graphics, half tone images etc. it is easily understood which limitations exist and will continue to exist for a considerable period of time.

To see what you get

On the screen

The electronic screen, mainly a cathod ray tube (CRT), is the basic device to create visible images.

A screen can display one single character, a part of a single line or a great number of lines (e.g. 72) with a given number of character positions (formatted displays). Formatting a display area to a given number of character positions and limiting the presentation to predefined characters reduces the amount of information to be stored, processed and transported. It also reduces the tasks which can be performed. Unformatted displays allow to address each single pixel on the screen and to assign different attributes (gray scale, color, blinking, etc.) to each pixel position. The usability of these screens is equivalent to the usability of paper, however the additional cost for processing and storing the data is much higher than by employing formatted screens. On the other hand, the programming effort for a given application is much lower if an unformatted display is used (Schnupp, 1982). Low cost screens display a poor image of 160,000 pels (picture elements, pixels) just sufficient to write 24 lines of 80 *coded* characters per line. More advanced screens, frequently used by system designers, display some 250,000 pels.

These screens can display 25 lines per 80 characters or limited graphics. Only a small number of systems use screens up to 1,2 Million pels mainly due to cost reasons.

Just to refresh their image at 70 frames per second to achieve a fairly flickerfree positive image an information of 84 MBit/s has to be processed. Normally the image is refreshed locally but still then an information rate of 7.2 MBit is to be transferred if additional 6 bits/pel gray scale is necessary to display "half tone" images with a limited scale of 64 gray shades.

In order to display images with smooth contours one needs a screen with approximately 12 Million pels. In this case a storage tube is to be used with poor contrast limiting the application to dark rooms. Thus there are severe technical, technological and cost limitations for screens. This is the reason why you do not see all what you will get on your screen. Even more technically based limitations rule the use of color screens. These display many colors with poor contrast, e.g. shades of red and blue, which makes them prone to disturbances by ambient light.

In addition, color displays create different colors by mixing three basic colors and thus can never create brown or shades of brown because this is physically not possible. Thus a designer who wants to create his product on a screen can not use brownish colors (but he can print them). Research results for computer generated maps e.g. show that there is great confusion if users are asked to discriminate among the colors RED and BROWN (Spiker et al., 1986). This is not surprising if one considers the disability of any device to create brown if it works with additive mixture of color stimuli.

The phosphors of mostly used color tubes have been made for commercial TV and are not flickerfree at refresh rates of 60 Hz which leads to the preference of negative images. The result of this becomes visible if you print the image, white is turned to black, black to white, yellow becomes virtually invisible. Thus creating your design on the screen you must *know what you get*. You do not see it. The systems lack consistency, one of the basic ergonomic requirements for any kind of system.

Due to cost considerations the "industry standard" works with poor quality screens which display 200 video lines per frame. This is not acceptable for most European users as it is not possible to display properly designed character fonts using 200 lines only. Present technology of creating working systems is based on hardware products in the conventional definition, offered by powerful companies which operate on the international market, whereas programs, procedures et al. are designed by smaller vendors. As the impact of the international suppliers of hardware products is incomparably higher the features, and also ergonomically relevant characteristics of the system are mainly determined by the relevant characteristics of hardware in the conventional definition. Thus "software" which can be bought is not *"soft"* at all, because the programmer must accept many limitations given by the supplier of the physical devices.

On hardcopy

Hardcopy can be created by using devices of very different quality and speed. In order to create a full fidelity color image with all the characteristics of good print a printer/plotter of unknown technical quality is needed.

The devices available on the marketplace start with type bar printers which can work at a speed of approximately 5 char/s and end with laser printers with about 20 million spots/sec. Even this is not the maximum feasible speed as the limitation is mere technical and not physical.

Unlike an electronic screen the color images on hardcopy are created by "subtractive mixture of color stimuli", a method with different physical rules than the "additive mixture of color stimuli". Therefore the exact match of visual characteristics (contrast, available colors, maximum resolution etc.) is physically not possible and thus technically not achievable.

Given the fact that a full fidelity color image with the resolution of a silver halide film with more than 5OO pels/cm is available both on screens and printers, the transport of the information between them for one single uncoded and unformatted A4-page will take many minutes and need very powerful and fast communication devices. Beyond it even the storage capacity of an optical disc (6OO MByte) will not be sufficient to store one book or report. One single A4-page of full fidelity print, stored without any loss in quality needs 5O MByte, if not processed and compressed. But the same optical disc can store a maximum of some 300,000 formatted A4-pages with approximately 2,000 coded characters.

For practical, technical and cost reasons the feasible quality and speed of hardcopy output devices is far below the available technology and mostly far below of what you really need. As color processing on printing devices is still an unsolved problem there are strict limitations to the use of color, the presentation of information is still going to be restricted to formatted pages and coded characters even if more convenient devices are already available e.g. for the applications in printing industry.

Unfortunately, despite substantially reduced demands the need exists to choose between different technologies. Printing devices with well defined characters and high contrast print (e.g. daisy wheel printers) are slow, noisy and expensive in use (film ribbon) because approximately 95 % of the "ink" is wasted. They can print a maximum of approximately 100 different characters without changing the wheel, with a limited height of about 4 mm. Their capability to print graphics is very limited. A set of rules enables them to print the complete character set of 310 teletex characters, however, with reduced speed and unfavourable character fonts. In addition, a text which is written in Germany does not appear in exactly the same shape in GB. You do not (always) know what your partner gets. Again the system lacks consistency.

Matrix printers solve this problem but unfortunately most of them are noisy too. The low cost matrix printers operate like a formatted screen with predefined characters which can be positioned on predefined spaces on the paper or film. The print quality and also the character definition are inadequate, but the printing speed is relatively high (300 char/s). Due to inadequate print quality (draft quality) these type of devices should not be used for correspondence.

Matrix printers with "near letter quality" are available, however, with reduced speed. Many of them are reversable in quality and speed (low quality - high speed and vice versa).

The printing techniques of matrix printers consist of impact and non-impact. Impact printers cause a noise level of more than 6O dB(A) and are not acceptable for ergonomic reasons if they are placed near the workstation. Non-impact printers are preferable due to noise considerations (less than 5O dB(A)). The most advanced technology is the desk-top laser printer which can create images with letter quality, print predefined character sets as well as unformatted images, variable character sizes etc. at a high speed.

The availability of these devices has revolutionized the typographic quality of printed information including the processing of text and graphics in one system with negligible limitations. The interdependence of hardware and software ergonomics can be easily understood by studying the impact of the laser printer - and the software needed to benefit from the abilities of this device - on the document quality.

To enter what you want to see

To enter more than text

Given the fact your system is well equipped with the best imaginable output devices, their benefits will be limited if it lacks powerful input devices to enter the information or devices to manipulate information already existing in the system. Unfortunately the existing devices like keyboards, mouse, light pen etc. have not been designed to perform all services the user needs both for input and manipulation, but suit different tasks with differing performance and convenience. The conformance of programs with ergonomic requirements cannot be evaluated without the knowledge of the usability of the physical devices. On the other hand the usability or the usefulness of a device cannot be evaluated without the knowledge of the program. Thus predicting that the only input and manipulation device would be a keyboard the programmer will design his product very differently from a programmer who determines that the system is going to be used with an electronic tablet and a pen. Creating a graph or table in the latter case may consume only 5 % of the time required without these devices if the program has been designed assuming the use of a tablet. Contrary to this, if only a keyboard is available, the system designer may create convenient and powerful search routines to overcome the limitations given by the keyboard - giving us one of the best demonstrations of the interdependence of hardware - and software ergonomics.

The keyboard issue

The consistency of the user interface of computer and office systems in the entire "organizational context" within an organization is regarded as a major goal in Germany. One of the secondary goals is to achieve an identical keyboard within the same company.

The background of this idea is the integration of different working areas within a company and the possibility of world-wide communication within a system or beyond the borders of isolated systems.

The reasoning is easily understood, however the method is not so, as more than 1,000 characters and symbols can be defined and used within a system whereas no existing keyboard can address them. Presently as many as four shift levels for keyboards are likely to be standardized and as many as seven levels are in discussion. There is a proposal for the standardization of labeling all seven levels. Putting seven labels on an area of approximately 13 x 13 mm^2 requires artistic skills from the ergonomist, whereas using these keys in addition to function and programmable function keys in the order between 20 and 200 requires even more skills from the user.

The keyboard *has been* the "hardest" of all hardware because even the most powerful organizations in the world did not succeed in changing its relevant characteristics for more than a century. The keyboards of the most advanced systems consist of a century old QUERTY-keyboard with numerous additional keys and keypads. The core of the layout is still the same, like the keys of the typewriter designed for input only, even if the task of entering text has a secondary role next to manipulating.

Today many problems occur with comparably simple keyboards which can be demonstrated by some of the critisism on the products of one manufacturer (SEAS, 1985): "European users of XXX hardware and software products *increasingly* find that these products do not meet their requirements in the areas of ... keyboards, *interproduct compatibility*. XXX hardware and software products are primarily designed for the English language and the 26 letter Latin alphabet. When installed in non-English-speaking countries most XXX products suffer a degradation in function and/or user-friendliness and/or performance ...". Reading the report mentioned above, the awareness of simple looking, but very severe problems of accuracy, consistency and convenience - mainly created by the keyboard - will expand. It is difficult to comprehend, why people speak of the "electronic cottage" in the era of world wide communications, while the users cannot transfer information from a data processing environment to a wordprocessing or PC environment consistently and without losing information. This occurs even, if *all* equipment has been bought from the same manufacturer. Reason: Inconsistent code points, and there is no consistent code table which is valid trough all systems.

Surprisingly, the former choice of a certain character set - due to hardware limitations of the keyboard - will affect the use of colors (SEAS), due to some cluster controllers, designed to handle this character set, can not be configured for 7 colors or graphics.

IMPACT OF LIMITATIONS ON ERGONOMICS OF HUMAN-MACHINE-INTERACTION AND ACCEPTANCE

The following examples demonstrate how limitations of physical devices including constraints on communication speed and accuracy can influence the ergonomics of systems with possible impact on their acceptance.

Telex (<u>telegraphic exchange</u>)

The telex system was designed at the end of the twenties mainly influenced by the former telegraphy system. The main goal was to achieve a *fast and robust* interactive communication system to be standardized and compatible in all components throughout the world and should be operable with low quality transmission facilities. Due to the fact that all goals were successfully achieved this system may survive its modern competitors.

The price of success was very high, as the system and its components remained unchanged for approximately 40 years. During this time period all local operators were "triggered" by the limited capacity of the transmission facilities (6 2/3 char/s) which made it necessary to construct a mechanical interlock for the keys. As this construction was very difficult to realize - and thus expensive - the application remained limited and required skilled operators. The operators of the computers of the 6O's and early 70's were forced to use the telex machines as terminals and forced to operate keyboards with unfavourable ergonomic features.

If the basic design of the system had taken the maximum typing speed into account which requires a transmission speed of 6O Baud instead of 5O Baud (= 6 2/3 char/s) the telex terminals would have been cheaper, the skills needed for their operation less, with possibly broader use in industry.

A second technical feature, the use of 5 bits per character, limits the character set to 31 characters either in upper or lower case mode. The code used in this system is not redundant, thus transmission errors cannot be detected. If the system worked with 8 bits per character all transmission errors would be detected. In addition, using the 8-bit-code allows the use of the "reflected copy mode" which means that the transmitting station can detect whether the received text is correct or not. You do not (exactly) know what your partner receives.

Even with highly advanced telex stations today, incorporating electronic screens, local editing functions, local text storage - it is not easy to write a commercial letter with an acceptable layout. The simple reason for this can be found in the main goal of interactive communication which is line oriented and not page oriented in addition to the limited character set.

Analyzing the method in which most installed computer systems operate the impact of the line oriented operation mode, (which was an answer to the character oriented mode of telegraphy) one can easily find essential influences of the telex system even in the architecture of computer programs.

This example demonstrates that a system which does not underlie to the control of user, meaning consists of hardware only, can be very useful and successful, if only it meets the needs of a target group. This system will put constraints on the user, which can also be unacceptable thus not ergonomic, and the spread of the implementation will be limited to the target area. It is not likely that such systems which lack any versatility can be established in this ever changing era. Thus the ergonomic requirement to establish efficient control of the user on the relevant characteristics of a system is also a vital interest for the system designer of a product of which the target area and group is not predictable.

The revival of the typewriter

The appearance of the (stand alone) wordprocessors in the seventies seemed to mark the end of the century old era of the typewriter. Experts predicted that by 1980 companies would invest in word processing as much as for data processing (Quantum Sciences, 1976). By 1986 the acceptance of the word processors continues to decline but the acceptance of the "typewriter" in comparison has not suffered at all. The typewriter, invented in the first half of the 19th century, is likely to keep its market share by the beginning of the 21st. Why and how?

The typewriter of our days incorporates the positive elements of its predecessors, high quality print and high quality keyboards, and plus new features of storing and editing text before printing. It has a display with very limited features and software considering the limitations of the whole system with regard to the well defined requirements of a limited target group.

Some traditional suppliers of typewriters, aware of the tasks of the target group, offer *a solution for a given task*. By connecting these products through the standard teletex interface a compatible system for world-wide (formatted and coded) text communication has been created. The basic goal of the teletex system is to minimize the impact of the communication systems on local functions and the habits of text generation.

Until the general implementation of communication systems with high throughput (>> 64 kBit/s) *formatted* text exchange will dominate this area (Ohmann, 1982). One should keep in mind that the implementation of 64 kBit/s-communication is just starting!

The difference of the system "typewriter + teletex" to telex from the point of ergonomics is enormous. The original telex system was a monolithic structure consisting of a communication system which ruled the entire operation. For example, local work had to be interrupted if a message was announced. Only a special device, the telex station was allowed to serve as a terminal. Contrary to this, within the new system any device which owns the capability of creating electronically readable textfiles regardless of the mode of its local operation can communicate with any others, and also with telex stations via converter. In this case the converted text may be shown to the originator. You know what your partner gets and the process of communication does not impair your local work.

The revival of the typewriter demonstrates how problems created by technical limitations of physical devices can be solved by optimizing software taking these limitations into account. The implication of teletex, with the function of an "interpreter" between not compatible machines, shows how to crack a non-versatile system (telex) into a controllable part, any typewriter or text originating system with desirable local functions, and a transparent communication network.

The entire system performs almost all additional work created by the properties of the system itself automatically according to the principle of "suitability for the task" in DIN 66 234 part 8.

The misery of interactive videotex (BTX)

The German version of interactive videotex (BTX) was believed "to change the entire (office) world" (Munter, 1983). Until now it failed to reach the target by 90 %, this means only 10 % of the predicted number of users have been attracted by this system. Ergonomic considerations may be among the reasons for this misery.

The target group during the planning of the system was non-commercial home users. They should be equipped with a general purpose communication system (text + graphics) using the home TVset and its keyboard as the human interface and the telephone line. The commercial partners should be able to use their computers for their input and updating.

Early on, it was apparent that the target group would be the commercial user. Unfortunately those do not want to use screens with 40 characters per line and 20 lines per frame. Regardless of the user's wishes, the TV screens do not comply with the German standards for visual display terminals which existed *before* interactive videotex started. The users also do not possess color printers for hardcopy.

The visual distance for the screens (recommended by the supplier) is 3 to 6 times screen diagonal (approx. 1,8 m to 3,6 m) whereas the visual distance in office environments is some 0,5 m.

Due to the limitations of throughput in the telephone network, transmission of one single page with a maximum of 960 character positions and with an average of 5OO characters lasts 6 to 12 seconds, hardly "task adequate". It is even too long for people who read slowly.

A microcomputer with color display (as monochrome is not accepted) is a minimum requirement for this system. Thus some companies use an ergonomic monochrome display to fit the needs of the user, and on the same desk a color display of poor quality to fit the technical system.

One day the BTX-system may serve as an excellent example for the disaster of a well planned interactive computer system, of which the planners have neglected the needs of the user at the very same point where the interaction takes place. In this case, the limitations by the physical devices are so rigid that it is unlikely to overcome them by software considerations. Unlike telex, BTX has to compete with many other systems, thus a failure seems to be likely if the system is not redesigned.

PERL or how to enhance hardware features by software

This last example demonstrates an intelligent software solution to the physical limitation of a screen. The designers of a CAD-workstation noticed that the user needs the resolution of a storage tube plus a color display which unfortunately lacks the high resolution. By using a color display the response of the system would be faster, the disturbing flashes of the storage tube while erasing would disappear and the improved contrast on the screen would be in favour of the user. They tried to combine the benefits of the storage screens with the benefits of a refresh color display. The result is PERL (perception enhanced resolution logic), a program that imitates a higher resolution display just for the human eye by manipulating the spatial luminance distribution of pixels or strokes on the screen.

A comparable but possibly less successful effort was made by another company to fit a software tool, which needs graphic presentation to systems which operate with formatted alpha-numeric screens and line printers (Kreplin et al.1983). In this case a variety of software functions (e.g. "logic zooming") have been created with the goal to achieve an acceptable presentation with no loss of relevant information.

In both cases the system designers perceived ergonomic requirements associated with the physical devices as important, however, existing devices did not comply with user's needs. Thus software solutions have been found, with more or less success to enhance the relevant characteristics of the equipment.

CONCLUSIONS

Human-machine-interaction and its ergonomic design is subject to severe limitations by the physical devices. The time scale for overcoming these is not predictable. A long time span from the availability of useful devices and their introduction in the workplace should be taken into consideration.

Therefore it can be recommended to define the design criteria *independently* from the state-of-the art technology and only limited by physical constraints like the impossibility of creating brown colors on active displays (CRT).

In a second step the requirements of the future tasks - as far as they are really predictable - should be defined, but also independently from current technology.

The third step should consider the limitations of the physical devices available and the best possible temporary solution for the software should be described in order to achieve a system behaviour which is regarded to be the best ergonomic solution to fit the system to the characteristics of the user. The awareness of the temporary limitations of devices may be helpful to overcome the problems by designing adequate programs or procedures.

The basic long-term goal of system design should be establishing and improving the control of the user in correspondence with higher order goals of the user, this means more "soft" features and less hardware. The technical infra-structure should not predict his or her goals.

REFERENCES

Bell, D. (1986). *The social sciences since the Second World War*, Frankfurt: Campus.

Cakir, A. (1986). Towards an ergonomic design of software. *Behaviour and Information Technology, 5*, 63 70.

Frese, M. (1985). *A theory of control: Implications for software design and training for computer aided work*. München: Department of Psychology, Univ. München.

Handelsblatt, 03.12.1986

IBM Deutschland (1978). *Englisch Deutsch. Fachausdrücke der Text- und Datenverarbeitung. Wörterbuch und Glossar*. Stuttgart: Ernst Klett.

Kreplin, K.-D., Schmidt, A., Wirtz, K.W. (1983). Erfahrungen beim Entwurf der Benutzerschnittstelle des mbp-tool-system. In: Balzert, H. (Ed.): *Software Ergonomie*, 240-253. Stuttgart: Teubner.

Munter, H. (1983). Bildschirmtext verändert die (Büro-)Welt. *Office Management 3/1983*, 80-82.

Ohmann, F. (Ed.). (1983). *Kommunikations-Endgeräte*, Berlin: Springer.

Quantum Sciences (1976). In: *BÜRO 1990*, Siemens, München.

Schnupp, P. (1982). Hochauflösende Rasterbildschirm-Systeme - eine neue Generation der Arbeitsplatz-Rechner. *Office Management 6/1982*, 614-617.

SEAS National Character Task Force. (1985). *White Paper on national character, language and keyboard problems*. SHARE European Association.

Spiker, A., Rogers, S.P. and Cicinelli, J. (1986). Selecting colour codes for a computer-generated topographic map, *Ergonomics 29*, 1313-1328.

Psychological Issues of
Human Computer Interaction in the Work Place
M. Frese, E. Ulich, W. Dzida (Editors)
Elsevier Science Publishers B.V. (North-Holland), 1987

USER ERRORS IN HUMAN-COMPUTER INTERACTION

Bert Arnold, Robert Roe

Department of Philosophy and Social Sciences, University of Technology
Delft, Kanaalweg 2b, 2628 EB Delft, The Netherlands

In this contribution it is observed that while user errors
are a highly important phenomenon in human-computer
interaction, little is available about their nature and
occurrence. It is argued that a systematic study of user
errors is required, based on general principles and
methods of error research. For this purpose a theoretical
framework and a scheme for the classification of errors
are presented, and some methods for the study of errors
are discussed. It is concluded, with reference to recent
research in human-computer interaction, that
standardized test environments for the analysis of errors
should be developed, and that error studies should be
carried out with regard to specific task domains, at
several stages of user learning and that techniques for
the prevention of errors and for improving error
handling should be developed.

INTRODUCTION

Within the domain of human-computer interaction there is growing
recognition of the importance of user errors (Henneman & Rouse, 1984;
Holt & Stevenson 1978; Norman, 1983; Rasmussen, 1984; Reason, 1985;
Rouse & Rouse, 1983). Examples of such errors are: typing errors, mistakes in creating and saving files, mode errors, or irreversible deletion
errors. The study of user errors is of interest for several reasons. First of
all, they affect the user's performance, effectiveness, efficiency, and cause
quality decline, while interaction time suffers. It has been shown (Davis,
1983; Magers, 1984), that system performance can drop drastically as a
result of user errors. In reported cases, which relate to a statistical analysis
task and an office task, 30 to 44% of the total interaction time was spent
on error recovery. Secondly, errors may have negative emotional and
motivational impacts on the user. Users tend to experience frustration and
anger when they are trapped in error-correction sequences. Futhermore,
the occurrence of errors will raise the user's work load, thereby demand-

ing an increasing mental and physical effort (Schönpflug, 1985). The study of errors is not only of importance because of such practical consequences. Instead, it is also of importance because of their underlying processes. E.g. errors may be seen as instances of inadequate man-machine interaction, that stem from a misfit between the user, the task, and the computer. And, more theoretically, they may be seen to offer important clues about cognitive structures and functions in human information processing in computer-aided work.

In order to know what types of errors users of computers tend to make, how frequently errors occur, which causes and conditions contribute to the occurrence of errors, how users react after having made errors, etc., a systematic inquiry into errors in human-computer interaction would be required. This would also help to find means for the prevention or at least reduction of errors and for the improvement of error handling. Although user errors have been studied on some scale, little systematic evidence is presently available about these matters. We are still far from a situation in which the aforementioned questions can be answered on the basis of a firm body of knowledge. Therefore, we have to resort to more general principles and methods of error research (Leplat, 1986; Norman, 1980, 1981; Rasmussen, 1982, 1983a, 1984; Reason, 1982, 1983, 1986; Rouse & Rouse, 1983), and consider their implications for the domain of human-computer interaction.

This defines the aim of this chapter. We will focus on the general questions of how errors in human-computer interaction can be studied, and how systems performance can be improved. We will start with the presentation of some basic concepts. Next we will present some relevant theories, a scheme for the classification of errors and a number of methods for the study of errors. Consequently we will consider possibilities of improving human-interaction by reducing errors and increasing error tolerance. Finally, we will briefly review recent research on errors in human-computer interaction, and draw some conclusions with regard to remaining research issues.

BASIC CONCEPTS

As Rasmussen (1982) has pointed out, it is very difficult to give a satisfactory definition of human errors. Basically, two positions can be taken, i.e. a technically-oriented and a user-oriented one. Technically-oriented definitions view an error as a violation of a specific rule and/or not meeting the normal system standard. According to user-oriented definitions one should speak of an error when a user's intention or goal is not attained and/or when a planned action or an action program is frustrated. Technically-oriented definitions have the advantage of being strictly operational. However, they preclude an analysis of errors in terms of underlying causes. On the other hand, user-oriented definitions are less sharply delineated, but they take antecedents and causes into account, making an in-depth analysis feasible.

It is clear that human error is a complex, multivariate phenomenon (Leplat, 1986; Norman, 1980). Rasmussen proposes (1982) to distinguishe between:
1. causes of human malfunction
2. mechanisms of human malfunction
3. internal human malfunction,
4. external malfunction.

Errors can be caused by a great variety of both internal and external factors. Examples of internal factors are limited perceptual capacities, or specific knowledge, or fatigue of the user. Environmental conditions, including climate, the presence of distracting stimuli, as well as interface characteristics (e.g. inconsistencies, lack of transparency) can be mentioned as examples of external factors. Factors like these, usually operating simultaneously, give rise to malfunction of cognitive and physical mechanisms, such as insufficient attention, inadequacies in discrimination of stimuli, faulty associations, etc. In turn these inadequacies lead to inappropriate action preparation and acting execution, thereby producing observable errors.

What types of errors are there? A common distinction is that between slips and mistakes (Reason, 1982, 1983). Slips are errors made by accident or lack of attention during the execution of very familiar actions. Well known examples are typing errors, errors in pushing function keys, etc. The notion of mistake, on the other hand, refers to failures occuring during action preparation, or the execution of problem solving tasks. Here, the person is fully aware of what he is doing, but he is erring in making bad predictions, drawing false conclusions, choosing wrong commands etc. A distinction frequently made in the area of human-computer interaction is that between semantic, syntactic and typing errors (Douglas & Moran, 1984). Several other, more refined distinctions can be made, depending on the theoretical framework adopted. This subject will be dealt with later on.

Errors are generally considered to be undesirable, and it seems evident that one should aim for their prevention. It should be noted, however, that errors may have great functionality for the user, especially during learning. When the user is able to find out what has caused the error and how to correct it, errors may be highly informative. This implies that one should not try to prevent all errors. Prevention should focus on frequently made errors and errors with serious consequences. Given the fact that errors can be useful, and that errors tend to be made with some frequency under almost any condition, systems should be made adaptive to errors. Rasmussen (1982) and Rouse (1985) advocate a general approach,

which combines error reduction with error tolerance, where error tolerance means observed and corrected for.

THEORETICAL FRAMEWORK

The literature provides two major approaches to the study of error
that correspond to the technical and user oriented definitions mentioned
before, i.e. the probabilistic and the causal approach (Rouse & Rouse,
1983). Within the probabilistic approach human error is analyzed in terms
of failure rates for particular types of tasks. Together with the failure
rates for hardware components an estimation of overall system reliability
can be made. An example of such an approach is the 'Sandia Laboratories
Method of Evaluating Human Reliability', called THERP (Swain et al.,
1975). This approach confines itself to directly observable empirical
events. It focuses on questions about the types of error that occur, error
frequencies etc. The causal approach takes the line that human errors are
seldom random and can be traced to causes and contributing conditions. It
is more theoretical by nature, raising questions about why an error has
occured, under what conditions, at what specific point in the interaction
sequence, etc. Here we will focus on this latter approach.

As the causes of human error are multivariate, several psychological
theories may be considered to be relevant for the study of error (Singleton, 1973). Under the assumption that human errors in the interaction
with computers are basically caused by a misfit between the user's mental
representation of the system and the actual properties of the system, one
would prefer theories that can throw light on the user's cognitive
structures and processes. Recognizing that making and correcting errors
can be considered as a form of human action, it would furthermore be
desirable to adopt a theory that can clarify the role that cognitive
mechanisms play in the production of the user actions. In other words, a
theoretical framework would be needed which describes human actions
and the underlying cognitive mechanisms in some detail. In our view such
a theoretical framework can be set up on the basis of action theory and
related cognitive theories (Hacker, 1978, 1985; Norman, 1981; Rasmussen,
1982, 1983b; Reason, 1982, 1984).

Action theory

The starting point of action theory lies in the axiom of the goal
orientation of human activity. The theory connects mentally represented
goals or intentions to observable human activities. It focuses on mental
processes, including goal setting and execution. Below we will summarize
action theory as formulated by Hacker (1978; 1985) and Rasmussen (1982,
1983b).

Hacker discrimates between acts, actions and operations. Acts are motivated and regulated by intentions, or higher-order goals, and are realized through actions. Actions are the smallest independent units of cognitive and sensory-motor processes, that are oriented towards conscious goals. Operations are action components, they do not have independent goals as counterparts. Actions and their constituent parts are mentally represented by action programs' (cf schemata). These programs are organized in a hierarchical-sequential fashion. Intentions and goals occupy a crucial position in the action programs. They serve to initiate and regulate action execution.

For the translation of an intention into an actual action, an action program has to be formed. This pre-execution phase is called 'action preparation'. The following steps in the preparation of an action program can be distinguished:

1. Goal setting
First, an objective goal (task) is translated into a subjective goal (task).

2. Orientation
In the next phase orientation takes place to conditions within the environment, such as the availability of information, tools, persons etc. and to personal conditions, such as knowledge, skills, capabilities etc.

3. Design of an action program
On the basis of an analysis of the goal and relevant conditions, variants of action programs are designed. Or an earlier designed program is reproduced.

4. Choice of a variant
Within given degrees of freedom, an action program is chosen from the available variants. Or an existing action program is actualized.

After completing these steps the action program, a mental representation of future action, is ready for execution. This execution can be described as follows:

- The action program is executed in a stepwise manner.
- During execution, feedback is obtained in order to guide and control the actions. At the highest level of the action hierarchy the (sub)results are compared with the anticipated results (goals or intentions) and the next steps are anticipated. When familiar actions are executed, there is no constant feedback to the top level of the hierarchy. The control is taken over by the specialized functional units responsible for the execution of the operations. The anticipated operation flow and the result are represented in these units. When a unit is triggered the operation cannot be stopped.
- Depending on the amount of practice, there is a tendency to execute more frequently at the lower levels of the hierarchy. In this way, new action steps can be anticipated and prepared at the higher levels during execution of an automized action (parallel processing).

Actions can be initiated and controled by various regulation mechanisms. Three levels of regulation (cf. information processing) can be distinguished. Rasmussen (1983a, 1983b) speaks of:
- knowledge-based regulation, (intellectual)
- rule-based regulation, (perceptual-conceptual)
- skill-based regulation, (sensory-motor).
These types of regulation will be clarified below.

A model of action regulation

Rasmussen (1982) has worked out a model of action regulation which is highly congruent with Hacker's theory, and shows in detail what information processes are involved at each of the three levels of regulation. The model distinguishes 5 'mental functions' that are required in any type of action regulation:
- observation
- identification
- interpretation
- task definition
- procedure formation
The model is presented in Figure 1.

The highest, knowledge-based level in the model is concerned with programming or redesigning action programs. The stimuli coming in from the perceptive system have a semantic value, or a conscious meaning. This level of regulation is characterized by problem-solving types of processes. After a diagnosis (identification) of the environmental conditions has been made, several solution strategies are developed on the basis of hypotheses about the creation of desired future results (interpretation). These strategies are mentally evaluated or tested, and the most optimal strategy is chosen (task definition). Next, this strategy is translated into new or (changed) existing procedures (procedure formation). The actual execution of these procedures takes place by delegation to the lower levels of regulation. Another function of this knowledge-based level is the guidance (anticipation and supervision) of actions. Only at points in the action program flow where conscious orientation is needed and under changed external and internal conditions, are results fed back to this level. Experienced persons will be switching back to this level less frequently than unexperienced persons.

The second, rule-based level actions are controlled by earlier stored rules or procedures. The incoming stimuli (observation), learned to be organized in 'signs' (cf. traffic signs), with some specific meaning, can trigger very complex actions. The signs are classified (identification), and a choice of a suitable procedure (task definition) is made. On the basis of this choice a procedure is recalled from memory (procedure formation), and after a check against the conditions stored in memory, is executed by delegation to the skill-based level. Feedback only takes place when the next procedure in the execution of the action program has to be started. At this level, control is theological in the sense that the rule is selected from previous successful experience (Rasmussen, 1983b).

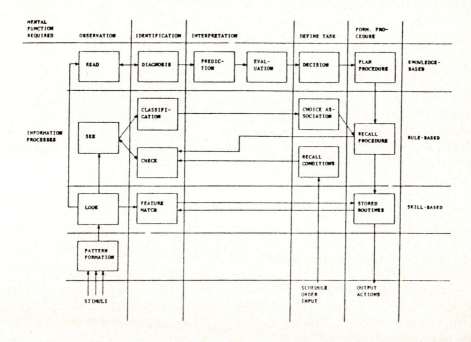

Figure 1: Model of action regulation
Adapted from Rasmussen (1982)

The third, or skill-based level is the one at which the actual execution of actions takes place. Stored operation routines are used for this purpose. These routines have a dynamic, active and specialized character. They are formed on the basis of experiences in similar situations. The operation routines are externally initiated and triggered by cues in the environment that are not consciously perceived 'signals'. After a process of pattern formation, the signals are matched with the sensory-motor representations. When a signal fits a related stored routine, this routine is triggered (procedure formation). When no fit is possible, the higher levels of regulation are activated. At this level there are at least two feedback mechanisms eg.:
- feedback after the operations have been completed (visual)
- feedback of the musculature (kinaesthetic)

However, these feedback mechanisms are too slow for very swift operations (Willems, 1981). Empirical data support the assumption that cognitive
processes play an important role in motor learning and control (Stelmach
& Szendrovits, 1981). Thus, the result of an operation must be represented
cognitively.

Additional theory

The action theory model seems very useful for the study of errors in
human-computer interaction, as it enables an in-depth analysis of
perceptual and cognitive processes lying behind errors as observational
phenomena. Specifically, it makes it possible to discriminate between
various error types related to inadequacies in human information processing at the stages of action preparation and execution. Of course, there
are other relevant theories like Reason's cognitive theory (Reason, 1982,
1983, 1984, 1985). Reason's theory stresses the dynamic aspects of
cognitive functioning. For example extensive consideration is given to the
so-called intention system, which is thought to play a role in the:
* assembly of plans
* monitoring and guidance of ongoing actions
* dealing with changes in circumstances
* detection and recovery of errors
Furthermore, it expands upon the properties of the 'attention system' and
its role in activating schemata. Taking account of the hierarchical organization of schemata, Reason's theory is able to explain the appearance of
various routine level errors.

ERROR CLASSIFICATION SCHEME

On the basis of the foregoing account of action theory, and other
relevant theories, a classification scheme has been set up. Rasmussen's
'model of action regulation' (see Figure 2) has been taken as a framework
for this scheme. The presented model slightly deviates from the original
one, i.e. the block 'pattern formation' has been added. Strictly speaking,
'pattern formation' does not belong to the skill-based level and is more of
a physiological nature. However, inadequacies in 'pattern formation' may
be important error sources. This classification scheme is clearly a be-
havorial-oriented scheme. It contrasts with task- and system-oriented
schemes (Rouse, 1983). The classification criteria within this scheme are
formed by the 'regulation levels' and 'required mental functions'. The cells
within the scheme relate to the blocks of the 'model of action regulation'.
These cells have been filled with information processing inadequacies from
various sources (Hacker, 1978; Rasmussen, 1982; Reason, 1982, 1983;
Rouse and Rouse, 1983).

Required mental functions	Levels of regulation		
	Skill-based	Rule-based	Knowledge-based
Observation	inadequate pattern formation: - stimuli not perceived - misperception looking errors: - patterns overlooked - inadequate looking	observation errors: - information not seen - information skipped - inadequate information reduction - patterns not recognized - insufficient information observed - inappropriate information observed	reading errors: - no reading by lack of information - inadequate reading - incorrect reading
Identification	feature match errors: - false match - false mismatch	checking errors: - inadequate check against conditions - no check classification errors: - stereotype error - stereotype fixation - classification criteria not recalled	diagnosis errors: - misinterpretation of correctly read data - no interpretation

Interpretation			prediction errors:
			- goal errors
			  • insufficient specification
			  • counter productive
			  • non-production
			  • goal not chosen
			- incorrect hypotheses
			  • inconsistent
			  • unlikely
			  • too expensive
			  • functionally irrelevant
			  • side-effects and conditions not considered
			
			evaluation errors:
			- erroneous hypotheses
			  • stopped before reaching a conclusion
			  • wrong conclusion
			  • not considered and tested
			  • false acceptance
			  • false rejection

Task definition		choice errors: - stereotype take over condition recall errors: - conditions not recalled - inadequate recall	decision errors: - choice would not attain goal - choice would attain incorrect goal - choice unnecessary for goal

Procedure formation/ execution	routine errors:
	- routine not available
	- inadequate routines triggered
	
	execution errors:
	- spatial misorientation:
	  • stumbling
	  • misgrasping
	  • spilling
	- motoric variability errors
	- slips:
	  • slip of the tongue
	  • slip of the pen
		recall errors:
		- forgotten isolated action
		- inadequate alternative procedure chosen
		
		procedure formation errors:
		- action-sequence(s) exchanged
		- required step skipped
		- unnecessary step inserted
			planning errors:
			- computation error

Figure 2: Error classification scheme

Within the context of human-computer interaction, these inadequacies can generally be seen as misfits between the user's mental representations of the system and the actual system features. The following types of misfit can be distinguished:
- given that the user's mental goal is adequate, a wrong software tool is used for goal realisation
- the appropriate software tool is chosen, but the strategy formed by the user is inappropriate
- an adequate strategy is chosen, but the translation into a procedure or an action program is inappropriate
- the created procedure is appropriate, but the execution is inadequate; the independent operations are in themselves correct, but there are flaws in the procedure as a whole.
- the operation of an independent operation is inadequate

The features of the human interface may play an important role in the generation of misfits. When vital information about the system is withheld from a user, errors are likely to occur. What kind of information is needed at certain points in the human-computer interaction, may be deduced from the errors actually made: loading file errors, file manipulation errors, mode errors, command errors, menu-choice errors, typing errors etc. A gross classification of these errors into slips (skill-based) or mistakes (knowledge-based) may be possible right away. However, for a more refined classification along the lines of the presented scheme, additional information is needed about the user's intentions, his action programs, his system knowledge, experience etc.

METHODS FOR THE STUDY OF ERRORS

The complex nature of human error has its consequences for the methods to be used in error analysis. Like in the analysis of human action in general (Zijlstra & Roe, 1987), one has to follow a strategic approach in which a combination of methods is chosen, taking account of the specific tasks, work setting, equipment, etc. We will only briefly indicate methods for observing and recording errors, and make a few remarks on research design issues.

There are several methods for observing and recording errors in human-computer interaction. These methods fall into two categories, i.e. objective and subjective methods. The distinction between the objective and subjective methods is based on the role of human judgement during the observation and recording of errors. Objective methods include:

- performance recording by usual means: stored lists, files, orders, messages, etc. (Hayes & Szekely, 1983),
- monitoring of the complete dialogue (Henneman & Rouse, 1984; Kraut et al., 1984; Neal & Simons, 1984), or the input part of it, by means of a computer log,
- video recording of the user's behavior during interaction (Gould, 1981),
- combined monitoring and video recording (Davis, 1983; Pinsky, 1983).
Subjective methods include:
- taking down a protocol of user verbalizations during the interaction (McCoy et al., 1984),
- stimulated recall interviewing (Davis, 1983),
- the use of questionnaires in problem areas and user satisfaction (Root & Draper, 1984).

It will be clear, in the light of the theory presented before, that both types of methods have their limitations. The objective methods can only record errors in terms of violations of specific system rules. They fail to indicate errors in terms of not reaching user goals or frustration during action execution. Furthermore, proper error diagnosis (identification and classification) solely on the basis of objective methods may not be possible; additional information is needed about the user's cognitive processes at the time of the error. The subjective data are better suited for these purposes, but they depend on the user's judgement. In this respect these data may be less precise and reliable. A specific problem with verbalization methods is that they affect the regulation level, forcing the user to execute his activities at a conscious level. This precludes an analysis of errors in terms of regulation levels. A fruitful approach seems to lie in a combination of objective and subjective methods. Interviewing the user on the basis of his interaction history, taken down by a log and video images, may provide good results.

Recording interaction data is of course only one step in the process of analyzing errors. The data should be interpreted in terms of error types, and antecedent conditions (causes, malfunctions, etc.) by using an adequate classification scheme and related theory. The classification scheme pre-sented above seems to satisfy this purpose.

It should be noted that the validity of the outcomes of error analysis depends on the conditions under which the study is performed. Here the distinction between field and laboratory research is relevant. From the point of view of action theory, actions should be studied under realistic conditions with regard to complexity of tasks, social and time pressures, interruptions, etc. However, this may lead to insufficient control of independent variables. Laboratory experiments offer far better opportunities for control, but they tend to suffer from lack of relevance. Again, a combination of both approaches seems preferable.

IMPROVING THE HUMAN-COMPUTER INTERFACE

The aims of reducing errors and increasing error tolerance can be accomplished by five basic measures i.e. 1) user or system selection, 2) user training, 3) system (re)design, 4) job (re)design and 5) aiding (Rouse, 1985). First, a better fit between the characteristics of the user and the system can be established by selection measures. Second, adaptation of the user to the system can be accomplished by training courses. Third, adaptation of the system to the user can be achieved by (re)design measures. Fourth, as conditions such as task content and structure, social climate etc. may play an important role in bringing about errors, job (re)design may be required. Fifth, the user needs to know how to achieve his goals. In other words, the user needs some support. The necessary support can come from various sources among which are system aiding facilities. The choice of a particular mix of measures in specific circumstances should largely depend upon knowledge about error frequencies and causes.

Here, we will focus on the option of system (re)design. Three issues are of special importance: prevention, error messages and error recovery. What can be said about these aspects on the basis of the proposed classification scheme?

Error prevention may be accomplished by supporting human action preparation and execution. For instance, during goal setting and strategy formation a user needs to know what to expect from the system in terms of end results. Further, knowledge is needed about the relations to other tasks in the user-task domain. For procedure formation a user must be informed about the structure and the syntactic rules of the system. Within the procedure execution phase, it is important for the user to keep track of the action flow. At this point, supervisory control information (feedback of past steps, actual status and anticipation) must be available. During operation execution the user must have detailed information about how to perform the operation and about the effect of the operation.

Since errors will always be made, attention should be given to error messages. Research in this field has revealed that designers' conceptions of error messages tend to be rather narrow (Isa et al., 1984). Quite often error messages do not offer the user information about action alternatives. In terms of the presented theory an error message should not only give the user information about the cause of an error, but also about how to continue in order to fulfil his action program. In this vein, the error must be interpreted and classified by the system, taking notice of the user's experience level. For instance, when an inexperienced user makes an error as a result of inadequate goal setting or strategy formation, information about the possibilities and limitation of the system should be given. When an error appears to be caused by inappropriate procedure formation, information about an alternative procedure should be given. And for the inexperienced user additional information should be given about how to execute this alternative, in terms of syntactic rules. An error apparently caused by inadequate procedure execution can be solved by supplying information about the actual position within the ongoing procedure, and about past and future steps. Detailed information about commands and syntactic rules are needed in the case of operation errors made by inexperienced users. In contrast, experienced users do not need this extensive information; a system sign that an error has occurred is sufficient here.

On the basis of the above, something can be said about error correction or recovery, too. First, it is very important that a user can return to previous steps within his action program. In other words, a system must allow reversibility of operations. Further, it is inconvenient for the user to be confronted with an error message during the phase of action preparation (goal setting, strategy formation and procedure formation). At that moment, an error message may block the train of thought. In this instance, error messages should be postponed until the action preparation is finished. The same is true for action execution. It should generally be tried to postpone error recovery to breaks in between independent operations or actions.

ERRORS IN RECENT LITERATURE

Within the field of human-computer interaction systematic research errors are scarce. First of all, errors are seldom studied per se. In as far as they are, they relate to classification of errors for specific task areas, rather than to underlying factors and processes (e.g. Hull & Brown, 1975; Galambos, 1984; Douglas & Moran, 1984; Pinsky, 1983; Gomez & Lochbaum, 1985). The study by Galambos may be taken as an example. According to Galambos an important part of communication is being able to point to an object (ostension) and this is an important error source within man-computer interaction. On the basis of observation of subjects' text-editing behavior a number of ostension errors are distinguished: 'the typewriter addiction error', 'the one-place off error', 'the missing the target error', 'the invisible trap', 'the no-man's land error'. Design implications were not offered in this study.

The majority of studies deals with errors as measures of performance. Errors are defined operationally, in terms of error rates, and employed as criteria for evaluating and improving user interfaces (Nawrocki et al., 1973; Ehrenreich & Porcu, 1982; Borenstein, 1985; Kraut, 1984; Leon, 1984; Ray, 1985; Villeges et al., 1985). A good example of this approach is offered by Kraut (1984). The aim of his study was the examination of command use in a UNIX software environment. In a field situation, 11,000 commands were monitored and command frequencies and command error rates were computed. No subjective measures were collected. On the basis of these data, some recommendations for improvement were made: 1) provide functional command organization, 2) provide relevant orienting information and feedback.

The empirical nature of the two cited evaluation studies is symptomatic of research on errors in man-computer interaction in general. In-depth analysis of errors in terms of errors or of contributing conditions and their psychological mechanisms are lacking in most studies. Consequently, generalization of results becomes problematic. Quite often design implications can only be drawn for the particular software package under study.

A more fruitful approach is offered by the work of Card, Moran and Newell (1983). They have developed a model (GOMS) which enables a formal description of the user's knowledge and operations, in terms of the following components: goals, operations, methods and selection rules. This type of model, which is related to the action theoretic framework, has been applied for evaluation purposes (Polson et al., 1985; Robertson, 1984). In our view it could be used for studying errors as well.

CONCLUSIONS

It appears that little systematic research effort has been spent on errors in human-computer interaction so far. In addition, most studies of error have treated errors as strictly operational criteria for evaluating users' performance. Thus a technical rather than a user oriented definition of errors has been applied. There are hardly any studies that offer an in-depth analysis of errors and underlying processes, as advocated by Rasmussen (1982).

Nevertheless the study of errors is of great theoretical and practical importance. It could offer insight into the regulation of interactive behavior, and supply a firm basis for the improvement of user interfaces, work procedures and aids, user training, etc. What would be required, in our view, is first of all the development of test environments for the study of errors. These should include standardized techniques and instruments for observing and recording errors, assessing users experiences, categorizing errors and antecedent conditions, etc. With the help of these test environments error studies should be undertaken in various task domains, aiming at a systematic description of errors (types, frequencies, causes, etc.). In addition, research should be done to find adequate measures for preventing and reducing errors, and for improving error handling, finally resulting in the formulation of design criteria, guidelines, and specifications.

REFERENCES

Borenstein, N.S.(1985). The evaluation of text-editors: a critical review of the Roberts and Moran methodology based on new experiments. In L. Borman & B. Curtis (Eds.), *Human factors in computing systems-II* (pp. 99-105). Amsterdam: North Holland.

Card, S.K., Moran, T.P. & Newell, A.(1983). *The psychology of human-computer interaction.* Hillsdale: Erlbaum.

Davis, R.(1983). User error or computer error? Observation on a statistical package. *International Journal of Man-Machine Studies, 19,* 359-376.

Douglas, S.A. & Moran, T.P.(1984). Learning text editor semantics by analogy. In A. Janda (Ed.), *Human factors in computing systems* (pp. 207-211). Amsterdam: North Holland.

Ehrenreich, S.L. & Porcu, T.A.(1982). Abbrevations for automated systems: teaching operators the rules. In A. Badre (Ed.), *Directions in human/computer ineractions* (pp. 111-135). Norwood, New Jersey: Ablex Publishing cooperation.

Galambos, J.A., Wikler, E.S., Black, J.B. & Sebrechts, M.M.(1984). How you tell your computer what you mean:ostension in interactive system. In A. Janda (Ed.), *Human factors in computing systems* (pp. 182-185). Amsterdam: North Holland.

Gomez, L.M. & Lochbaum, C.C.(1985). People can retrieve more objects with enriched key word vocabularies. But is there a human performance cost? In B. Shackel (Ed.), *Human-computer interaction* (pp. 257-261). Amsterdam: Elsevier Science Publishers b.v. (North-Holland).

Gould, J.D.(1981). Composing letters with computer-based text editors. *Human factors, 23 (5),* 593- 606.

Hacker, W.(1978). *Allgemeine Arbeits- und Ingenieurpsychologie, Psychische Struktur und Regulation von Arbeitstätigkeiten.* Bern: Verlag Hans Huber.

Hacker, W.(1985). Activity: a fruitful concept in industrial psychology. In M. Frese & J. Sabini (Eds.), *Goal directed behavior: the concept of action psychology* (pp. 262-283). Hillsdale, New Jersey: Lawrence Erlbaum Associates.

Hayes, P.J. & Szekely, P.A.(1983). Graceful interaction through the COUSIN command interface. *International Journal of Man-machine Studies, 19,* 285-306.

Henneman, R.L., & Rouse, W.B.(1984). Human performance in monitoring and controling hierarchical large-scale systems. *IEEE Transactions in systems, man and cybernetics,* vol. smc-14, no.2, 184-191.

Holt, H.O. & Stevenson, F.L.(1978). Human performance considerations in complex systems. *Journal of System Management ,* October.

Hull, A.J. & Brown(1975). Reduction of copying errors with selected alphanumeric subsets, *Journal of Applied Psychology, vol. 60*, no. 2, 231-237.

Isa, B.S., Boyle, J.M., Neal, A.S. & Simons, R.M.(1984). A methodology for objectively evaluating error messages. In A. Janda (Ed.), *Human factors in computing systems* (pp. 68-71). Amsterdam: North Holland.

Kaczmarek, T., Mark, W. & Sondheimer (1984). An integrated interactive environment. In A. Janda (Ed.), *Human factors in computing systems* (pp. 98-102). Amsterdam: North Holland.

Kraut, R.E., Hanson, S.J. & Farber, J.M.(1984). Command use and interface design. In A. Janda (Ed.), *Human factors in computing system* (pp. 120-124). Amsterdam: North Holland.

Leplat, J.(1986). *Human error in new technologies: methods of analysis.* Presentation held on symposium 'Optimierung geistiger Arbeitstätigkeiten, Dresden.

Leon, L. de, Harris, W.G. & Evens, M.(1984). Is there really trouble with UNIX? In A. Janda (Ed.), *Human factors in computing systems* (pp. 125-129). Amsterdam: North Holland.

Magers, C.S.(1984). An experimental evaluation of On-line HELP for non-progammers. In A. Janda (Ed.), *Human factors in computing systems* (pp. 277-281). Amsterdam: North-Holland.

McCoy, K.F.(1984). Correcting misconceptions: what to say when the user is mistaken. In A. Janda (Ed.), *Human factors in computing systems* (pp. 197-201). Amsterdam: North-Holland.

Nawrocki, L.H., Strub, M.H. & Cecil, R.M.(1973). Error categorization and analysis in man-computer communication systems, *IEEE Transaction on Reliability*, vol R-22, no. 3, 135-140.

Neal, A.S. & Simons, R.M.(1984). Playback: a method for evaluating the usability of software and its documentation. In A. Janda (Ed.), *Human factors in computing systems* (pp. 78-82). Amsterdam: North-Holland.

Norman, D.A.(1980). *Errors in human performance.* San Diego: University of California, report no.8004.

Norman, D.A.(1981). Categorization of action slips. *Psychological Review, volume 88*, number 1, January.

Norman, D.A.(1983). Design rules based on analysis of human error. *Communications of the AMC, volume 26*, 254-258.

Pinsky, L.(1983). What kind of 'dialogue' is it when working with a computer. In T.R.G. Green, S.J. Payne & G.C. van der Veer (Eds.), *The psychology of computer use* (pp. 29-40). London: Academic Press.

Polson, P.G., Kieras, D.E.(1985). A quantitative model of the learning and performance of text editing knowledge. In L. Borman & B. Curtis (Eds.), *Human factors in computing systems-II* (pp. 207-212). Amsterdam: North Holland.

Rasmussen, J.(1982). Human errors. A taxonomy for describing human malfunction in industrial installations. *Jounal of Occupational Accidents*, 4 , 311-333.

Rasmussen, J.(1983a). *Human errors in process control*. Italy, Bellagio: Position paper for NATO Workshop on the origin of human error.

Rasmussen, J.(1983b). Skills, rules, and knowledge, signals, signs, and symbols, and other distinctions in human performance models. *IEEE Transaction on systems, man, and cybernetics*, vol. smc-13.

Rasmussen, J.(1984). *New technology and the effects of human errors*. Bad Homburg: workshop.

Ray, H.N.(1985). A study of the effect of different data models on casual user performance in writing databases queries. *International Journal of Man-Machine Studies, 23*, 249-262.

Reason, J.(1982). *Slips, lapses, blases and blunders*. Liverpool: British Association.

Reason, J.(1983). *On the nature of mistakes. Manchester*: University of Manchester, Department of Psychology, internal report.

Reason, J.(1984). Absent-mindedness and cognitive control. In J. Harris & P. Morris (Eds.), *Everyday memory, actions and absentmindedness* (pp. 113-132). London: Academic Press.

Reason, J.(1985). *Recurrent error forms in nuclear power plants and their implications for the design and deployment of intelligent decision aids*. Pisa, Miniato: NATO Advanced Study Institute.

Reason, J.(1986). A framework for classifying errors. In J. Rasmussen, J. Leplat & F.K. Duncun (Eds.), *New technology and human error*. John Wiley.

Robertson, S.P. & Black, J.B.(1984). Planning units in text editing behavior. In A. Janda (Ed.), *Human factors in computing systems* (pp.217-221). Amsterdam: North-Holland.

Root, R.W. & Draper, S.(1984). Questionnaires as a software evaluation tool. In A. Janda (Ed.), *Human factors in computing systems* (pp.83-87). Amsterdam: North-Holland.

Rosson, M.B.(1984). Patterns of experience in text editing. In A. Janda (Ed.), *Human factors in computing systems* (pp.171-175). Amsterdam: North-Holland.

Rouse, W.B. & Rouse, S.H.(1983). Analysis and classification of human error. *IEEE Transaction on system, man, and cybernetics*, vol. smc-13, no.4, 539-549.

Rouse, W.(1985). Optimal allocation of system development resources to reduce and/or tolerate human error. *IEEE transactions on system, man and cybernetics*, vol. smc-15, no.5, September/Octobertem.

Schönpflug, W.(1985). Goal directed behavior as a source of stress: psychological origins and consequences of inefficiency. In M. Frese & J. Sabini (Eds.), *Goal directed behavior: the concept of action psychology* (pp. 172-188). Hillsdale, New Jersey: Lawrence Erlbaum Associates.

Singleton, W.T.(1973). Theoretical approaches to human error. *Ergonomics, vol. 16*, no.6, 727-737.

Stelmach, G.E. & Szendrovits, L.D.(1981). Error detection and correction in a structured movement task. *Journal of Motor Behavior*, vol. 13, no.3, 132-143.

Swain, A.D. & Guttman(1975). Human reliability analysis applied to nuclear power. *Proceedings 1975 annual reliability and maintainability symposium.*

Villeges, R.C., Elkerton, J., Pittman, A.J. & Cohill, A.M.(1985). Providing online assistance to inexperienced computer users. In: B. Shackel (Ed.), *Human-computer interaction* (pp. 765-769). Amsterdam: Elsevier Science Publishers b.v. (North-Holland).

Willems, P.J.(1981). *Inleiding in de psychologie van menselijke verrichtingen*. Holland, Deventer: Van Loghum Slaterus.

Zijlstra, F.R.H. & Roe, R.A.(1987). Arbeidsanalyse ten behoeve van (her)ontwerp van functies: een handelingstheoretische invalshoek. In J.A. Algera (Ed.), *Analyse van arbeid*. Lisse: Swets & Zeitlinger.

Psychological Issues of
Human Computer Interaction in the Work Place
M. Frese, E. Ulich, W. Dzida (Editors)
© Elsevier Science Publishers B.V. (North-Holland), 1987

OPTIMIZING INPUT DEVICES OF COMPUTER AIDED DESIGN SYSTEMS

Ekkehart Frieling, Jürgen Pfitzmann, Foad Derisavi-Fard

Dept. of Ergonomics, Gesamthochschule Kassel, Heinrich-Plett-Str. 40,
3500 Kassel. Federal Republic of Germany

The following article shows how menu tablet devices (MTD) can be improved considerably by modifying the arrangement of functions. As manufacturers of CAD-systems generally do not attach great importance to the design of menu tablet devices, the communication between user and system often causes problems. The aims of our project were to develop an MTD that should be structured systematically and designed in such a way as to meet the requirements of psychological graphic design. Thus, both the training phase and the subsequent use of the system should be simplified. The results of our study show the importance of an improved MTD-design. An appropriate selection and grouping of functions as well as a standardization of symbols improve the user's communication with the system. It also helps to remember the functions and their appropriate symbols.

INTRODUCTION

In Computer Aided Design (CAD), different kinds of connections between system and user exist, such as menu tablets, dials, mouse, roll-balls, keyboards, electric pens, light pens, joysticks, etc.

Different data input devices can be connected with different CAD-systems. As far as we know, no studies have been made on how the combination of input devices and CAD-systems can be optimized from the ergonomical point of view (Encarnacao, Straßer, 1986).

The lack of homogeneous set of input devices is due to the fact that every manufacturer uses different input devices in connection with specific software systems. As long as it will not be possible to standardize input devices so that they may be combined with different kinds of hardware and software systems for CAD, an ergonomically oriented research is unlikely to be successful.

Today, considerable differences exist in the evaluation of screen display menus (for example IBM/CATIA) and tablet menus (for example Control Data/CD 2000 or Contraves/Concad 2). People preferring for example the IBM-system believe that the fact of changing the field of vision too often causes stress for the system-user. We do not agree with this argument as it is also necessary to change the field of vision from time to time while using screen display menus. The fact that the user of a tablet menu system has to look at his keyboard, the dials and the mouse at the same time cannot be considered a disadvantage from our point of view. In addition to physiological aspects, one has to take into consideration that frequent changes of the field of vision trains the eye muscles which prevents them from being overstrained after a short time (Krüger & Müller-Limmroth, 1979, p.17).

But we do not want to continue the debate about advantages and drawbacks of screen display menus. On the other hand, we think it to be justified to go into detail as far as the design of menu tablets is concerned. Thus, an analysis of existing menu tablets was carried out. As a result of this, a series of design guidelines have been worked out that will be presented here with the aim of giving some advice as to how existing MTDs (Menu Tablet Devices) could be optimized in the future by improving working conditions.

The following points support the introduction of menu tablets as an input device:
- a survey of all the functions is offered on the MTD; though, the number of functions should be not too big;
- the individual functions can be grouped according to their different kinds of application;
- menu tablets are always present; thus, the learning process of functions connected with symbols is facilitated;
- after a period of time, the user has less difficulties in getting used to the system again as the functions/symbols only have to be remembered and not to be reproduced actively.

After having made some general statements about existing MTDs, we will now discuss the possibilities of modifying and redesigning menu tablet devices.

System "CD-2000" by Control Data is used as an example to show the limits of inflexible CAD-Systems. "Concad 2" by Contraves demonstrates the problems of redesigning.

The modification of the "CD-2000" MTD was sponsored by the BMW-group in connection with a feasibility study about work structuring in the research and development department (granted by the Federal Department of Research and Technology).

The evaluation and redesigning of the MTD (from Contraves Concad 2) was sponsored by the manufacturer himself.

DESCRIPTION OF EXISTING MENU TABLET DEVICES-PROBLEMS

Contrary to conventional designing processes where the designer uses separate instruments, the CAD-designer uses an instrument with several hundred functions and commands.

The commands used for producing lines, circles and other graphic elements are represented by different functions or function groups depending on the given circumstances. Now, the designer's task consists in the identification of the different functions or function groups.

A systematically designed MTD that corresponds to the requirements of perceptional psychology supports the user during his training phase on a new CAD-system and in his later work with it. The menu tablets vary according to their field of application and from manufacturer to manufacturer.

Differences exist in the description and representation of functions, in colour coding and in the size of the room available for symbols.

Generally, the description of functions and their representation can be divided into four categories:

Verbal Function Listing

Every function is described with a word or an abbreviation that can either be German or English. Generally, different abreviations are used for the same functions, depending on the manufacturer.

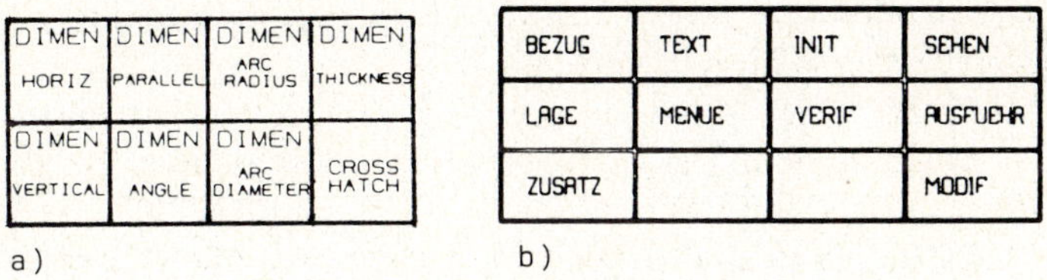

DIMEN HORIZ	DIMEN PARALLEL	DIMEN ARC RADIUS	DIMEN THICKNESS
DIMEN VERTICAL	DIMEN ANGLE	DIMEN ARC DIAMETER	CROSS HATCH

a)

BEZUG	TEXT	INIT	SEHEN
LAGE	MENUE	VERIF	AUSFUEHR
ZUSATZ			MODIF

b)

Fig. 1: Example for same function groups dimension menu,
a) system Anvil 4000
b) system Matra Datavision

CAD-users who do not speak English have considerable difficulties in understanding the meaning of the abbreviations that sometimes seem to be illogical.

Due to the considerable amount of functions as well as to the smallness of the different areas on the MTD, the user has problems in reading or finding functions on the menu tablet especially when the functions are only partly grouped into functional categories so that users need a lot of training to find the functions they are looking for (Wessells, 1984).

During the training phase, the user often is unable to connect certain verbal descriptions with the appropriate functions, a fact that is mainly due to the abstractness of descriptions.

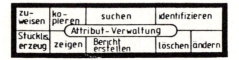

Fig. 2: Attribute-menu, system CD 2000, Control Data

Symbolically Coded Functions

Most of the functions are represented by graphic symbols. There are only few MTDs that prefer graphic symbols without any verbal descriptions. These MTDs are often used for specific purposes, as for example fig. 3.

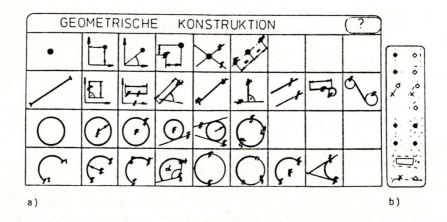

a)   b)

Fig. 3: a) Section of geometric construction-menu, system Concad 2,
*   Contraves*
*   b) Line menu, Medusa, AGS*

The symbols used here refer only partly to standardized symbols as used for technical drawings. In case that the graphic symbols are too small or cannot be grouped into categories, similar problems appear as described under verbal function listing.

As far as the graphic design of symbols is concerned, it is not always clear what kind of elements needed for the execution of functions are present respectively have to be generated.

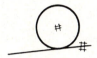

Fig. 4: Graphics

In our example, it is not clear whether a circle is to be drawn near to a tangent or vice versa.

Verbal Descriptions and symbolically coded functions

In general, the following combinations are used:

Symbolically coded functions are used together with verbally coded functions and/or functions are coded symbolically as well as verbally.

The combination of symbols and verbal descriptions facilitates the finding of functions in case they are clearly arranged. The more abstract certain functions are as for example "attributes" or functions such as "fading in" or "fading out", the more difficult they are to be represented graphically.

Thus, functions that are relatively clear should be represented by symbols.

Ambiguous functions should be completed by verbal abreviations whereas abstract functions should only be described verbally.

As far as existing MTDs are concerned, there are only first signs of adequate systematics.

Colour Coding

With many MTDs, similar functions as for example creation of lines, points and circles are represented in connection with colours, which, it has to be said, are used unsystematically for the grouping of functions. Thus, the colour red is used for critical functions such as "delete" as well as for functions that are not problematical, for example "creating point/line". The use of saturated colours reduces the legibility of functions so that the

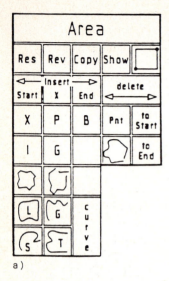

a)

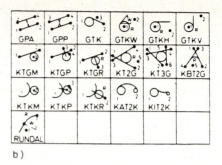

b)

Fig. 5: a) Face-element-menu, system Digital AV-DQ 70 A-TH
b) Part of line-menu, system Procad 2D

complex process of understanding and perception is complicated with certain MTDs, for example by using black letters on a red background.

Problems in Handling the MTD

Based on studies of working conditions, interviews and our own experience in working with CAD-systems, especially system CD 2000, the following drawbacks have been discovered:
- size of the room available on the MT; available menu areas on MTs are sometimes too small (less than 1 cm^2) so that verbal descriptions of functions are hardly recognizeable;
- difficulties in fixing sub-menus; in order to fix sub-menus to the menu tablet, adhesive tape is needed. This is caused by considerable tolerances in production of digitizer tablets. Submenus must be held with the left hand;
- damage of the MT-surface; as considerable pressure is required to touch the MT with the light pen, the surface gets damaged after a short time due to frequent usage;
- kind of printing used; words that are written vertically or in capital letters are difficult to read. As most of the functions are represented by words, their selection tend to be difficult.

Suggestions for Modification (CD 2000)

This is due to the fact that manufacturers do not seem to be interested in modifying their systems. In addition to this, users accept changes of MTDs only to an extent that makes relearning unnecessary as well as the modification of manuals or other literature.

Despite of all these restrictions, the following modifications could be realized for the CD 2000:

The printed MTD-copies are put into plastic foil that is about 0.5 to 0.8 mms thick. It is fixed to the digitizer with the help of buttons so that displacement is impossible and holding unnecessary.

Many functions that are represented verbally can be made clearer and easier to learn by using graphic symbols. For the development of suitable symbols, the following method was applied:

A group of 10 students from the department of mechanical engineering was asked to relate graphic symbols to certain verbal descriptions. Then, the most frequent symbols were selected. For the redesigning of functions, we agreed on the following symbols:

```
o      a circle symbolizes an existing point or
       a pick-point (with cross hairs)

●      a filled circle marks a point to be created

----   a dashed line represents an existing line (element)

━━━━   a thick continuous line marks a line (an element)
       still to be created

───    a thin continuous line represents an auxiliary line,
       especially for dimension, distance, ....

─·─·─  a dot-dash line represents a vanishing line or a
       construction line
```

Fig. 6: Symbol agreements of representation

As a consequence of this, the user is now able to distinguish between existing elements and those to be created. The new symbols were created with regard to existing standards (ISO or DIN). In connection with this, we started to create a collection of symbols that is generally applicable.

In order to gain a more reasonable colour coding, all functions were classed in 19 function groups and a specific colour was related to each of them. This was made with regard to the following aspects:

- optimum degree of colour reflection (50 to 80 per cent)
- harmony of colours
- legibility of symbols
- contrasting colours for important functions (delete, reset, return to main menu).

In written descriptions, the words are normally capitalized at the beginning which improves their legibility. As a consequence of this, the use of small letters was introduced as well as to reduce the exclusive use of capital letters. Despite of obvious disadvantages, vertical columns had to be preserved which is due to the system's inflexibilty (Schmidtke, 1981).

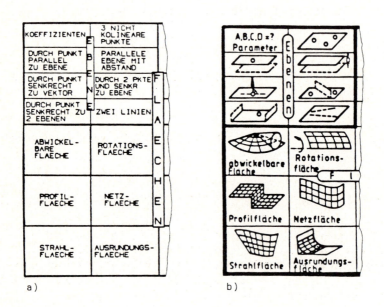

Fig. 7: Selection of CD 2000 - a) old, b) new

As a result of our study, it can be said that the users generally welcomed our modifications. The system has become clearer and relating symbols to their appropriate functions during the training phase is easier now.

In order to improve the effect of the training phase, it is necessary to use the same symbols on the MT as well as in the training manuals. In practice, manufacturers do not seem to attach considerable importance to them - didactical aspects are practically ignored. Based on the results obtained during the modification of existing MTDs, a collection of universally applicable functions will be created for the most important functions normally contained in CAD-Systems. Then, they can be used whenever new MTDs are to be designed.

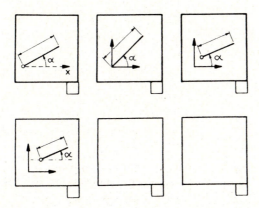

Fig. 8: Example: creating a line with a distance to an existing point and an angle to the x-axis

CONCEPTION OF A NEW MTD-SYSTEM CONCAD 2 - CONTRAVES

For redesigning an improved MTD, we used the results obtained during the process of modification of the CD-2000 MTD. As the digitizer field is much larger (1,000 x 1,280 mms^2) in comparison with the CD-2000 (about 280 x 280 mms^2), there are no technical restrictions for using appropriate /suitable symbol areas.

Design of Symbols

In creating new symbols, we used our collection of symbols as well as the symbols provided by the manufacturer of the Concad 2 system. Altogether, we created more than 400 symbols. Sometimes, several symbols were related to the same function. The agreement about the designing of symbols was the same we used in connection with CD-2000 MTD (see above). For the most difficult functions, two or more versions were created with the aim of finding the best one with the help of a selection test.

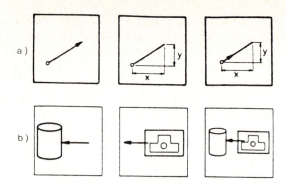

Fig. 9: Example of alternative symbols
a) creating a line in vector direction
b) saves the drawing

Realization of a Perception Test for the Selection of Suitable Symbols

From a total amount of 400 functions, we chose 55 which were difficult to be represented graphically. We created 149 versions for them, with two to six graphic symbols for each of the 55 functions. Then, they were divided into two series of slides:

Group A consisted of 27 functions and 77 versions for the creation of points, lines, circles and arcs.

Group B consisted of 28 functions and 72 versions for the following operations: trimming, dividing, grouping and management of drawings.

Each slide presented 9 symbols of which one had to be related to an explanation read aloud by the examiner. The symbols on the slides were arranged unsystematically in order to avoid unwanted preferences in rating, with the exception of identical symbols which always appeared in the same position. This was made to exclude differences in selection time.

Group A was shown to a group of 20 students, group B to a group of 10 students from the department of mechanical engineering without special knowledge in CAD. The average test time was between 35 and 40 minutes including some time for introduction and preparation.

During the test, the following parameters were registered:
- reaction time between presentation and identification;
- registration of how frequent a symbol was related to the right description (of functions);

- registration of how often symbols were mixed up: it was for example registered how often the description "creation of line with angle and length to a straight line" was related to the symbol describing the function "creation of line with angle and length to the x-axis";
- registration of how frequent the description of functions could not be related to any of the given symbols; for example, about 50 per cent of the test persons were not able to relate any of the symbols shown to the description of the function "creation of line in direction of a vector".

The length of reaction time was an indicator for the difficulties the test persons had in identifying the right functions or commands. As for the identification of symbols, the reaction time varied between 3,8 sec and 31 sec.

By analysing the average selection time for every function, the following values were determined:

Table 1:

FUNCTION	REACTION TIME	FUNCTION	REACTION TIME
point	10.3 sec.	dividing	14.8 sec.
arc line	8.5 sec.	grouping	14.1 sec.
line	8.2 sec.	trimming	13.9 sec.
circle	6.5 sec.	draft managing	11.5 sec.

The following figure demonstrates which symbols per group were recognized very quickly and which caused problems. The process of relating functions to symbols is marked by "x", as shown in figure 10 below.

Evaluation of the Experiment: Consequences

The results gained out of the previous experiment were analyzed with the help of arithmetic methods free from parameters, the Friedmann-Analysis. For the designing of new symbols, only such functions were selected that showed a significance level of $1 < 0.10$. Besides the reaction time, we also took into consideration, which symbols were clear, i.e. that have always been related to their respective functions as well as those that were related to the wrong functions and those that have not been selected at all.

The knowledge gained out of this experiment is of considerable importance as to the redesigning process of existing MTDs. It leads to an arrangement of functions that is clearer than before. Furthermore, the

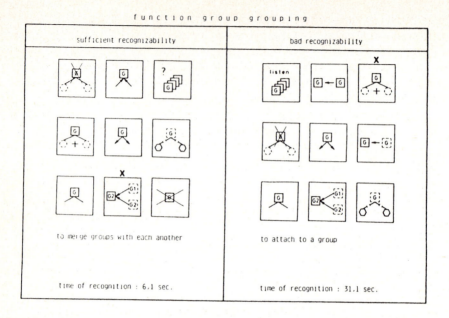

Fig. 10: Example for function groups

user's communication with the system is improved by an unambiguous representation of functions so that the user has less difficulties in remembering the arrangement of functions after some time.

Our next step consisted in the necessity of arranging the most suitable symbols of every function group in such a way that the CAD-user will be able to find them as quickly as possible. A specific colour was given to every function group contained in our collection of symbols. The standardization of colour coding contributes to the design of new MTDs in a positive way - it facilitates the identification of symbols.

In the selection of colours the following aspects were taken into account: (Frieling, H., 1968, p. 150ff):

- sufficient contrast between the colours and the symbols/letters (i.e. only such colours were selected that showed a degree of reflection between 50 and 80 per cent);
- general harmony of colours: no use of too many different colours;
- avoidance of simultaneous contrasts and
- consideration of colour blindness (especially red-green blindness of male users).

Nr.	Colour-Code	Function Group	HKS-K	Colour-Scale Euro Y, M, C	DIN 6164
17	green	help function	67 K 100 %	100, -, 60	24 : 6 : 2
18	orange	delete	7 K 100 %	100, 65, -	5 : 5 : 2
19	light-blue	geometrical construction	50 K 30 %	-, -, 20	18 : 1 : 1
20	blue	line - attribute	50 K 55 %	-, -, 40	18 : 2 : 1
21	light-yellow	modify	3 K 30 %	50, -, -	
22	yellow	command option	3 K 55 %	70, -, -	
23	light greenish-blue	surface symbol form- and position tolerance	64 K 30 %	30, -, 25	23 : 1 : 1
24	greenish-blue	surface data	64 K 55 %	60, -, 50	

Y = yellow ; M = red ; C = blue

Fig. 11: Colour table of function groups (selection)

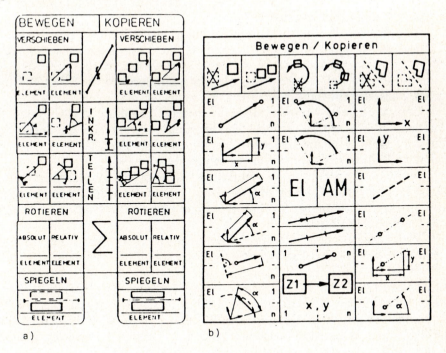

a)   b)

Fig. 12: Menu move / copy from MTD System Concad 2 - Contraves
a) old menu, b) modified menu

As Fig. 11 shows, the groups contain about 30 different functions connected with different colours. The distribution of colours takes into consideration the relationship that exists between functions belonging to the same group. The same colour coding is used with the different sub-menus. The colours are standardized.

We are convinced it is possible to introduce a similar colour coding procedure for different CAD-systems that use about the same functions.

Several alternative tablets were developed by varying dimensions, relation of symbols, size of letters, headlines and so on. The different tablet menus were tested by CAD-users as well as the manufacturer. The best one was selected and printed afterwards.

The functions were grouped in such a way that they could be arranged within reach of the hands so that frequent arm movement should be avoided.

CONCLUSION

MTDs are an important connection between user and system. They have to be carefully designed in order to facilitate and not to complicate the work of designing engineers.

Together with the respective training manuals for each CAD the MTD should form an integrated whole. If the same graphic symbols are used in the training manuals as well as on the MTD, it facilitates the use of the system as well as the relearning of functions in case that the user has not worked with the system for some time.

Compared with screen display menus, graphic MTDs have the advantage of immediate access of functions that makes an active reproduction of the menu structure unnecessary, so that the user does not need to reproduce actively the menu structure.

A "logical" grouping of functions as well as systematical colour coding facilitate the finding of functions; especially if the user has little training. As a consequence of this the time needed for finding is reduced during the training phase.

The consideration of aspects that follow from the study of perception and psychology leads to the development of new concepts.

Moreover, the use of verbal and graphic descriptions that are standardized facilitates the transfer of knowledge between different CAD-Systems. This transfer would not be limited to CAD-Systems with MTDs, but could also exist to some extent in connection with screen display menus, in case they would also use graphic symbols in training manuals for the explanation and illustration of functions.

As CAD-systems are very expensive, the consideration of certain ergonomical basic rules should be quite natural (as for example non-reflecting surfaces, no damage of MTD-surface with electric pens, possibility to fix MTD so that it needn't be held with the left hand, and so on).

REFERENCES

Encarnacao, J. & Straßer, W.(1986). *Computer Graphics*. München: Oldenbourg.

Frieling, H. (1968). *Gesetz der Farbe*. Göttingen: Musterschmidt.

Krueger, M.; Müller-Limmroth, W. (1979). *Arbeiten mit dem Bildschirm - aber richtig*. Hrsg. Bayerisches Staatsministerium für Arbeit und Sozialordnung. München.

Schmidtke (1981). *Lehrbuch der Ergonomie*. München: Hanser.

Wessells, M.G. (1984). *Kognitive Psychologie*. New York: UTB Harper & Row.

Psychological Issues of
Human Computer Interaction in the Work Place
M. Frese, E. Ulich, W. Dzida (Editors)
© Elsevier Science Publishers B.V. (North-Holland), 1987

A WORK PLACE FOR COMPUTER SUPPORTED STATISTICAL CONSULTING

Gerhard Dirlich[1], Hermann Federkiel[1],
Viola Strube[2],
Alexander Yassouridis[1] and Erwin Hansert[1]

[1] Max-Planck-Institute for Psychiatry, Munich, F.R.G.

[2] Department of Psychology, Technical University Munich

Statistical consulting is centered around a dialogue between the consultant and the client. Client and consultant seek to combine their differing bodies of expert knowledge. A computer may play different roles in this process, especially that of an integrated work place. We describe aspects of our work place from the points of view of the designer, of the consultant, and of the client, and discuss the danger of focus.

INTRODUCTION

Statistical consulting

The work place discussed in the present chapter is highly specialized. It is designed for a consultant for methodological aspects in project planning and statistics in a research institute in the biomedical domain. Researches, who encounter methodological, and, in particular, statistical problems when planning their studies or during the evaluation of observational data consult experienced statisticians in order to understand, solve or circumvent the difficulties.

The statistician (consultant) and the researcher (client) meet one or several times and work jointly on the problems. Typically, neither the knowledge of the client alone nor the knowledge of the consultant alone provide a sufficient basis for a solution of the problems. Only through a constructive combination of the client's and the consultant's knowledge the problems can be solved (Miyake, 1986; Hansert, 1979; Hansert and Federkiel, 1982).

Statistical consulting is centered around a dialogue between the consultant and the client. Client and consultant seek to combine their differing bodies of expert knowledge: the first contributes his expertise in his field of research, the latter his methodological and statistical knowledge (Zahn and Isenberg, 1983).

Different phases can be discerned during the dialogue: at first, the client tries to communicate the difficulty or the problem that he has encountered to the consultant. Then, the consultant and the client seek to develop a common understanding and representation of the problem. Once this goal is reached the next phase begins: the search for strategies to solve the agreed upon problem and the execution of plans that lead to a solution.

Statistical consulting is characterized by a wide spectrum of essentially different types of tasks some of which are standard, and others are novel, sometimes requiring the creative development of new concepts, problem solving strategies, and algorithms.

Although statistical consulting is concerned with highly specific problems some features of our consulting situation are shared by a variety of other consulting situations encountered in e.g. medical consulting (Feinstein, 1977), travel consulting, financial consulting, project planning. All these consulting situations have in common that pieces of knowledge of the client must be combined with pieces of knowledge of the consultant.

Consulting situations are an interesting domain for designers of computer software because they require high standards of functionality and usability of the systems. Consulting situations are rather difficult with respect to computer support because there are two users, consultant and client, with different goals and different knowledge about computers. Moreover, the client's problems can in general not been completely anticipated by the system designer. Therefore, only partial computer support appears to be possible (Dirlich et al., 1986 a; Wingert, 1986; Schiff, 1986).

Possible roles of the computer

Let us briefly outline possible roles of the computer in statistical consulting situations.

(1) The computer as a computing tool for simple tasks, e.g. arithmetic tasks: hand-held computers which are today found on almost every office desk.

(2) The computer as a computing tool for complex tasks, e.g. multivariate analyses of large bodies of data by means of statistical software packages such as SPSS. Two factors, however, essentially reduce the attractiveness of such systems during the consulting dialogue: limited interactivity and insufficient transparency of the computations.

(3) Integrated work places for statistical consulting:

With personal computers it is possible to avoid some disadvantages mentioned under (2). Integrated work places must be equipped with tools that are easy to use and tailored to the special functional requirements of the consulting situation.

(4) Work places with "intelligent" tools:

We can envision integrated work places equipped with "intelligent" tools which - comparable to assistants - intelligently perform certain subtasks in the process of consulting, e.g. the automatic generation of graphical representations according to rule based knowledge.

(5) Expert systems:

Still more ambitious is the enterprise to develop expert systems which are capable of carrying out some of the major decisions that have to be made in the consulting process, e.g. the selection of appropriate statistical procedures given a hypothesis and a set of data with certain formal properties. Research along these lines is flourishing in recent years (e.g. Thisted, 1986).

(6) The "artificial statistical consultant":

A system which could replace the knowledge and the skills of an experienced consultant for statistics and methodology. Due to our present understanding of the consulting process and the given technological standards this appears to be an unrealizable dream.

Our goal is to explore the possibilities for computer support of the consulting dialogue beyond the limits set by programming packages, multi-user systems and the presently popular type of personal computers: We develop an integrated work place equipped with special tools on a so-called workstation. Our approach is best characterized by alternative (3).

Overview

The present chapter has three parts. In the first, we discuss little scenes from consulting dialogues in order to familiarize the reader with the heterogeneous task domain of statistical consulting.

In the second part, we look at the computer based work-place from the differing points of view of the three people who are concerned with the system: the system designer, the consultant, and the client.

In the last part, we briefly point out the "problem of focus" encountered in psychological research on man-machine systems while taking a close look at one of the tools available at the work place.

A special feature of our chapter needs to be mentioned here: it is "a case description" rather than a report of results from psychological theorizing or experimentation. Yet, several psychological factors have been considered in the conception of the integrated work place described here.

WHAT IS STATISTICAL CONSULTING ?

The following scenes from different consulting dialogues shall illustrate what statistical consulting is, which kinds of tasks occur, and which strategies can be used to solve the encountered problems.

Gaps in knowledge structures

In the beginning of the consulting dialogue the client describes the difficulties or problems that he has encountered in his research to the consultant. It is a frequent experience that the client in his description does not mention certain facts which are crucial prerequisites for a correct understanding by the consultant. These facts are so familiar to the client that he does not recognize that they constitute essential prerequisites for a correct problem representation and understanding. Thus, he does not mention them. Sometimes, it is quite difficult to discover such gaps in the knowledge structures of the dialogue partner.

Scene 1:

> The client, a neurobiologist, has measured nerve growth factor concentrations (NGF) in brain tissue of rats. He explains: "The main goal of my study is to obtain a 'map' of the rat brain with respect to NGF. The interpretation of my empirical data, however, requires some statistical comparisons. According to our theory I expect that all areas of the cortex should show similar NGF concentrations." He adds: "an analysis of variance would perhaps be an appropriate statistical treatment for the data".
>
> The consultant agrees that an analysis of variance is indeed a suitable test for the statistical hypothesis "there are no significant differences between the mean values of several samples of NGF values in different cortical areas".

At this point, there was, however, an important piece of knowledge lacking in the mental model of the problem that the consultant had conceived, namely, that the values observed in the subcortical areas were without exception essentially smaller than the values measured in the cortex (The client had not mentioned this). The client's statement that "similar values in the cortical areas were expected" gained its meaning mainly from the context that there were essential differences between values from subcortical and values from cortical areas. He should have explained: "In comparison to the essential differences between subcortical and cortical values the differences between cortical values are negligible."

The client assumed that the statistical proof of the existence of insignificant differences between the cortical areas would objectify his subjective impression of "negligible differences in the cortical data as compared to the essentially smaller subcortical values".

Obviously, here existed a significant misunderstanding between the dialogue partners. The scene demonstrates that decisions about appropriate statistical procedures are critically dependent on sufficient knowledge about the empirical facts. It is a major objective of the consulting dialogue to convey sufficient knowledge between the client and the consultant in order to build up a common understanding and representation of the problem. Presently, no essential computer support for this type of task, the building of statistical arguments, is at hand.

Explorative modeling

It is not always the best strategy in statistical consulting to attack problems in a straightforward manner. Detours may sometimes circumvent difficulties and shed light onto a problem from new perspectives:

Scene 2:

The client, a psychologist, investigates ultradian rhythms in memory performance. In a pilot study subjects had to do a recognition test (16 items) every 20 minutes for 12 consecutive hours. The observed hit frequencies formed time series. The data showed fluctuations which in quite a few cases seemed to be rhythmical. The working hypothesis "memory function is subject to cyclic ultradian modulations" combined with the visual impression of the first data favored an explorative analysis of the data by means of spectral analytic methods.

The results were ambiguous. At this point of the consulting process two strategies could be chosen: (a) more extensive data analysis, or (b) explorative modeling.

Explorative modeling starts out from a representation of functional relations between important factors influencing the data. In the present case, a binomial probability distribution with $p = 0.5$ provides a rough model for the hitrate in each test capturing "randomness" as a factor influencing the observed hitrate. A computer program which according to the binomial random model produces different time series of simulated hit-frequency values yields a simple working model of the experiment.

Working models can be regarded as representations of theories or hypotheses. Data obtained from Monte Carlo studies with working models can be visually inspected and compared with observed data, and/or be analysed by the same procedures as the experimental data.

In the present case, the simulated time series obtained by explorative modeling showed similar rhythmical fluctuations as the real data. The client understood that on the basis of the given knowledge the observed rhythmical phenomena in his data could not be discerned from mere random fluctuations.

Explorative modeling can be a useful tool in statistical consulting. It can support the planning of empirical studies, help to avoid unproductive empirical work and support the understanding and interpretation of observed phenomena. Presently, however, explorative modeling is not widely used in statistical consulting because suitable tools integrated into the work environment are not yet available.

Statistical data analysis

The preceding scenes were selected in order to demonstrate the wide spectrum and the heterogeneity of the types of problems encountered in statistical consulting. The following scene captures a standard type of problem, namely the investigation of bodies of data with respect to statistical features and statistical hypotheses.

Scene 3:

> *The client, a developmental psychologist, has observed the interaction of 17 parents with their 2 month old children. Episodes of a duration of 3 minutes from video recordings were analysed with respect to sequences of recurrent parental behaviors, e.g. repeated head nodding. 12 variables were evaluated for about 300 behavior sequences. Two tasks were conceived: (a) The conception of graphical representations which should make the data transparent, and (b) descriptions of the data by statistical parameters such as mean values, medians, standard deviations, and quantiles as a basis for an exploration of quantitative features.*

In contrast to the problems pointed out in the scenes 1 and 2 for tasks of this kind effective and efficient computer support by graphical and statistical systems is available today. The present prototype of our work place can be regarded as an integration of such resources, namely graphics tools and statistical procedures, into a user-friendly work environment. It is a major objective of the work place to support tasks of the kind just described.

A WORK PLACE FOR STATISTICAL CONSULTING

Our computer based work place can be compared with an office of the kind presently used by statisticians: there are stacks of paper, pencils, hand-held computers, statistical procedures, graphic tools, statistical tables etc. Presently, our computer based work place does not offer qualitatively new functions beyond the classical work environment. An important difference to a real work place, however, is the fact, that the tools are now integrated into an environment which allows easy and extensive interaction between the computer system and the user and between the different tools. The integration combined with a significantly altered mode of human-computer interaction has an impact on the consulting process: its efficiency rises, goals can now be conceived which, for practical reasons, have been unreachable before, and the subjective qualities of the consulting work change (Dirlich et al., 1986 b). In order to clarify these statements we look in the following at this work place with the eyes of those who design it and those who work with it: we describe aspects of our work place from the differing points of view of the designer, of the consultant, and of the client.

The designer's point of view

The hardware used for our work place is a workstation, a personal computer with a powerful processor, a 19 inch high resolution screen with about 1 million pixels, a keyboard, and a so called mouse as pointing device. Under a UNIX operating system several higher programming languages are available. Our system is mainly written in C. The most striking advantage of workstations over conventional computers, however, is the window system combined with the mouse: different windows can be created and utilized for different tasks. Windows assigned to different types of tasks can for instance be used in programming (Fig. 1).

The programmer can now organize his task and activity structures in the form of a network which is tailored to his personal working style. This liberates him from boring, stressful and error-subject side tasks and allows him to focus on the implementation task as such. Window systems significantly modify the task of implementing software as compared to conventional multi-user systems. The efficiency is greater, and some subjective qualities of programming appear to be modified (Goldberg, 1984).

The system software provides several types of control elements which allow the system designer to equip application programs with direct manipulation interfaces (Hutchins et al., 1986). There are labelled buttons, pull-down-menus, choice-strings, and sliders available which can be integrated into the operating panels assigned to functions that have been specified by the designer (SUN, 1986).

Figure 1: Screen while modifying a program Arrows indicate the subtask cycle. Windows starting counter clockwise from upper right are assigned to: (1) editing source code, (2) compilation, (3) execution, (4) input data, (5) output (graphical), (6) additional output for debugging. Pull-down menus: (in background) generation of various types of windows, (at black bar on top of (1)) window handling, (in window (5)) handling content of the window. Icons near upper left corner of the screen: temporarily closed windows.

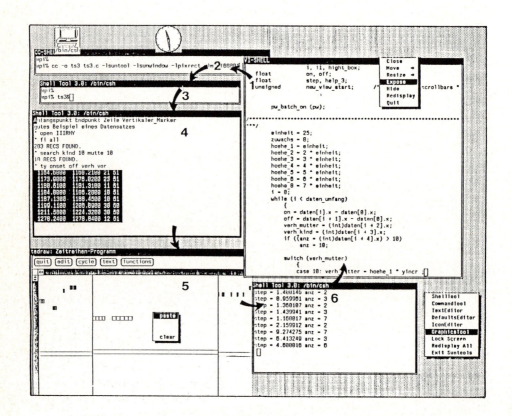

The different surface of application programs is linked to a different type of control structure. In conventional programs the programmer had to establish a global control structure which transformed user actions into internal signals which triggered procedures. In programs which engage direct-manipulation elements on our workstation, special components of the system software organize the communication between the user-interface and application procedures. The programmer merely needs to specify (a) the system surface with its operating panel, (b) the procedures which shall be controlled through the panel, and (c) the relations connecting operating elements and procedures. With these software resources it is possible to equip our work place with consistent and application-independent human-computer interfaces (cf. Dzida, in this book).

The process of implementing software is no longer a bottleneck in system development. It has become much more attractive and efficient. Therefore, we can work with an "open systemapproach": when the need of new functions is discovered during the consulting, it is in many cases possible to create new system components fast enough - in one or several days - to support ongoing consulting processes.

The consultant's point of view

Most important for the consultant is the functionality of the work place: which types of tasks encountered in statistical consulting are supported by the system? How effective and efficient is the support? Is the system easy to operate? Are the actions and the output of the system transparent? Is the collective acting of client, consultant and computer system successful?

The basic structure of the work place and some presently available tools are schematically depicted in Fig. 2.

A central principle in the design of our work place is modularity (Dirlich et al., in press): there are different types of tools each of which has a "simple" function, e.g. data retrieval or statistical procedures or graphical functions. In order to accomplish a "complex" task it is in general necessary to engage several tools.

We discuss the structure and the utilization of the work place by describing how the task outlined in scene 3 can be carried out. We can distinguish four subtasks, namely the retrieval of a set of data, its graphical representation, the performance of statistical computations and the graphical representation of their results.

The tool for data retrieval at the work place is a QUERY LANGUAGE: a window is assigned to the communication with a data base system, which is actually located in a central computer to which the workstation has access. The sample has to be specified and the output format must be determined. Respective retrieval and formatting commands

Figure 2 :   Basic structure of the work-place. Boxes represent the objects
which are manipulated at the work place. Arrows represent tools.
The labels in shaded ovals indicate the functions of the tools.

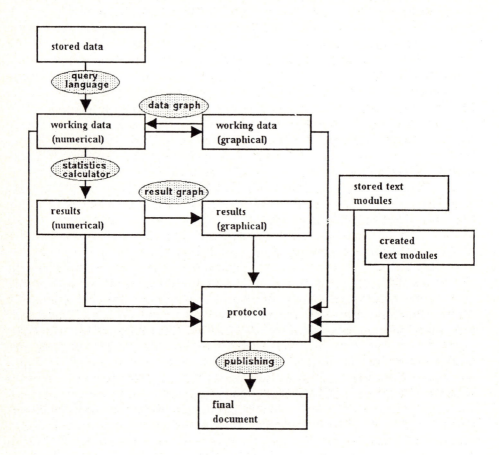

trigger the search, transformation and output procedures: The data appear
in the form of a table in the window (WORKING DATA).

A fundamental design principle of the work place is the dual representation of information: numerical and graphical representations should
always be visible at the same time (Dirlich et al., 1986 b). For this purpose
there are different tools labelled DATAGRAPH. Besides general purpose
tools, e.g. a tool which generates 2-dimensional scatterplots, there are
special purpose DATA-GRAPH tools which produce problem specific
graphical representations. A tool of this kind for the data mentioned in
scene 3 is described below.

Statistical procedures are available through a set of tools labelled STATISTICS CALCULATORS. A tool of this type is discussed after these remarks concerning general features of the work place.

The graphical representation of results obtained by statistical computations requires another type of tool labelled RESULTGRAPH.

Data and results in numerical form, as well as graphical representations of data and results are materials out of which a PROTOCOL can be composed. In addition, STORED TEXT modules with explanatory texts and FREE TEXT created during the consulting session can be incorporated into the protocol. The protocol can then be used as raw material for a FINAL DOCUMENT created by a desk-top PUBLISHING system.

It is an important rule for the use of our work place that, in general, the consultant operates the system. This simplifies the system design essentially since it is not necessary to provide system support for unexperienced users. New users are introduced to the system by experienced users. This principle matches with another principle, namely, that the consultant, in cooperation with the client makes the decisions which tools should be applied to which objects. Our work place in its present version has no built-in intelligence to support automatic reasoning processes. It is rather a tool than a partner in the sense of artificial intelligence.

Let us now describe, how complex functions can be specified by combining different tools which are accessible through different windows: there exists a powerful system function by which the user can establish a direct communication between windows (CUT AND PASTE). The central component of this function is the SHELF, an (invisible) device which can be used as a temporary storage: portions of the content of a window can be marked by the mouse, this action transfers a copy to the shelf. When the mouse is moved to another location in the same window or in another window, the content of the shelf can be copied to this location. A user controlled transparent communication between different windows is enabled by this CUT AND PASTE tool. Different tools are accessible through different windows, thus different tools at our work place interact with each other by means of the CUT AND PASTE function.

Our tools are operated by means of direct-manipulation interfaces with labelled buttons, and other types of control devices.

For example, the statistical computations required in our sample task can be performed by the STATISTICS CALCULATOR tool with such an interface shown in figure 3. Data are transferred to the calculator by a CUT AND PASTE action. Then one or several statistical procedures can be triggered by activating the respective buttons in arbitrary order. The results appear in the output window. Explanatory texts, which can support an understanding of the strategy of analysis and of the results can be merged with the results by using pull-down menus available at each button. Moreover, free text created during the consulting session can also be

Figure 3: Statistics calculator in working environment. The two windows
show: dialogue with database system, working data in the form of
a table with two columns of numbers (left), *STATISTICS CAL-
CULATOR* tool for two-sample problems (right): operating panel
(upper part), input window (lower left part), output window lower
right part). Statistical procedures are triggered by activating the
labelled buttons, results are displayed in the output window (1).
Pull-down menus for each button allow the display of stored text-
modules containing explanations (2).

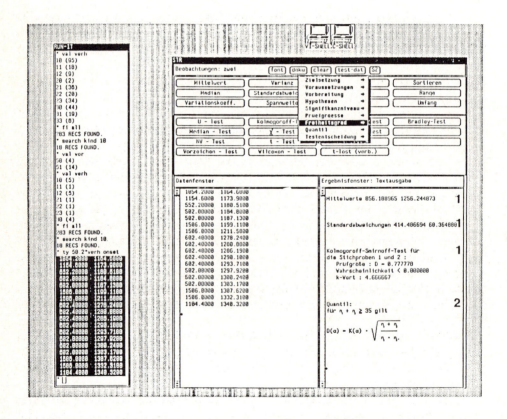

edited into the output window.

The structure of the work place outlined here requires that the users, i.e. the consultant in cooperation with the client, determine goals and appropriate action structures. Difficult decisions can be discussed extensively and a wide spectrum of possible actions can be considered. The simple and appealing mode of operation of the tools reduces the cognitive effort required for the human-computer interaction and enhances in this way the problem solving capacity of client and consultant.

The client's point of view

The client is in general neither an experienced user of a workstation nor an expert in statistics. The big high resolution screen with multiple windows, the direct-manipulation interfaces of the tools, the short reaction time of the system often surprise our clients. The natural curiosity in the workstation as such, however, should not distract from the central expectation of the client: he wants to get effective and efficient support with respect to the problems that caused him to seek the consulting.

We want to focus here on the client's expectation of transparent and problem specific support. In order to elaborate on this we once again return to scene 3 and describe an initial step in the consulting process with the developmental psychologist: the conception and realization of special graphical representations for his data.

As already mentioned above the source of the data was a relatively small number of episodes from video recordings of parents interacting with their 2-month old infants. We wanted to create graphical representations which should have as much similarity as possible with the familiar video recordings. Therefore, they had to capture the most important features of the experimental situation and the variables of interest, namely the temporal structure of the episodes, and the behavior of both partners, parent and infant (fig. 4).

The concept of this representation emerged during the consulting dialogue. The realization within the framework of our "open system" approach mentioned above required only few hours of implementation, testing and prototyping work.

In addition to descriptions by statistical parameters such problem specific graphical representations of the data can support the exploration of the material. The representation demonstrated here contains much information and is easy to understand. It makes the data transparent, because it preserves important features of the empirical situation. It is "natural" for it can be related to the video recordings from which the data were acquired with little cognitive effort. With such highly specific graphical representations we pursue the guideline that problem specific DATA-GRAPH tools should be available at the work place in order to bridge the cognitive gulf between the observed phenomena and the stored data.

Figure 4: *Problem specific graphical representation. The two windows show: dialogue with database system, working data in the form of a table with 5 columns (left), special purpose DATAGRAPH tool (right): the horizontal axis represents time, segmented rectangles represent parental behaviors (onset time, offset time, duration, the type of behavior is coded by the vertical position, frequency of repetitions coded by segmentation), parallel horizontal lines represent the behavior of the infant (the type of behavior coded by the vertical position), vertical lines represent changes of the infant's behavior. On top of the graphic: operating panel with labelled button for graphics editing.*

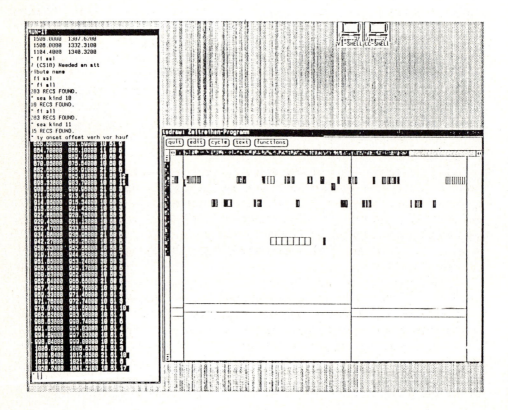

For our clients a large cognitive distance between the observed phenomena and the results is a major obstacle on the way to a fully satisfying evaluation of empirical data. Computer support which reduces this problem is an essential accomplishment.

THE DANGER OF FOCUS

In the preceding parts of this chapter we have introduced the heterogeneous task domain of statistical consulting. For tasks concerned with computations computer support already exists or is realizable. In contrast, for many frequent and important tasks in statistical consulting we still need to explore how computer support should be provided in the future. Obviously, our work place in its present form is both, a work environment employed in routine tasks, and also a tool in the search for new approaches to computer supported statistical consulting. The present structure of the work place, the set of tools, and the form of human-computer interaction are determined by several factors, namely, by the specific functional requirements encountered in statistical consulting, the philosophy of desk-top office systems, and the subjective experience of the three groups of people who work with our system.

The concept of our work place has emerged during several proto-typing cycles. In each cycle we focused on few aspects of the system. At the same time we pursued the principle to have prototypes of the tools available at each time which could be used in routine applications. Therefore, our system emerges as a compromise taking into consideration a wide spectrum of requirements, constraints and relevant factors. We conclude this description of our approach by taking a close look at one of the tools from an earlier prototyping cycle which demonstrates nicely such a compromise (fig. 5).

This tool can be used to perform a complex task in the sense defined above, because it combines several simple functions, namely (a) the creation of a scatterplot by means of a direct graphics editor or by 2-dimensional external data, (b) a direct manipulation dynamic dichotomization of the two axes, (c) the computation of frequencies in a 2-by-2 table, and (4) a parameter required for a statistical test procedure. The tool can be used in the planning phase of experiments for simulation purposes and during the phase of data analysis.

Figure 5: *Surface of a tool for simulation and data analysis operating
panel (top), subwindow for the graphical representation of data
(scatterplot) (bottom left), subwindow for the graphical representation of results (frequencies of dots in the four quadrants defined by the crosshair) (bottom right). The crosshair can be moved
by the mouse. Icons in the left part of the operating panel are used
for direct graphics editing ("create", "read-in", "move", "erase" of
dots). The frequencies and the the chi-square statistics are computed dynamically, the actual values are displayed in the 2-by-2
table (top right) and the narrow subwindow below.*

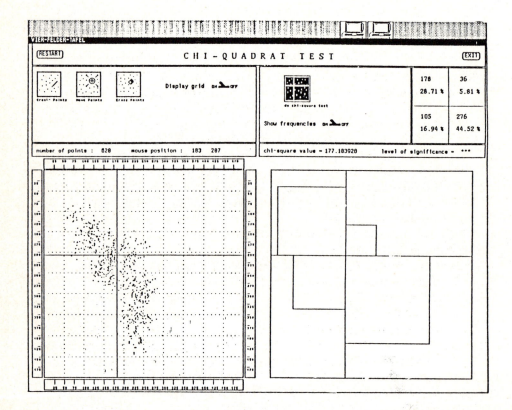

Apparently, it is not easy to evaluate its utility and its psychological qualities. Why is this difficult? System designers, consultants and clients, as well as psychologists who study computers at the work place must focus on certain aspects of the work situation and the system. However, according to our experience such necessary focussing brings about the danger to loose the context out of sight. Norman (1987) labels this difficulty in system design the "danger of focus" and explains: "focus on one variable and there is apt to be neglected another. Focus on utility, and functionality is apt to suffer. Focus on functionality and utility will suffer. Focus on cost and everything else will suffer, focus on aesthetics, and other things suffer. So it goes."

REFERENCES

Dirlich, G., H. von Benda, C. Freksa, U. Furbach, A. Müller, und K. Wimmer, (1986 a). Computerunterstützte Planung von Ferienreisen - ein fiktives Beispiel. In: *Kognitive Aspekte der Mensch-Computer-Interaktion*. Workshop, München, April 1984. G. Dirlich et al. (Hrsg.). Springer, Berlin.

Dirlich, G., H. Federkiel, G. Gleixner, E. Hansert, P. Kremser, and A. Yassouridis, (1986 b). Direct graphics manipulation in a system for explorative statistics. *COMPSTAT 86*, Short Communications and Posters. F. de Antoni, N. Lauro, A. Rizzi (Eds.). Physica, Heidelberg, 73-74.

Feinstein, A. R. (1977). *Clinical Biostatistics*. The C. V. Mosby Comp., Saint Louis 1977.

Goldberg, A. (1984). *Smalltalk -The Interactive Programming Environment*. Addison-Wesley, Reading, Mass.

Hansert, E. (1979). Statistik als Methodik zur Konstruktion von Wissen. In: I. Dahlberg (Ed.). *Klassifikation und Erkenntnis I*. Gesellschaft für Klassifikation e.V., 99-116.

Hansert, E. und H. Federkiel (1982). Computer-Aided Statistical Consulting in a Research Institute - Methodological and Research Aspects. *COMPSTAT 1982*.

Hansert, E., H. Federkiel und G. Dirlich (1979). Statistikprogramme oder programmierte Statistik? Eine Analyse und ein Versuch. *Stat. Software Newsletter 5*, 3-7.

Hutchins, E., J. D. Hollan and D. A. Norman (1986). Direct manipulation interfaces. In: D. A. Norman and S. W. Draper (Eds.) *User centered system design: New perspectives on human- computer interaction*. Erlbaum Associates, Hillsdale, N.J.

Miyake, N. (1986). Constructive interaction. *Cognitive Science, 10*.

Miyata, Y. and D. A. Norman (1986). Psychological issues in support of multiple activities. In: D.A. Norman and S.W. Draper (Eds.), *User centered system design: New perspectives on human-computer interaction.* Erlbaum Associates, Hillsdale, N.J.

Norman, D. A. (1986). Cognitive Engineering. In: D. A. Norman and S. W. Draper (Eds.) *User centered system design: New perspectives on human-computer interaction.* Erlbaum Associates, Hillsdale, N.J.

Norman, D. A. (in preparation). *The Psychology of Everyday Things.*

Schiff, J. (1986). Funktionsverteilung in Mensch-Computer-Systemen am Beispiel Reiseberatung. In: *Kognitive Aspekte der Mensch-Computer-Interaktion.* Workshop, München, April 1984. G. Dirlich et al. (Hrsg.). Springer, Berlin.

Sun Microsystems, Inc. (1986). *SunView Programmer's Guide.* Mountain View, Ca.

Thisted, A. R. (1986). Representing statistical knowledge for expert data analysis systems. In:. *Artificial intelligence and statistics.* A. W. Gale (Ed.) (1986) Addison-Wesley, Reading, Mass.

Wingert, B. (1986). Reise nach irgendwo - Anmerkungen zu einem Reise-Buchungs-System. In: *Kognitive Aspekte der Mensch-Computer-Interaktion.* Workshop, München, April 1984. G. Dirlich et al. (Hrsg.). Springer, Berlin.

Zahn, D. A. and Isenberg, D. I. (1983). Nonstatistical Aspects of Statistical Consulting, *The Am. Stat. 37,* 297-302.

TRAINING FOR
HUMAN-COMPUTER INTERACTION SKILLS

Psychological Issues of
Human Computer Interaction in the Work Place
M. Frese, E. Ulich, W. Dzida (Editors)
© Elsevier Science Publishers B.V. (North-Holland), 1987

FIVE GAMBITS FOR THE ADVISORY INTERFACE DILEMMA

John M. Carroll

IBM Watson Research Center Box 704
Yorktown Heights, New York 10598 USA

A key research and development issue for advisory
interfaces is identified. Five technical approaches to
managing it are illustrated.

For several years, our research group has been concerned with characterizing the learning problems of new users, and addressing those problems with new training designs. Through this work we have become aware of what might be called the Advisory Interface Dilemma: advances in help and training are constrained by advances in information management and user interaction with respect to both the user problems that require help and training support and the means to deliver help and training to the user. This is a key issue for the developer of advisory facilities. Their time is often spent discovering, and then designing advice for, problems that might have been more properly addressed in the design of information management and users interaction. And the delivery vehicles available to them for help and training often slightly lag the leading edge of users interface technology.

In our own work we have worried sometimes that we are over-studying a collection of interface design problems that we will only exit until currently new interface paradigms are better consolidated. For example, users are often stymied by integrated applications that provide little real integration, and by integration unsuited to their needs (Nielsen, Mack, Bergendorff, and Grischkowsky, 1986). This makes it very difficult to identify and address user problems in understanding and using integration *per se*. The same point arises in other interface arenas. We are very interested in point-and-select user interaction, but find that people are frequently confused by a clutter of windows, menus, and icons for even simple tasks (Carroll and Mazur, 1986). This confusion is probably not inherent in the point-and-select interaction style, so it undermines any investigation of how people learn and use point-and-select skills.

In this chapter, I describe some recent projects of the Advisory Interfaces group at the IBM T.J. Watson Research Center. This group includes Amy Aaronson, Robert Campbell, John Carroll, John Checco, Randy Eckhoff, Richard Herder, Donald Kirson and Donald Sawtelle. Our work is focussed on understanding and developing approaches to user assistance and education, that is, on help and training-- or what we call *advisory interfaces*. I have structured my review of our research program into five gambits for managing the Advisory Interface Dilemma. I have tried to include many pointers to the related papers we have already published so that the reader can use this brief chapter as a guide to more detailed reports.

It is very appropriate for this discussion to appear in a volume addressed to psychological issues of human-computer interaction *in the workplace* because we have always made the assumption that direct relevance to real workplace problems is a fundamental requirement for our research. We have specifically eschewed the study of idealized laboratory models and toy systems -- in fact we have become dedicated critics of such approaches (Carroll and Campbell, 1986).

BACKGROUND

One view of current developments in computing is that of a "race" between powerful function and ease of use. We are witnessing the extremely rapid introduction of new and powerful function: larger screens and more powerful processors, handwriting and speech input, intelligent services for help and training, and a great variety of new applications. Despite the fact that at least some of these enhancements are specifically directed at *improving* ease of use, there is no clear indication that learning to use the system of today is any easier than was learning to the systems of ten years ago. In an absolute sense, it may be harder. Those people who have already put in enough time and effort have become initiated. But the vast majority of people in the workforce remain *un*initiated. They are losing ground in the race between more powerful function and better ease of use.

This is not merely because more powerful systems present more function to learn about. It is also because functional innovations in computing systems quite often address existent usability problems while at the same time creating new usability problems. Examples of this evolutionary process of old usability problems developing into new usability problems can be seen in the contrast between the IBM Displaywriter (introduced 1980) and the Apple Lisa (introduced in 1983), as revealed in our own empirical usability studies.

In the Displaywriter, the user must specify a name for a document *before* that document can be created, that is, before the system will allow the user to enter or edit any text (Carroll, Smith-Kerker, and Mazur, 1986). This struck many user as a contradiction: How can something that not yet exists already have a name? The Lisa addresses this problem by allowing unnamed documents. Not only could one enter and edit text prior to assigning a document name, but in fact one *never* had to assign a document name. This approach, however, led new users to carelessly create many unnamed and undistinguishable documents which cluttered their workspaces and confused them (Carroll and Mazur, 1986).

The Displaywriter distinguishes between several different kinds of removal operations (Backspace for single characters, Delete for strings and blocks of text, Reply for prompts, Cancel for panels). We found that such "fine distinctions" often confuse and frustrate new users (Mack, Lewis, and Carroll, 1983). The Lisa collapsed some of this distinctions into a single operation of dragging an object's icon to a trashcan icon for disposal. This more general approach, however, allows to discard applications as easy as they could discard practice documents. In fact, one of our subjects did this and was unable to accomplish simple tasks because the function was literally no longer there (Carroll and Mazur, 1986).

These contrasts appear in the area of training and help designs as well. The Displaywriter, in its initial releases, provided no on-line training for users. It provided a fairly good training manual, but many user problems stemmed from the lack of coordination, or integration, between information and information users encountered while they actually used the system (Carroll, Smith-Kerker, Ford, and Mazur, 1986). The Lisa addressed this sort of problem by providing an on-line training package which was designed to appear to the user to be integrated with the real system function (that is, appeared to allow one to learn by really using the system). In fact the tutorial provided *only* an appearance of the system which the user could "break" by failing to follow tutorial instructions precisely. Moreover, the tutorial function had to be loaded, using a procedure which was both difficult and risky (Carroll and Mazur, 1986).

HOW CAN WE STUDY ADVISORY INTERFACES?

Our motivation in selecting the Displaywriter and the Lisa for study was that these seemed to be highly "representative" systems. In this time (1980-4), Displaywriter was the best-selling stand-alone office system in the world. For this reason it seemed to be an excellent choice of a representative system interface for studying usability and training issues for office systems. The Lisa, in its time (1983-1985), created extraordinary excitement in the trade press as a new interface look for office systems (e.g., Merkin, 1983; Williams, 1983). Accordingly, it too was an excellent choice of a representative state-of-the-art system. We wanted to study representative systems to avoid the methodological pitfalls of focussing too much attention on simple, highly-controlled laboratory situations that may have little or nothing to do with problems in real world.

The strategy of focussing attention on commercial systems trades off unfavorably with other research priorities. for example, by definition a commercial system - no matter how widely distributed or up-to-date - cannot be truly "leading edge". Leading edge interfaces by definition don't quite exist in the sense that they are not robustly implemented, not well integrated with existent system utilities and databases, and not supported, distributed or installed in real workplaces. This re-raises the Advisory Interface Dilemma: if we work on state-of-the-art commercial systems we are forever just one step behind leading edge work on users interfaces and advisory interfaces. The Displaywriter and the Lisa were real systems; we were able to study their usability and design new training approaches for them (Carroll and Carrithers, 1984; Carroll, Mack, Lewis, Grishkowsky, and Robertson, 1985; Carroll, Smith-Kerker, Ford, and Mazur, 1986). But by the time we had completed this work, the leading edge had already moved on.

A second unfavorable tradeoff in focussing attention on commercial systems is that one constantly risks being caught up in the details of *those particular* interfaces. It is not that the details don't matter; they do. Effective advisory interfaces require attention to user interface details. But analyzing details is unlikely to lead to cumulative science and engineering; it is unlikely to contribute much to what we need most, a theory of help and training. Our deepest worry is that as we progress through a research program of understanding usability problems with real, representative systems, to its culmination in the design and evaluation of new instructional technology, that the details, the quirks, whatever they are, of the specific interfaces we investigated might increasingly intrude on the generality of our conclusions. We have often asked ourselves weather we have spent too much time analyzing specific interface problems which are fundamentally ephemeral.

The Advisory Interface Dilemma is indeed a dilemma. We need to focus attention on real, commercial-scale system problems, but we also have to keep our attention on the horizon of new user interface technology. We need to appreciate the details of user interfaces in order to design effective help and training, but must avoid getting bogged down too much in the particulars of particular interfaces if we hope to learn anything general. We can not "solve" the Advisory Interface Dilemma; the best we can do is to manage it sensibly. But it is important to learn how to do at least this well, for if we don't, we really will continue to face a choice among unacceptable alternatives (understanding clearly what we should have done yesterday, studying irrelevant toy-scale situations in the laboratory and then having to embellish them with creative interpretations, endlessly predicting that each new interface style in its turn has finally provided an ease of use panacea, etc.).

In the balance of this paper, I discuss five gambits our research group is pursuing. Most simply, we have tried to codify our on-going state-of-the-art empirical assessment into a practical model for the design of advisory interfaces - not a formal deductive model, for no such model is likely ever to exist, but a model that designers can use. We have tried to work within the design process, developing our own advisory materials and systems, and working with other groups. These two initial gambits allow us to provide better starting points for the design of advisory interfaces and help to guide the design progress.

To really manage the Advisory Interface Dilemma, we need to control future technology development. We have, to this end, worked on runnable user interface models to demonstrate new advisory possibilities to developers *before* these possibilities have been overlooked or preempted by other decisions. We have discovered and created behavioral simulations of technological possibilities that cannot yet even be implemented as runnable interface models. These two gambits push on the technological frontiers of user interface development, and indeed try to anticipate where the frontier will be some years from now.

Our fifth gambit is to back off from technology development to examine issues which are so poorly understood, and yet so fundamental, that providing even a technology-free characterization can advance the state of the art in advisory interfaces. We now turn to these five gambits.

GAMBIT 1: PROVIDE STARTING POINTS - PRACTICAL MODELS

A key on-going activity in our group is the empirical analysis of state-of-the-art interfaces ranging from traditional character-boxes, menu-based styles (Mack, Lewis, Carroll, 1983) to raster graphics, direct manipulation styles (Carroll and Mazur, 1986). Our goal is to inventory and describe the most critical usability problems at appropriate level of detail to provide guidance for interface and training designers. To a great extent, the problem people have learning computing systems depend on idiosyncratic details of the particular system. However, we have found that from a moderate level of abstraction, a class of fairly general problem types emerges (e.g. Carroll, 1984).This on-going analysis led us to a view of human learning that questioned well-established ideas in instructional science.

We find that users are always fundamentally motivated to get something done. Both the organizational context for learning new computer software and the internalized standards that adult learners have for determining what is worth spending time on bias user against a "learning for the sake of learning" attitude. New users want to get started fast; they like to jump the gun (executing a procedure when it is merely mentioned in a overview); they like to skip around on their own in a training sequence. People want to learn by doing, to reason things out instead of merely reading about them. They resent rigidly structured exercises that often compel them to copy text character for character and then subject them to insincere praise for these forced accomplishments: "Excellent!"

They like to test hypotheses that they generate on their fly and to make use of their prior knowledge and reason by analogy. This "active" orientation to learning often badly misfits training design which are predicated on instructional models that begin with a logical analysis of what needs to learned and then successively decomposes each learning object into a step by step learning sequence of preview, practice test and review (for example, see Gagne and Briggs, 1979).

These findings called for a new approach to online training, one that seeks to provide an "explanatory environment" for the new user, an environment that affords active involvement in the learning process, one that encourages initiative and hypothesis testing. A major consideration in this approach is user error. Error is a major consideration for any training model, but the standard rote-practice model typically just ignores the problem, printing steps in bold-face and imploring learners to be careful. From an active learning perspective the problem is completely different: errors are expected; they are unavoidable; they are opportunities to learn. If learners are going to take initiative in directing their own learning, they are going to make errors. The problem for designers of training is to manage the consequences of errors so that the greatest possible learning benefit obtains.

A training model appropriate for active learners simply cannot demand that the learners sit at the interface and read. People don't want to do this, and they in fact don't do it. The Minimalist training model we developed takes this hard reality as a starting point (Carroll, 1984). The sheer volume of training material must be minimal: the ever-present sales pitch should be cut (the user has already bought the system), section overviews, previews, and reviews should be drastically cut (users often try to execute them), far less how-it-works information should be presented (new users don't have to know details of magnetic recording to use diskettes). Installation should be simple (e.g., loading a single diskette). System and tutorial screen should differ as little as possible (tutorial screen often get confusingly cluttered). The overhead of learning the jargon of the training itself should be minimized (e.g., eliminating fine distinctions between "topics" and "chapters" or between "message lines" and "information lines").

None of this is to say that Minimalist design for active learners is easy design. The Minimalist approach requires that we take a very hard position. We will put a higher premium on what can be eliminated than on what can be included. We will deliberately not explain everything we can, but rather explain only what we must. We will incorporate testing with real users to determine what tasks are initially important, interesting and attractive, and we will use that information to direct the development of training. When we find a problem with a training package, we will not automatically build additional modules to clarify, but quite possibly remove the material that caused the problem. This is a radical alternative.

It is not easily implemented from an organizational standpoint, because it fundamentally conflicts with the standard practice of providing overly thorough training material and of remedying observed user problems with the addition of further training material. It is not easily implemented from a technical standpoint, because there are very few examples to draw upon and few developers of user assistance and education have any direct experience with Minimalist designs.

GAMBIT 2: WORK WITH THE PROCESS - REAL SYSTEMS

Working with other groups to apply Minimalist advisory designs has emphasized for us the importance of understanding (and of working to improve) the development process. Indeed, Minimalist training and help requires a design process that is different from common practice. For example merely throwing away modules and screens would make materials briefer but not necessarily better. Designing Minimalist training is a process of refining and rejecting interim solutions based on empirical evaluations carried out within the design process itself. The Minimalist model is not deductively strong enough to generate good advisory materials in a single pass from product specifications. In our view this is not a limitation in the model, but a recognition of what the facts of life are in the arena of system design. (Carroll and Rosson, 1985).

We have tried to develop a framework for engineering usability in the design of advisory materials and to apply that framework in our own development case studies. Two case studies of this sort were the Training Wheels interface and the Minimal Manual, both for Displaywriter. In both cases, our starting point was a detailed qualitative understanding of what people did when they tried to learn the system. We inventoried and analyzed the most typical and most serious errors. We noted the tasks that users wanted most to be able to do. We designed to these analyses as usability requirements.

Our Training Wheels interface was designed to block the consequences of major new-user errors. Thus, if a user prematurely selected an advanced function the keystroke would be intercepted and thrown away. Instead of suffering the tangling consequences of such an error, the user was merely informed by a special system message that the function or choice had been disabled in the training system. The Training Wheels design simultaneously allows a reduction in the sheer amount of training material (i.e., error consequences that cannot occur need not be explained) and supports error recovery (by attenuating the consequences of certain serious errors). Most importantly, it accomplishes this by making learning by doing more attractive and more feasible (Carroll, 1984; Carroll and Carrithers, 1984a,b; Catrambone and Carroll, 1987).

The Minimal Manual also stressed brevity, error recovery and learning by doing. It was less than a quarter the length of the standard Displaywriter manual (we eliminated repetition, all summaries, reviews, and practice exercises, and all material not related to doing office work). However, we significantly *increased* error recovery material (like most self study manuals, the original Displaywriter manual had virtually none). For example we had found that learners had trouble with the diskette name concept and often typed an incorrect diskette name when prompted, which had the effect of leaving the system hung up. The system in fact had a specific recovery procedure for this problem, but the commercially developed training manual failed to mention it, and learners did not manage to find it in the ancillary documentation. The Minimal Manual included the specific error recovery information for this error.

One of our chief goals was to help users edit and print out their own documents as quickly as possible. Procedural details were deliberately specified incompletely to encourage learners to become more exploratory, and therefore, we hoped, more highly motivated and involved in the learning activity (e.g., the function of the cursor step-keys was introduced with to "try them and see"). Stress was placed on real familiar tasks. Chapters has titles as "Printing something on paper" instead of "Menus, Messages and Helps" (the latter a real and notorious example). Learners create their first document only seven pages into the Minimal Manual. In the commercial manual the creation of a first document is delayed until page 70, yet this is perhaps the overriding goal of new users. Of course, what is most important is that these ideas do not merely sound right, they have been demonstrated in usability studies (Black, Carroll and McGuigan, 1987; Carroll, 1984; Carroll, Smith-Kerker, Ford, and Mazur, 1986).

We have worked in a consulting role with a wide assortment of system development projects and have been successful in applying the Minimalist advisory model and, to some extent we think, in changing the development process that produces users interfaces and advisory material.

Some of our most recent work is directed at the development of help systems: we see no useful distinction between help and training, but we need to demonstrate that a successful help system loses nothing in being designed to be appropriate for learners. Our approach is to present online help as hypertext (Nelson, 1981): the text is structured as a network instead of as a linear string. Hypertext embeds text at multiple levels in a hierarchy and makes extensive use of crossreferencing. The user can get access to more detailed information by selecting highlighted keywords in the help text. This text design allows the user to control the level of detail accessed and to optionally explore cross-references as well. We are studying the performance of a help system developed by Robert Campell for a popular PC editor in both learning studies and longitudinal monitoring of experts. We hope that this work will enable us to develop a more articulated view than now exists about what on-line help is good for - both *how* it assists new users and the "natural history" of help use over time by experienced users.

GAMBIT 3: PUSH TECHNOLOGY - USER INTERFACE MODELS

Working in the context of system development tightens the lag of the Advisory Interface Dilemma: one still has to wait on the development of new systems, but being a participant in that activity, one is better assured of being able to respond quickly to the results of the system development effort. How can one tighten the lag down to zero? or even get ahead of the development of systems? The answer lies in discovering and developing techniques to get ahead of the real world, to lead the technical future. This is not easy to do.

One approach is to construct "interface models", programs that provide the appearance and some skeletal function for a system that does not yet exist (the term "user interface model" is due to John Richard, I think). Developing interface models, and then studying user performance with these models, allows us to work in an environment we can control, even to get ahead (to some extent) of what *could* be conveniently implemented now if we were only to work on fully functioning systems. As an example, I will briefly describe our current work with the Task Mapper and the Personal Planner interface models.

TaskMapper is a prototype office information system we are implementing in Smalltalk-80 (Goldberg and Robson, 1983). The key interface idea is to represent a task scenario as a path in a two dimensional map. Instead of a messy desk, in which documents and applications can become lost in the active workspace (Carroll and Mazur, 1986), we are investigating an organized desk (Malone, 1983), a task oriented graphic interface. User sessions are initiated from an origin menu in the center of the display. As new applications and documents are selected they are opened along a path, clearly indicating what is related to what. Several paths can be open at a given time, thus addressing "the many small things" phenomenon described by Nielsen, Mack, Bergendorf and Grishkowsky (1986).

In this system, applications are views on collections of objects drawn from a single database. Any piece of data is a document that can be viewed through various editors appropriate to the task at hand. We apply the powerful concepts of database manipulation to documents, as the elements of this office-oriented database, that can be accessed, sorted, and managed according to the structure of the current task rather than stored in a fixed file hierarchy. (See Bobrow and Stefik, 1986, and Williams, 1984, for discussion of the "object oriented" and "query by reformulation" programming paradigms that this work rests upon).

TaskMapper provides some unusual opportunities for us to research on advisory interfaces of the future. We are convinced, based on our prior work, that Minimalists learning-by-doing instructional designs will become typical in the future. TaskMapper, by incorporating some of the leading interface ideas we are aware of, allows us to begin studying learning by doing in an interface style that does not yet exist in the commercial world. We have outlined new approaches to ask oriented help, to training wheels interfaces, and to coordinating tutorial presentation with learner activity for the TaskMapper interface style (Carroll, Herder and Sawtelle, 1986). We can begin now to understand the difficulties users will have with these systems when they become more common.

A second interface model we have developed has allowed us to investigate the role of new media and intelligence in user interfaces. The Personal Planner models a planning application with calendar, to-do list, phone directory, address book, electronic mail, notes, and public bulletin board. It is written in the authoring language Handy (developed by Don Nix at the Watson Research Center), which permits the incorporation of media peripherals like speech synthesizers and video signal. One line of work with the Personal Planner has developed the notion of a scenario machine: a computer application that has coded into it a sequence of user tasks. (Carroll and Kay, 1985).

In the case of Personal Planner, we have designed a scenario in which each task provides intrinsic motivation for the user to undertake the succeeding task. Thus, at the login, the user receives an alert that a mail item has been received, which motivates the goal to read the mail item. The mail item is from a colleague who informs the user that an interesting Bulletin Board item came up that morning, which motivates the goal of going to the Bulletin Board and reading the item, and so on. Such a scenario machine allows us to write "intelligent" error messages: We prescribed the scenario, we know the appropriate goals, hence when the user strays from the path we can deliver intelligent advice. We have shown that dynamically task-oriented advice can help progress through basic user tasks more quickly (McKendree and Carroll, 1987). We also have used the Personal Planner to contrast different approaches to intelligent advice, for example, "step" level advice (e.g., "Select Browser") and "goal" level advice (e.g., "You need to look at your new mail").

Since Handy permits a convenient interface to peripheral output devices, we are also using the Personal Planner to anticipate advisory interface research question in that area. We have constructed a "what is this?" speech help system that explains what a currently pointed at object is. We believe it is important to get some experience with such media, since their increasing availability and lowering costs will create opportunities to incorporate them in systems in the near future. In the particular case of the "what is this?" speech help, Don Kirson, Randy Eckhoff and I are investigating the motivational variable of user control: the spoken help texts are presented contingent on a keypress (User controlled) or contingent on the systems recognition of user pointing (System controlled). We plan to develop an analogous project with integrated video presentation of advisory information.

The gambit of developing interface models is an extremely exciting one. Perhaps the most aggressive response to the Advisory Interface Dilemma is to become a prime mover, to push the interface developers instead of waiting to react. Anticipated requirements for training and help could set user interface requirements. Nevertheless, we do not yet know what our prospects are in pursuing this gambit. In the next of couple years we should be able to see weather we have been able to catalyze new user interface possibilities by presenting existence proofs (in the form of interface models) of new advisory possibilities.

GAMBIT 4: ANTICIPATE TECHNOLOGY - BEHAVIORAL SIMULATIONS

In some cases, creating a user interface model may be inconvenient or infeasible. Another approach is to use behavioral simulations that model some aspect of an imagined system or to contrive a situation that does. Though as mentioned above, some of our work on intelligent advisory systems has been developed in the context of the Personal Planner interface model, most of our work on intelligent help has taken the gambit of investigating behavioral simulations.

One of our projects in this area began by collecting transcripts of human advisors providing computer consultant help to human clients, face to face, via electronic mail, and over telephone. Only very fragile and limited examples of intelligent help systems now exist, and none has been demonstrated to be successful (Carroll and McKendree, 1987). Human advisors actually exist, are robust, and have a record of at least passable success (Coombs and Alty,1980).

Some of our findings could indeed be useful to designers of intelligent help systems. For example, we inventoried and described the many types of roles that the advisors play in these interactions (McKendree and Carroll, 1986). Some of the predominant roles are also the least cognitively demanding (e.g., informing the user about a single piece of information, like a correct command form). In the protocols we have analyzed, the majority of user queries described a result, asking how to achieve or avoid it (Aaronson and Carroll, 1987a). We noted that many dialogs never reached resolution in an "answer" and yet were apparently helpful to the client.

We described the advisors' planning and interfaces in these interactions. For example, in the electronic mail interactions, the advisors clearly planned their advice to preempt the need for the client to ask a follow-up question. The first answer given often added conditional information or pointers to other information sources (Aaronson and Carroll,

1987b). Advisors regularly answer questions other than those explicitly put to them; they answer the question they infer the user really meant.

Some of our findings raise serious questions for the design of intelligent help systems. In our face-to-face advisory dialogs the clients typically articulated specific hypotheses about what was happening in the program, possible sources of the problem and steps in a candidate solution (Aaronson and Carroll, 1987a). We think this serves a variety of useful purposes for the client (e.g. it is a means for elaborating and consolidating an understanding and solution). However, the intelligent help demonstration systems that exist today are generally prepared only to deal with question-answer structures, *not* with dialog structures in which the client poses an answer to which the advisor responds.

To have more control over the advisory dialogs available to us for study, we have developed an apparatus linking two workstations, one of which can take control of the other's display (Carroll and Checco, 1986). Amy Aaronson and I are using this apparatus to simulate intelligent help. We selected a popular database and report application and inventoried the most typical and serious errors for users. We designed advisory dialog for these errors and for situations in which we observed users to hesitate (indicating uncertainty about what to do). We then had people use the system while we remotely monitored their session. When a serious error or hesitation occurred, we sent an intelligent help message - advice that inferred what the user was trying to do based upon the context in which the error occurred.

This sounds easier than it is. In many cases, despite our pre-testing, we had to construct intelligent help messages on the fly - people are very creative in the errors they make. But the most surprising outcome of this work is that it has helped us to see several usability problems for intelligent help. For example from a naive standpoint it is easy to assume that if intelligent help is offered, people will take it. This is not so. Users have their own agenda of goals and there is no way in principle of reliably determining what that agenda is (as people, we cannot always tell what others want to do). Yet if the advice does not perfectly match the current goal, it will very often be ignored. In many cases, our users saw the help, saw the problem, acknowledged that the help was relevant to the problem, and then decided to go on with what they wanted do at that moment, often saying that they would get back to the deferred problem (and often never doing that). What should intelligent help do in this situation?

Intelligent help will also have credibility problems. When the user misexecutes a correct suggestion from the help system, it is natural for the user to consider the possibility that the help system was wrong. This may be unfair, but we saw it happen. What can intelligent help systems do about this? A user who begins to question the authority and the competence of the help system will be even more likely to defer or ignore its suggestions, may thereby risk further tangling errors, and as a result make it more difficult for the help system to provide competent help! This work is very exiting. It raises the possibility that by anticipating technology with behavioral simulations we might be able to redirect the development of new technology so that it produces advisory systems. In the specific case of intelligent help we might be able to help determine what is worth building *before* the investment.

GAMBIT 5: EXPLORE ISSUES THAT ARE FUNDAMENTAL

The nub of the Advisory Interface Dilemma is that new technology must in some sense exit before we can begin to worry about how to instruct and assist people in using it. However, one approach to this is to question the presupposition: aren't there technology-free issues? One has to be careful. As a cognitive psychologist by training, I am well aware of the limited impact basic psychology has had on applied questions. Nevertheless, it seems that particularly in areas where there has been little prior work or in which any understanding would have pervasive implications for the design of user interfaces and advisory systems that being fundamental can be a very practical approach.

We have taken this gambit in several areas. For example, we have tried to understand how prior knowledge can be codified in interface metaphors to help people learn appropriate models of the system function (Carroll and Thomas, 1982; Carroll and Mack, 1985). The use of the "typewriter" metaphor in the design of word processing applications and the "messy desktop" metaphor in integrated packages like Lisa are well known. The logic behind these designs is simple: if the user already understands desktops and the appearance and operations of the electronic desktop is similar to that of a real desktop, then there can be a savings in learning and skill.

Our studies of people learning and using systems have convinced us that metaphors can be conceptual aids as much because they *mismatch* their targets as because they match. Pressing character keys elicits glowing dots on a TV screen rather than of lines of ink on a paper; these are really very different effects. And typing over characters on the screen replaces the prior characters or inserts the new characters, although *both* outcomes are unpredictable on the basis of literal metaphor projection. Indeed, given a simple view of metaphor, it is remarkable that neither of these metaphor misfits has a very troubling consequence for the learners. In fact, encountering these misfits can afford a concrete opportunity for developing an enhanced understanding of the electronic medium (e.g., the concept of dynamic storage).

However, for a metaphor mismatch to be an efficacious learning tool it is critical that it occurs in the context of obvious consistency. Learners want and need to solve problems in order to learn actively, but to do this they need to be able to discern what the problem is. There must be a background of predictability for them to notice what is novel. A new user of the Lisa was trying to create a document and was prompted to "tear off paper", in the context of an icon representing a pad of paper. The user took the prompted quite literally and tried to devise some action of "tearing" or sweeping the cursor across the desktop and the icon representing a pad of paper. The metaphor in this case was a mismatch: actions applied to objects like files (or applications) must be selected from menus which describe the actions in the Lisa. The metaphor was not a failure however. The experience provided a key insight - not only into how to select actions in this interface, but about the boundary conditions for the interface metaphor (see also Carroll and Rosson, 1987).

Another fundamental project is our effort to better understand the roles that motivation and emotion play in user interfaces and advisory systems. It is a puzzle that while few would debate the claim that motivation and emotion are first order factors in usability (perhaps more potent than the cognitive factors which are so widely studied), very little research has yet been directed at these factors (Carroll, 1982; Malone, 1981). In fact, it is quite common to find that experiences like "fun" are systematically confused with properties like "ease of use" and hence undermine the conceptual integrity of usability (Carroll and Thomas, 1987).

Software can evoke a variety of strong reactions from people. Terms such as "fascinating", "fun", "interesting", "entertaining", even "addicting" are often used when people describe their positive reactions to software. These terms reflected cognitive/emotional states that have strong implications for the quality of users' experience with software. We are using the Conceptual Encounter interview technique of de Rivera (1981) to collect protocols on what it means to be fascinated, interested, entertained, etc. by software; what it is about specific events that evokes these experiences; how different emotional experiences can interact (Kirson and Carroll, 1987) Unfortunately, current software practice can evoke positive emotional experiences for users only inconsistently. There are no guidelines for creating software that elicits these positive reactions. Our goal is to provide an understanding of the emotional concomitants of software that could help designers more deliberately evoke these experiences.

PROSPECTS

I think it is useful for researchers interested in user education and user assistance to worry about the Advisory Interface Dilemma when they select and design projects to work on. My belief is that much current research is out of date before it is ever completed. This is just not acceptable. Just as we have found that it is often impossible to scale up basic psychology laboratory studies to make them relevant and useful in settling system design questions, I think we will find that studying usability and advisory problems of old technology will frequently not be relevant or useful in settling design questions for new technology. We cannot expect to be seers and magicians; we cannot do empirical research on figments of someone else's imagination. But we can try to do the best we can do.

I have outlined a five-pronged attack on this problem. We can provide practical models, like the Minimalist training model, models with less-than-deductive strength, but models that provide useful abstractions and guidance for designers. We can work with the design process: we have to since our practical models will have to function within that process and since the new technologies we need to use and to develop for new advisory interfaces emerge from it. We need to push technology ahead of itself too, to develop interface models as existence proofs of new possibilities. We need to anticipate things that can not even be modeled, where possible to help set constraints on technologies that do not now exist, to help determine what technologies will be available in the future for advisory interfaces. Finally, we need to break ground on fundamental issues, to investigate questions that will be good questions whatever our technological futures.

These are not alternatives, they are complementary modes of attack on the Advisory Interface Dilemma. Are there other gambits? I hope so - this list isn't long enough. I think the approaches I have outlined are promising. I am personally encouraged by the progress our group has made and directions in which we have begun to move. I hope that the many pointers I have included to our other published work will be useful to others in confronting these issues. I think I am worrying less about Advisory Interface Dilemma than I was two years ago, but I still keep my eye on it.

FOOTNOTE

I am grateful to Amy Aaronson, Robert Campbell, Rick Herder, Don Kirson, and of course to Mary Beth Rosson for helpful discussions and comments while I was preparing this chapter.

REFERENCES

Aaronson, A.P. and Carroll, J.M. (1987a). The answer is in the question: A protocol study of intelligent help. To be published in *Behavior and Information Technology*, 1987.

Aaronson, A.P. and Carroll, J.M. (1987b). Intelligent help in a one-shot dialog: A protocol study. In J.M. Carroll and P.P. Tanner (Eds.), *Proceedings of CHI+GI'87 Human Factors in Computing systems and Graphic Interface.* (Toronto, April 5-9) ACM New York.

Black, J.B., Carroll, J.M., and McGuigan, S.M. (1987). What kind of minimal instructional manual is most effective. In J.M. Carroll and P.P. Tanner (Eds.), *Proceedings of CHI+GI'87 Human Factors in Computing systems and Graphic Interface.* (Toronto, April 5-9) ACM New York.

Borow, D.G., and Stefik, M.J. (1986). Perspectives on artificial intelligence programming. *Science, 231,* February 28, 951.

Carroll, J.M. (1982). The adventure of getting to know a computer. *IEEE Computer, 15/11,* 49-58.

Carroll, J.M. (1984). Minimalist training. *Datamation, 30/18* (November 1, 1984), 125-136.

Carroll, J.M., and Campbell, R.L. (1986). Softening up hard science: Reply to Newell and Card. *Human Computer Interaction, 2,* in press.

Carroll, J.M. and Carrithers, C. (1984a). Training wheels in a user interface. *Communications of the ACM, 27,* 800-806.

Carroll, J.M. and Carrithers, C. (1984b). *Human Factors, 26/4,* 377-389.

Carroll, J.M., Herder, R.E., and Sawtelle, D. (1987). TaskMapper. *IBM Research Report.* (shortened version to appear in Proceedings of INTERACT'87).

Carroll, J.M. and Kay, D.S. (1985). Prompting, feedback and error correction in the design of a Scenario Machine. In L. Borman and B. Curtis (Eds.), *Proceedings of CHI'85 Human Factors in Computing Systems.* (San Francisco, April 14-18). ACM, New York, 149-154.

Carroll, J.M. Smith-Kerker, P.A., Ford, J.R., Mazur, S.A. (1986). The minimal manual. *IBM Research Report 11637.*

Carroll, J.M. and Mack, R.L. (1985). Metaphor, computing systems, and active learning. *International Journal of Man-Machine Studies, 22,* 39-57.

Carroll, J.M. and Mack, R. L. (1984). Learning to use a word processor: By doing, by thinking, and knowing. In J.C. Thomas and M. Schneider (Eds.), *Human factors of computing systems.* Ablex, Norwood, NJ.

Carroll, J.M., Mack, R.L., Lewis, C.H., Grischkowsky, N.L. and Robertson, S.R. (1985). Exploring a word processor. *Human Computer Interaction, 1,* 283-307.

Carroll, J.M. and Mazur, S.A. (1986). LisaLearning. *IEEE Computer, 19/11,* 35-49.

Carroll, J.M. and McKendree, J. (1987). Interface design issues for advice-giving expert systems. *Communication of the ACM, 30,* 14-31.

Carroll, J.M. and Rosson, M.B. (1987). Paradox of the active user. In J.M. Carroll (Ed) *Interfacing Thought: Cognitive aspects of human-computer interaction.* MIT Press, Cambridge, MA.

Carroll, J.M. and Thomas, J.C. (1982). Metaphor and the cognitive representation of computing systems. *IEEE Transactions on Systems, Man, and Cybernetics, SMC-12,* 107-116.

Carroll, J.M. and Thomas, J.C. (1986). Fun. *IBM Research Report 12267.*

Catrambone, R. and Carroll, J.M. (1987). Learning a word processing system with training wheels and guided exploration. In J.M. Carroll and P.P. Tanner *Proceedings of CHI+GI'87 Human Factors in Computing systems and Graphic Interface.* (Toronto, April 5-9) ACM New York.

Checco, J.C. and Carroll, J. M. (1986). SmartHelp. *IBM Research Report 12371.*

Coombs, M.J. and Alty, J.L. (1980). Face-to-face guidance of university user--II: Characterizing advisory interactions. *International Journal of Man-Machine Studies, 12,* 407-429.

de Rivera, J. (Ed.) (1981). *Conceptual encounter: A method for the exploration of human experience.* University Press of America, Washington, D:C:

Gagne, R.M. and Briggs, L.J. (1979). *Principles of instructional design.* Holt, Rinehart, and Winston, New York, 2nd Edition.

Goldberg, A. and Robson, D. (1983). *Smalltalk-80: The language and its implementation.* Addison-Wesley, Reading, MA.

Kirson, D. and Carroll, J.M. (1987). The emotions of software. To appear in Proceeding of *INTERACT'87.*

Mack, R.L.,Lewis, C.H., and Carroll, J.M. (1983). Learning to use a word processor: Problems and prospects. *ACM Transactions on Office Information Systems, 1/3,* 254-271.

Malone, T.W. (1981). Toward a theory of intrinsically motivating instruction. *Cognitive Science, 4,* 333-369.

Malone, T.W. (1983). How do people organize their desks? Implication for the design of office information systems. *ACM Transactions on Office Information Systems, 1,* 99-112.

McKendree, J. and Carroll, J.M. (1986). Advising roles of a computer consultant. In M. Mantei and P. Orbeton (Eds.), *Proceedings of CHI'86 Human Factors in Computing Systems* (Boston, April 13-17), ACM, New York, 35-40.

McKendree, J. and Carroll, J.M. (1987). Impact of feedback content on initial learning of an office system. To appear in Proceeding of *INTERACT'87.*

Merking, M. (1983). In love with Lisa. *Creative Computing,* (October), 12-17.

Nelson, T.H. (1981). *Literary Machines,* Swarthmore, Pa.

Nielsen, J., Mack, R.L., Bergendorff, K.H., and Grischkowsky, N.L. (1986). Integrated Software Usage in the Professional Work Environment: Evidence from Questionnaires and Interviews. In M. Mantei and P. Orbeton (Eds.), *Proceedings of CHI'86 Human Factors in Computing Systems* (Boston, April 13-17), ACM, New York.

Williams, G. (1983). The Lisa Computer System. *BYTE*, (February), 33-50.

Williams, M.D. (1984). What makes Rabbit run? *International Journal of Man-Machine Studies, 21*, 333-352.

Psychological Issues of
Human Computer Interaction in the Work Place
M. Frese, E. Ulich, W. Dzida (Editors)
© Elsevier Science Publishers B.V. (North-Holland), 1987

MENTAL MODELS IN LEARNING COMPUTERIZED TASKS

Yvonne Waern

Dept. of Psychology, University of Stockholm, S-106 91 Stockholm
Sweden

A mental model has two characteristics: 1) it represents some part of reality and 2) it is to some extent similar to that part of reality. The model may resemble reality in three respects: 1) as regards functions in which case only the output of the process is modelled, 2) as regards process, in which the steps in the processes are mapped, and 3) as regards structure, in which case the structure generating the process is mapped into the model. A user of a computer system needs a mental model for planning, problem solving, communicating ideas and stimulating creative thinking. Different empirical examples of these functions are presented. It is suggested that a computer system can facilitate learning by mental models in three different ways: 1) by presenting a model which is an analogue to some prior task, 2) by creating a consistent model for new concepts, and 3) by facilitating the learners' exploratory creation of own models.

INTRODUCTION

The reader may wonder what is so distinctive about the learning of computerized tasks, to warrant separate consideration. I'll argue here that there are at least two reasons which make the learning of computerized tasks different from learning new languages, or mathematics, or the capitals of the African countries.

The first difference is related to the fact that the learners are not school-children. In schools we usually encounter children or young adults who expect to be taught. In the computer learning situation, we generally encounter adults who are experts at a particular task, who want to go on being experts at this task and who want to perform it as well as possible. They are usually not particularly interested in the computer system for any reason except that it may help to improve their performance of the central task.

The most important difference between young pupils and adult experts lies in the learning strategies. In a new learning situation adult learners will most certainly try to rely as far as possible on prior knowledge. This means that adult experts will plan their actions with the system, will expect particular things to happen, and will interpret what happens with respect to how it fits into their knowledge of similar tasks which they have performed before.

The second reason relates to the arbitrary and unconventional relationship between computer systems and the world outside of computers. People who meet a new computer system have very little chance to know in advance how this system relates to their prior knowledge, be it the outer reality or other computer systems. Not only do different program systems to some extent perform different functions, but they also require that their users interact with them in ways which may be very different from system to system. This arbitrariness is very different from the arbitrariness of for instance mathematics or natural language. Computer systems are neither based on any common reality, neither on any agreed upon consistent set of concepts. They therefore require that their users acquire a new set of concepts as well as a new set of designations of these concepts.

These two factors combined, i.e. the need to use prior knowledge in situations where it may not be applicable, and the need to acquire unfamiliar concepts, lead to a situation where confusion easily can arise. In the workplace this situation can be handled in several different ways. The user can be carefully instructed in the details of each new concept. The user can be offered only a subset of concepts and functions in the system in order to keep the complexity within reasonable limits. However, to enable users to develop their competence in extending the use of the system to new tasks something more is necessary. The users have to acquire (by themselves or by instruction) some conceptual tool which helps them to overview those parts of the system which they need in order to perform both routine tasks and those nonpredicted exceptions, which always occur.

The suggested tool to help computer users to place the new concepts in the context of their prior knowledge is the "mental model". (Halasz & Moran, 1983, Norman, 1983). A mental model may be explicitly taught by the system designers or system trainers, or it may be developed by the users themselves. Each meaningful learning will in some way or other involve a mental model.

This need for a conceptual tool does not only pertain to the user. System designers need tools, both to understand the user's task and how to perform it in the computer system. Instructors about computer systems need tools to describe the system to the users.

This chapter aims at analyzing the role of the mental model in learning computerized tasks. The problem will therefore be dealt with from the point of view of the user. The system designer and instructor may have different problems, and for them the mental models may be different and even play different roles.

SOME CHARACTERISTICS OF THE "MODEL" CONCEPT

Definitions

The concept of mental model as currently used by researchers in the field of human-computer interaction is prescientific. It is used to explain observations and to stir imagination, rather than to test hypotheses. There is no agreement on the definition of the model, on what it refers to or how it functions in the thought processes of the individual.

The dictionary definitions of the word "model" does not give us much help with understanding the concept, by examples as:
- A person who poses
- A copy
- The original pattern according to which other items are made
- A miniature representation of a thing (selected examples from Webster's unabridged dictionary).

In psychology, the following definitions may be more useful, the first one suggested by Craik (1943):

> *"By a model we ... mean any physical or chemical system which has a similar relation-structure to that of the processes it imitates. By 'relation structure' I ... mean ... the fact that it is a physical working model which works in the same way as the processes it parallels, in the aspects under consideration at any moment ..."*

The second is put forward by Chapanis (1961):

> *"Models are analogies. Scientific or engineering models are representations, or likenesses, of certain aspects of complex events, structures systems, made by using symbols or objects which in some way resemble the thing being modelled".*

Two points are essential in both definitions: the idea that a model represents reality, i.e. is symbolic, and the idea that the model has a structure similar to that of reality.

That a model should represent something which is to be modelled is unlikely to cause much trouble (except if we believe in pure idealism). The similarity aspect, however is much more difficult to capture. What is similar between a model and the thing modelled?

Different kinds of modelling

In a computer situation, the reality to be modelled is dynamic, i.e. it consists of goals to be reached and actions to be performed. Then there are at least three aspects, in which we can envisage some similarity between model and reality. These aspects correspond to the questions: "WHAT is performed?", "HOW is it performed?", and "WHY does the thing modelled function as it does?". In an individual's mental model of a computer situation all these questions may be included.

The WHAT question refers to superficial performance: a music cassette gives us music as does a gramophone record. The output is the same, although the medium whereby the music is stored and retrieved in the two cases is quite different. In a computer situation, a model based upon performance similarity contains enough information to enable a user to understand the functional properties of a system. When a wordprocessing system is compared to a typewriter, only superficial characteristics are considered. The keyboard is similar to a typewriter's keyboard, the text on the screen is similar to a text on paper. This does not mean that the typewriter is a sufficient model of all the functional properties of a wordprocessing system, but it suffices to cover some of the functions. It should be noted that this functional similarity does not include the processes by which actions are performed, nor the underlying structure of the systems.

The next aspect of similarity concerns the HOW question, i.e. the processes by which an action is performed. For any particular function it is much more difficult to find a model which is similar to reality in its processes than to find one possessing functional similarity only. This difficulty indicates that a user may go through several different answers to the HOW-question, before arriving at an answer which is valid for the system concerned.

We can take an example of human-computer interaction: The user of different wordprocessing systems can find some functions which could be based on similar processes, but which are not. The functions of inserting and overwriting are two good examples. Inserting means that you always put the text typed in at the place where the cursor is, and push the rest of the text towards the end (rightwards and downwards). This means, that if you want to delete anything in the text, you must issue a specific delete command. Overwriting means that the text typed writes over the already existing text. This means that no particular delete command has to be issued for the text typed over. In some systems, inserting is default, in others overwriting. In others again, you can switch easily between "insert" and "overwrite" mode. This means that the user has to be very careful about the processes used for inserting and overwriting, when changing systems. One system cannot be used as a model of the other where the process aspect is concerned. As regards the functional aspect, however, they are sufficiently similar to allow one to be modelled by the other.

Lastly, the WHY question concerns the structure of reality. Only a model which is structurally similar to reality can answer the question WHY. This is an aspect of systems modelling, which few users have to bother with. It concerns the actual implementation of a system. The programming language, the methods for addressing memories, and allocating resources, as well as the particular hardware employed all answer the question WHY. We know that these details do not usually affect the functions a system can offer. They do not generally affect the processes either (from the point of view of the user). But they concern those who have to get the systems to work. Even the users of small PCs must have at least some sort of fragmentary model of the apparatus they are using. They have to understand that disks may get full, that files may get overwritten and that it may not be possible to run some programs on their own particular computer. All these matters to some extent call for a model of structural aspects.

Users thus need and will develop models which embrace functional and process similarities in relation to the reality being modelled.

What reality is covered by a system model?

The reality to be embraced by the user's mental model is the computer system. This reality is by no means well defined, and we have to ask what is meant by the "computer system". First it must be recognized that a computer system's reality differs from user to user; it can vary because of the way the computer is actually used. We can distinguish here between "application tasks", such as wordprocessing, book-keeping, data base processing, and "system tasks", concerned with handling the computer system itself. To a user engaged in an application task, the computer reality is contained in the concepts and procedures required to perform the particular task. This means that a user of a wordprocessing system will be primarily concerned with the reality of concepts such as words and lines, paragraphs and pages, and with corresponding activities such as typing, deleting, inserting, justifying, etc. An application user should in a well designed system not note any difference between the "system" and the "task in the system".

The distinction between "application" and "system" tasks is not quite clear and allows for some overlap, particularly when subtasks are concerned. For instance, what would we call the task to create a "macro" to perform a wordprocessing subtask quicker? And would we be willing to call the handling of workstations, such as positioning of windows and pulling down of menus, "system" tasks? Particularly when workstations are concerned it is obvious that many tasks are preparatory to the actual work with the application task. A user's "mental model of the task in the system" will then have to include such preparatory actions as well as the actions aimed at performing the task.

Allowing some fuzziness, we can say that systems programmers are mainly working with "system tasks". For them, the distinction between the different kinds of actions, system actions, operating system actions, work station actions and application task actions is likely to be very relevant. Their computer reality is very different from the reality encountered by an "ordinary" user. The application task to be performed by a potential user involves just one of several possible functions which could be realized by the computer structure created by the system designers. Since they know several systems, several programming languages, several operating systems, etc., they can make a choice about which reality to present to the users on a basis of this knowledge. The system task will consist of getting the system to perform the functions specified by this reality and to allow the user to use some particular processes in order to get these application functions done.

Reality does not only differ in its content, but also in its scope. We should be very cautious in speaking of a "system model". Virtually no user will possess a model of the system as a whole (not even a systems programmer). Each user selects his own part of the task in the system reality for modelling. For instance, the user of a wordprocessing facility on a mainframe computer may need to use some parts only of the whole operating system, i.e. those that are concerned with handling files and getting files printed. Nonetheless the user may have to handle a very involved reality in terms of wordprocessing. The system operator, on the other hand, may be more concerned with the operating system's reality and less concerned with the distinctions necessary in a wordprocessing task. Thus a system programmer may be familiar with many different inner tasks, but remain rather ignorant about the outer tasks.

This difference between the realities of system users engaged on different tasks, and even more between "end users" and system designers, gives rise to a corresponding disparity in their system models and their task models.

We can thus conclude from the above that any consideration of users' "system models" must also take into account the reality to which the model refers.

The conceptual status of a mental model

When researchers and systems designers create models of systems or of users, the models are explicit. But what about users? Is the model an entity of which the users are aware? Or is it an implicit reality which represents unknown obstacles as well as invisible support?

Researchers and systems designers have used the concept of the mental model in different ways. But when it is claimed that users need system models in order to learn new systems (Carroll & Thomas 1980, Carroll & Mack, 1985, Halasz & Moran, 1983, Mayer, 1981), it is explicit models that are meant. Given that a model can resemble its modelled reality in different ways (in terms of functions, processes, or structures), one model can also enjoy varying conceptual status with respect to the different aspects. A model may be explicit in the functional dimension without being explicit as regards processes or structure. It may be explicit as regards processes but implicit as regards structure. It is also possible that people who can represent the structure of reality in a model are nevertheless unaware of the consequences in terms of processes and functions.

In the following pages I will focus on mainly the effects of models as distinct conceptual entities. I thus look upon computer users as "creating" models, "understanding" models, and "comparing" models and observations. The explicit comparison may concern different aspects. At the same time I do not exclude the possibility that people simply act, without making any conscious representation of the relevant reality.

Functions of Mental Models.

Models are not the same as reality. They are simply similar to reality in certain respects. Models can even be partly false, and still be useful. Which immediately evokes the question: useful for what?

In the introduction I suggested that mental models functioned as a conceptual tool to handle the arbitrariness and nonconventionality of concepts related to computerized tasks. Now let me develop that suggestion a little further.

Mental Models For Planning

One important function of models relates to planning, which is expressed in the following quotation from Craik (1943):

"If the organism carries a 'small- scale model' of external reality and of its own possible actions within its head, it is able to try out various alternatives, conclude which is the best of them, react to future situations before they arise, utilize the knowledge of past events in dealing with the present and future, and in every way to react in a much fuller, safer, and more competent manner to the emergencies which face it."

This function of a mental model is related to its symbolic nature. Without a model we should have to act out all possible actions, and we should not be able to predict their outcomes. Thus models give a shortcut to action. If they are valid, of course.

Mental Models For Observation And Interpretation

There are two important ingredients in learning: observing the situation and the outcomes from actions, and interpreting the effects of actions. In both cases models serve important functions. The mental models will determine what a user observes on the screen. Quick, flashing messages will not be observed if the user cannot fit them into his mental model. Some systems for instance indicate that they are working internally by a very small signal, which is easily overlooked by a user who has got the mental model that the system does what he tells it to do and nothing else.

When something unexpected happens, the mental model will determine how the user interprets the event. Since the event is unexpected, it cannot be totally explained by the existing mental model. However, only minor changes may be necessary in order to incorporate the event in the existing model. If the mental model seems totally out of place, the person will feel confused and cannot make any sense of the event. Due to the circumstances, a user of a computer system can in this situation either give up trying to understand the event or continue to work towards another model, which eventually can embrace the event.

A mental model will thus have an important function for both observation and interpretation. Without a mental model, important events may not be noticed, and if noticed, their importance may not be appreciated.

Mental Models For Problem Solving

When a novice encounters a new computer system and wants to perform a task he/she has not performed before, the situation is very much similar to a problem solving situation. There is a goal (the accomplished task), an initial situation (the current situation as perceived by the user) and the user does not know how to proceed from the initial situation to the goal situation.

An analysis of the problem solving situation for the computer related task is the following: The user has to understand what kinds of concepts the task involves in order to be performed by the system. He also has to understand what can be done in order to change the current situation to some other, i.e. what operations he can perform in the situation. The understanding of relevant concepts and operations is equivalent to what in problem solving terminology is called the "problem space" (cf. Newell & Simon, 1972).

The understanding is not enough, however. The user also has to try out different ways to proceed, i.e. what sequences of operations to perform in order to go the whole way from the initial situation to the goal. This trying out is in problem solving terminology called the "search in the problem space" (Newell & Simon, 1972).

In the creation of the problem space, a model facilitates the finding of adequate concepts and operations. Some researchers have even suggested that the model can be regarded as the problem space, in which the problem solver operates (Halasz & Moran, 1982, Young, 1983). As an example, we can take the model of a typewriter given to a user of a word-processing system. This model furnishes the concepts of letters and lines and the operations of typing in and deleting, as well as moving over the text by the space bar, the tabulator, or the linefeed key.

An important property of a model is its ability to simplify reality by leaving out irrelevant details, or by chunking concepts and procedures. A really good model would allow the user to overview the whole problem space at once, thus eliminating the need to try out different alternatives, i.e. the need for search. In some computer interfaces, the need for extra search due to the system is drastically reduced by making the system as similar to reality that it almost feels as if you were working with reality. Direct manipulation interfaces allow for such analogical models.

However, sometimes search in the problem space is necessary. This is the case when the system requires long sequences of operations, and the user does not know yet what sequence will perform the job. This is also the case when the problem is complex and involves several different natural steps. In both cases, the problem space is big enough that the user cannot review it as a whole. The bigger the problem space, the more search is necessary, and the greater the risk of getting lost. Here a more abstract model than the analogical one can facilitate by suggesting different ways to search the problem space. Heuristics, or thumb-rules can be contained in the model, as well as explicit algorithms.

We can thus agree that models serve important functions in problem solving. Quite different questions concern how models can be transferred from one person to another (the educational problem) and how users create helpful models themselves. The later question will be covered to some extent below.

Mental Models in Skilled Performance

Expert users of particular computer systems for particular tasks do not encounter problems in the system as often as novices. Instead, the models they use can be regarded as facilitating their skilled performance. In this case, the models provide the user with efficient procedures by rules which specify what methods to use in order to achieve a particular goal in a particular situation. For instance, expert users of a wordprocessing system can have rules to decide when to use the overwrite mode (when the new word is shorter than the one to be changed, for instance), as well as rules to decide what particular method to use for "cut and paste" operations. They will probably have rules to decide what names to give to different texts and different versions of the text, as well as rules to decide how many versions to keep.

It is possible that some of these rules are automated in order to speed up performance (Card, Moran & Newell, 1983). In such a case, the user is not aware of the model while performing the actions (awareness would slow down performance). The users can then "trigger" and "run" the models automatically. This does not prevent the user from being able to think about the model before performing the action (in planning) or afterwards (in explaining to somebody else).

Mental Models In Communication

Another important function of models stems from the need for communication. People do not only work on problems or take actions, they also talk to each other about actions and problems. Communication represents one important way of getting to know about the world. If people are to understand one another, messages should be based on agreed and unequivocal concepts, and it should be possible for everyone engaged in the communication to handle the complexities of the problem.

A model which can perform these functions has to fulfill more severe requirements than one which is employed for personal purposes only. The model must be simple, yet expressive, it must be comprehensive, yet understandable, it must use conventional means of expression, yet cover the relevant aspects of the problem.

These characteristics of models are usually covered by natural language. In most ordinary life circumstances we can convey what we mean by natural language, even though natural language is vague and rather informal. This is due to the fact that we in an ordinary human conversation almost always talk about things which refer to a common reality or at least to a common set of concepts. If the understanding breaks down, we further can change our ways of expressing things.

Communicating system models may be much more difficult, however. First the system models may not refer to a common reality for different kinds of users, particularly not for so called "end users" and system designers. Second, the natural language may not have words which correspond to the concepts necessary. We find for instance difficulties with how to express the concept of "files". For a word-processor, the concept of "text" could be more appropriate, for a mail system the concept of "letter".

This makes the need for models pertinent for communicating concepts which are foreign to computer-naive users or which have no unambiguous translations in natural language. By finding up a model which covers several concepts communication can be facilitated. Even if the single word is not quite adequate, according to the natural use, it can be understood by the context which the model furnishes. Again the direct manipulation systems by analogies can be taken as example of models which fulfill the communication purpose. Users can talk to each other as well as to the system designers with terms taken from the analogy. It is much easier to tell somebody who is not used to computer concepts that "you can have only one text at a time at the clip-board" than to explain the meaning of "the buffer can only accomodate one file".

Models In Creative Thinking

The last function of models to be discussed here is that of providing a spur to creative thinking. Two factors can be seen as responsible for creating new outcomes. One factor relates to generalization. The other relates to conflicts.

Creativity by generalization results when ideas which are relevant in a particular context are applied to another context. Sometimes such generalized applications do not function due to the restrictions of nature. Sometimes they are so common that the resulting result seems trivial rather than creative. This applies to children saying "childs" instead of "children" or "cutted" instead of "cut". A similar transcendence of boundaries can however lead to what is regarded to be big creative leaps, as when for instance Descartes detected the relationship between geometric and algebraic concepts and thus created analytic geometry. A model can thus lead to creative results, when it is applied to a new context, and when it works in that new context.

The factor of conflict is another important impulse to creative thinking. How can models function by conflict? We must remember that models are similar to, but not the same as reality. Some disparity will always remain between the model and the reality modelled. The difference may be less serious as regards some parts of reality and more serious as regards other. One model may be entirely appropriate to certain tasks, and quite unapplicable to others.

Since people often try to simplify things by using the same model in different situations, models are sometimes applied to parts of reality for which they were not originally intended. If a model does not fit a particular section of reality, the person will perceive a conflict. Conceptual conflict of this kind triggers conceptual activity. Different ways of resolving the conflict will be tested, both mentally and in practice. This is one of the chief ways in which science proceeds. But even our everyday thinking depends on this sort of conceptual activity. We have to question the range of application of models as well as the models themselves, and this in turn may mean that the range of reality represented and thus the models used will have to be changed.

The present-day computer user is quite likely to encounter conflict between the model he employs to understand the system and the output of the computer system. This may be due to inconsistencies in the system itself or inconsistencies between the system and its documentation, or to unwarranted assumptions on part of the user. Whatever its cause, this kind of conflict can start the user off on a creative train of thought about the system. He may ask himself: What if... and: Why not? Conflict may trigger exploratory activity, as well as attempts at creating new and better models.

SOME EMPIRICAL DATA ON THE ROLE OF MODELS IN LEARNING

The reader might now be persuaded that mental models have important functions for human planning and interpretation, for problem solving, communication and creativity. Since learning includes all these different activities models should indeed be important in learning. The interested reader should however deserve some empirical demonstrations of the role of models in learning.

In order to make the points quite clear I have chosen a very particular, seemingly simple task. We can regard this example as just one small particle in the whole jungle of tasks which an office worker encounters in learning a new computer system. The task is chosen as an illustration because it represents a new challenge to the users. The users have been taught a particular word-processing system, but they have not been explicitly taught how to perform this particular task. As we shall see, the task turned out to be much more difficult than expected, and the users' struggles with the task are illuminating as to how mental models are used and developed.

This is the situation studied. Students, who had no experience with wordprocessing were trained in a very simple screen-oriented word-processing system, containing only seven commands (except the cursor movements). After this training, they were given a table, where some numbers were displaced. They were asked to fix the table so that all columns were straight. The system did not allow them to perform automatic column alignments. An example of one task is given in the table below. The subjects were asked to think aloud while performing the tasks.

Table 1. Example task

	Grade 3		Grade 4		Grade 5	
Question 1	2.07		1.53		1.37	
Question 2	2.28		2.11		0.63	
Question 3		3.13		2.96		2.59
Question 4	2.67		2.19		1.59	

The commands which the users had been taught contained "insert" and "delete". The insert command took the signs to be inserted as argument, and caused the signs to the right of the insertion position to be moved rightwards. The delete command took the number of signs to be deleted as argument and caused the signs to the right of the deletion position to be moved leftwards. Thus the most efficient way to perform this particular task is to position the cursor immediately after "question three" and give the command to delete three signs. Thereby three blank signs are deleted, and the row moved three steps towards the left. For rightward movements, an "insert" command can be issued, by inserting three blanks, produced by the space bar. Further details about this investigation can be found in Waern & Rabenius (1986).

Models Used For Planning

Due to the empirical data collected it is impossible to tell whether or not the subjects would have performed an explicit planning. Since they were required to think aloud, they expressed their plans and actions. What is more interesting to note is the type of planning performed. The following comments were typical in the beginning of the session:

(Subject 43)

"The easiest way must be to take the numbers out and then write them back in again. But I can't delete the whole row, because then I won't remember what to write. So let me start at the 3, delete it, and write it there instead. And then I'll take the next."

(Subject 8)

"So I take away this 3, and put it here instead, and I take away next, and put it here."

We see that the comments refer exclusively to procedures to perform the task. The model then can be regarded as a direct reflection of the actual procedures performed. This kind of model does not serve well for any other of the functions (interpretation, problem solving, communication or creation).

The procedural orientation is quite natural to planning. Therefore it can be interesting to see what happens when the subjects have encountered some more tasks. Here is one example:

(Subject 4)

"I don't want to write each digit. It should be possible to take all at once. But then you have to tell it where to start..."

The plan here is related to a dissatisfaction. The subject has however not yet developed any model which can help her to find a good procedure for her new plan. This model cannot be found until the subjects notice what happens and interprets the events. Let's look at the functions of models in those situations.

Models Used For Observation And Interpretation

It was suggested above that models were important in observing results of actions and in interpreting these results. The empirical data indicate that models are not be as important for observation as expected. It was found that many subjects did not notice the movements caused by their actions. But many of them noticed the movements, even though they did not have any models, within which to place the observations. The following comment is an example of observation without interpretation:

(Subject 4)

"Interesting that they move. Here, they're very close, the columns, and then you find that they move to the right."

However, observations of the movements were necessary to form interpretations about the effects which in some way hinted about a process model:

(Subject 4):

"Hmmm ... is that why they move? That they push a whole row? Well, I'll have to figure that out later..."

(Subject 33):

"Whether or not there is a sign, the machine will look at it as if I took away 3 signs, and then everything jumps, the text is displaced the same number of signs as I put there."

We see in the comments of Subject 4 that interpretations are not always performed. Thus we can say that explicit models are not always worked out. Sometimes the subjects are so eager to continue their work that they do not stop for reflecting. Subject 33 has however formed an interpretation, which reflects a useful model. The model is formed in terms of a process, with some anthropomorphic accent.

Models Used For Problem Solving

The interpretations which the subjects give of the effects of their actions give us a hint of their problem space. Some comments indicate that subjects during their work with the tasks changed the concepts, i.e. their problem space. One change relates to the concept of "separate numbers" to the concept of "a row as a whole". This change is evident in the following comment:

(Subject 46)

"I never dreamt that you really could move all the columns in a row. It took a while before I found that out."

This changed problem space helps the user to find a method to perform the task, which is related to the idea of rows:

(Subject 46):
"To move it to the left I push Esc and then the number of ... eehhh ... let's call them marks ... which are needed to move the row to the left and then I push D, and then you give the command. Then the whole text on the row is moved to the left - I think. Because it's not just the remaining text after the cursor which is moved."

In this comment we see that the subject did not quite understand the problem (the operation and its effect was still unclear) The most difficult thing to understand in the problem is that blanks are equivalent to other signs (letters, numbers). This difficulty is clearly evident in the following comment:

(Subject 47):
The experimenter demonstrated the effect of deleting three blanks.
Experimenter: *"I took away three signs. What did I take away?"*
Subject: *"Three squares on that screen."*
Experimenter: *"Yes, you could say that you take away three empty signs."*
Subject: *"But that sounds so stupid: empty signs! People would think you were empty in the head!"*

From the data it was evident that the subjects worked with different models in order to carry out the problem solving. However, it seemed to be very difficult to derive an adequate model. This is due to several factors. As was mentioned above, some subjects did not observe the moving effects, and those who did, often did not try to interpret them. Another factor which prevented them from using their observations was their forgetting. Here is one example comment:

(Subject 33)
"What did I do last time, when everything jumped so easily?
I took away a word, and everything moved one step to the left.
I'll move the cursor in any case.
What did I do?
I moved the whole row so easily.
(Makes a new attempt, moving the cursor backwards)
No, everything stays in the same place.
I can always try to move as usual."

Another factor which prevented the subjects to form an adequate model of the task in the system was their orientation towards procedures. Since the main difficulties lay in understanding the problem space (particularly the role of the blank signs), an exclusively procedural orientation was detrimental. One example is the following comment:

(Subject 46)
*"I would like to have a command (to move the row to the right),
like the one I used to move to the left, another Esc, but you don't
use D."*

Looking for a command does not help in this situation, if the relationship between the command and the objects on which the command
works is not understood. Since this subject worked with the concept of
"rows" instead of single signs, the procedure could not be used to create a
general model.

Models Used For Communication

After the learning and task sessions the subjects were asked to
describe their experience of the system in terms of advice to a novice
user. Some examples may serve to illustrate the contents of the systems
models which users consciously employ and their ability to communicate
these models to other people.
(Subject 45)
"It is important to remember that it really works like a typewriter."
(Subject 46)
*"You can look at the system like this: imagine you have some blocks
lying here, and then you take away one block and push in another."*

These descriptions indicate that the subjects communicate a
metaphor, with very little processing details.
Other comments are a little more specific, but concern mainly the
functioning of the system:
(Subject 47)
*"It's different from a typewriter because you can't just type over on
a typewriter; you have to rub out first. And you can move lines
sideways, and you can make empty lines and move lines downwards, and all kinds of splendid things you can't do on a
typewriter. And it goes much faster, because you can rub out whole
words directly, and whole rows you can rub out just by pushing
some keys."*

Still more specific descriptions concern the process by which the
functions are performed and contain more procedural details.

(Subject 44):
"It says in the manual that a sign may be a letter, a figure or a blank. But then the problem is, what is the blank? I realized that I should put in a blank, but I did'nt not know which key to press."

These comments suggest that novice users talk about (and probably also think about) systems models at different levels. This was also stressed by an investigation performed by van der Veer, Felt & van Muylwijk (1986).

They may have caught the metaphor way of describing the system because they were given a metaphor to start with. Metaphors have usually been considered as a rather efficient way to present computer concepts to novices. (Douglas & Moran, 1983, Mayer, 1981). However, it is not self-evident that the users will continue using the metaphor given. Take subject 46 as an example. She was taught the wordprocessing system by a typewriter metaphor. Her experiences with the system induced her to develop another model instead, a "building block" model. Thus it was important for her to communicate this insight in her description of the system. The other examples indicate that at least some users understand that they have to communicate not only metaphors, but also actual procedures. The relationship between the metaphor and the procedures may not be that easy to communicate.

It should be pointed out that the subjects found it rather difficult to describe their idea of the system. When asked to suggest some guidelines for novice users, some of them could only think of advice like: "just try as many different alternatives as you can think of!" or "work slowly and systematically". And even these comments came after considerable prodding on the part of the experimenter. These difficulties suggest either that the model was not conscious enough to be communicable, or that it is difficult to communicate a model of the system without describing a particular task.

Models Used For Creativity

The task as such can be regarded to require creativity in order to be solved in the most efficient way. (See above, under the presentation of the task.) However, it was found that very few subjects actually solved the problem in this efficient way. They were prevented from finding the solution by several different factors, and their use of invalid models was one of the preventing causes.

One example of a creative solution derived from the attempt to generalize the (partially valid) model can however be described. It relates to subject 46, at a point in her learning, when she had detected that she could move a row leftwards by deleting signs. She then tried to move the row rightwards in another task, by positioning the cursor to the right of the row and giving the "delete" command at that position. We can interpret this action as an extension of the model of "moving by deletion" to the task of moving rightwards.

Creation by generalization is an important activity, and should be encouraged in the models of computer systems.

It is also evident from the comments of the subjects that conflicts are not enough in order to trigger creative activity. Most subjects found that they performed the task in an inefficient way. Many of them observed the conflict between their way to look at the system and the actual behaviour of the system. In particular, they were very concerned by the fact that some numbers moved, when they tried to correct some others:

(Subject 19)
"It's quite awkward this - I get furious! Now it jumps out again - it doesn't do as it should!"

One of the main reasons that this observation didn't lead to any insight or creative activity is the feeling of time pressure:

(Subject 19)
"Now I'll never try anything quicker - it just takes longer!"

It can be concluded that creativity based on conflicts can only result under very particular circumstances. In an ordinary work situation it is most probable that the need to get work done within a certain time will prevent attempts at solving problems creatively, even when models are close and conflicts are perceived.

FINAL WORDS

The relationship between learning computerized tasks and mental models of the tasks is fairly complex. It is easy enough to say that a model which is compatible with the learner's prior knowledge, and which is applicable in the new situation implied by the computer system will facilitate users' learning in performing tasks in this system. However, there are some definite problems in finding situations, where optimal models for learning and using a system can be created.

Let us suppose that the computer system really complies with the user's prior knowledge of a particular task. Analogical models with direct manipulation are an example of such systems. We find such systems in computer games and some office automation systems. Analogical models restrict the users to tasks which are analogue to tasks performed without the system. It may be easier and quicker to perform the task in the system than without the system, but the system is not utilized to more than a small part of its capacity. Computer games may be fun to play, but they certainly do not foster any models of computer systems which are useful outside that application domain. If nothing else is needed than quicker and easier performance of the same tasks as were performed before, analogical models certainly are sufficient.

Often, however, we want to utilize the capacity of a computer for some new tasks. If we want to integrate wordprocessing with information retrieval, if we want to combine calculations with presenting their results graphically and communicate these to others, and if we want to repeat some actions in some circumstances but not in others, new concepts have to be introduced. These new concepts may be incompatible with the model previously used for the task. This situation requires great ingenuity of the system designer. The new task (in the system) should preferably be worked out with concepts and operations which form a consistent whole. Otherwise, the model may as well cause confusion (cf. Halasz & Moran, 1982). This requirement applies to the designations of the concepts as well.

Even if the system is designed with a consistent and workable model, the problem of communicating the model to the user remains. From the empirical data above we saw that models need both an overview level to indicate the general idea of the system, (for instance in terms of a metaphor) and a detailed level, in order to indicate what procedures to use. In a complex system, it may not be possible to communicate the relevant model in a way that is easy to understand and learn.

Whether an adequate model can be communicated or not, it is very probable that users create models of their own, for instance to serve a subpart of the system or to invent new tasks, which were not predicted when the system was designed. Explorations of the systems possibilities and active learning will lead to spontaneous model creation. A good systems design should allow for such activities too.

FOOTNOTE

The empirical investigation referred to has been supported by a grant from the Swedish Board for Research in the Humanities and Social Sciences.

REFERENCES

Card, S.K., Moran, T.P. & Newell, A. (1983). *The Psychology of Human-Computer Interaction.* Lawrence Erlbaum, Hillsdale, New Jersey.

Carroll, J. M. & Mack, R. L. (1985). Metaphor, computing systems, and active learning. *International Journal of Man-Machine Studies,* *22,* 39-57.

Carroll, J.M., & Thomas, J.C. (1980). Metaphor and the cognitive representation of computing systems. *Report RC 8302, IBM Watson Research Center*, May.

Chapanis, A. (1961). Men, machines, and models. *American Psychologist, 3*, 113-131.

Craik, K. (1943). *The Nature of Explanation*. Cambridge: Cambridge University Press.

Douglas, S.A. & Moran, T.P. (1983). Learning operator semantics by analogy. *Proceedings of the National Conference on Artificial Intelligence*, Washington D.C.

Halasz, F. & Moran, T.P. (1982). Analogy considered harmful. *Proceedings from the Conference Human Factors in Computing Systems*. ACM: Gaithersburg.

Halasz, F. & Moran, T.P. (1983) Mental models and problem solving in using a calculator. In A. Janda (Ed.) *Proceedings of the CHI'83 Conference on Human Factors in Computing Systems*, New York: ACM, 212-216.

Mayer, R.E. (1981). The psychology of how novices learn computer programming. *Computer Surveys, 13*, 121-141.

Newell, A. & Simon, H.A. (1972). *Human problem solving*. Englewood Cliffs, New Jersey: Prentice-Hall.

Norman, D.A. (1983). Some observations on mental models. In: Gentner, D., & Stevens, A.L. *Mental models*, Hillsdale, N.J.: Lawrence Erlbaum Ass.

Waern, Y. & Rabenius, L. (1986). On the role of models in the instruction of novice users of a word processing system. Paper presented at a MACINTER meeting in Stuttgart, September, 1985. *HUFACIT reports No.8*, Department of Psychology, University of Stockholm, 1986. Submitted for publication.

van der Veer, G.C., Felt, M. & van Muylwijk, B. (1986). Development of mental models of office systems. *Paper presented at the Third European Conference on Cognitive Ergonomics*, Paris.

Young, R. M. (1983). Surrogates and mappings: Two kinds of conceptual models for interactive devices. In: Gentner, D. & Stevens, A. (Eds.) *Mental models*. pp. 35-52. Hillsdale, NJ: Lawrence Erlbaum Assoc.

Psychological Issues of
Human Computer Interaction in the Work Place
M. Frese, E. Ulich, W. Dzida (Editors)
© Elsevier Science Publishers B.V. (North-Holland), 1987

WHEN THE INTRODUCTORY PERIOD IS OVER: LEARNING WHILE DOING ONE'S JOB

Stephan Dutke and Wolfgang Schönpflug

Institut für Psychologie, Freie Universität Berlin,
Habelschwerdter Allee 45, 1000 Berlin 33,
Federal Republic of Germany

The concept of advanced learning is emphasized, and the task requirements which the users of a text processing and -communication system encounter after their initial training are examined. The importance of advanced training is substantiated by arguments relating to changes of tasks and of the work environment. Results from a questionnaire study and two laboratory studies are reported in order to describe organizational conditions as well as cognitive and motivational features of advanced learning. The use of external sources of information such as the system itself, manuals, or expert colleagues is characterized as a salient problem in advanced learning. Learning how to use an external source of information is stressed as a central goal of advanced training.

Training in human-computer interaction develops into a well established paradigm for psychological research. The computerization of traditional work and the implementation of new hardware and software raises many psychological problems. Wexley (1984) e.g. estimates that office workers have to be retrained for new computer systems five to eight times during their career. Whereas Schindler & Schuster (1986) discuss general features of user training from a psychological point of view, Fischer (1986) and Schmalhofer & Kühn (1986) investigate the effectiveness of training programs based on different teaching strategies. Frese, Schulte-Göcking & Altmann (1987) extend their studies of training by the incorporation of the additional variables "learning strategy" and "kind of human-computer interaction". Learning processes in using a text processor are studied by Carroll & Mack (1983, 1984) and Carroll & Carrithers (1984); these authors propose to adapt training and software design to a basically active style of learning. Computer training as a method of preventing stress in the workplace is emphasized by Greif (1986). Helmreich (1986) states the importance of training for user acceptance. Manufacturers seem to be aware of the fact that a product can only be highly appreciated if it is appropriately applied to the tasks it was designed for. With regard to this aspect, user training plays an important role in economical considerations, both of manufacturers and customers. Efforts in developing and conducting user instruction seem to be greater the longer and the more frequently the system is supposed to be used in work.

This paper does not deal with the learning tasks during the "first hour" (Schmalhofer & Kühn, 1986) of getting familiar with a system. It treats learning after the first stage of introduction, or the problems of the advanced learner. The problems of the advanced learner have at least two facets which are elaborated in separate sections: the social and organizational conditions of learning, how to use a text communication device, and the process of acquiring explicit or verbalizable and implicit or practical knowledge on how to operate the system. A special feature of advanced learning is how to acquire, integrate and utilize available supports; this feature is considered in the final section.

TRAINING FOR THE ADVANCED USER

Most scientific and practical endeavours in this field are restricted to the very beginning of the learning process, to the introduction of a new system or the arrangement of a new working environment. A less prominent issue to be outlined here, is the training of those users who already have some experience concerning their tasks and the means to solve them. The learning process does not stop after the successful introduction of a new computer system and the initial practicing of basic functions: "Training does not simply mean practicing operating procedures. Usually it is possible to work with an office system after a few hours of practice. Real learning starts when an attempt is made to incorporate the technology into existing tasks." (Helmreich, 1986, p. 923). In the following paragraphs some arguments in favour of the necessity of a training for advanced users will be discussed.

Most introductory training procedures are to provide the user with some basic operating knowledge. Teaching and acquiring this knowledge often take place without any specific relation to the demands and tasks the user will encounter later in his job. After this initial period it is up to the user to adapt this operating knowledge to this job's tasks and to develop a satisfying level of competence. Having this period of learning in mind, Helmreich (1986, p. 923) states: "Then it is no longer a question of which key to press when, but of the advantage the individual can gain from his work in the office system. In this phase users need encouragement and support." To put it more precisely: There is not only the chance to gain advantage, there is also the danger to make work more complicated, more stressful and less satisfying if this phase of learning process takes an adverse turn.

During the initial training, the user is not able to anticipate the changes in work organization, flow of information and social relations caused by the new system (Oborne, 1985). Encountering time limitations, the instructors have to cope mostly with the more basic problems such as giving an idea of the system's general features and teaching operating procedures. Therefore, problems arising from changes in the work environment are no substantial topic in a training program. Besides organizational limitations the trainers are often not familiar enough with the individual work place to anticipate such developments. On the other hand, the standard of performance is usually the same or even higher after the introductory period (Carroll & Mack, 1984). After the instruction users are often expected to be familiar with the system and feel obliged to come up to this expectation. The above mentioned knowledge to specific tasks, have to be met in spite of potentially worsened conditions: changing work environment and at least constant performance standards.

Especially if a system is supposed to be easy to operate the need for both the initial and advanced training is often underestimated. New technical equipment being not as salient as a complete new office system, is often regarded as the feature of a smooth, evolutionary development. This way a text processor is diminished to a device belonging to a "new generation of typewriters" and modern telecommunication facilities are treated as an extension of the "old telephone". In these cases the new quality of work organization is often neglected, so that training, especially after the introduction is appraised as a desirable but not necessary measure. Sometimes this leads to the paradox that just the simple and only temporarily used systems cause more problems than the complex systems claiming the largest portion of working time. This may also be due to a matter of aspiration level: If a system is introduced as a quite simple device which is allegedly easy to learn, the level of aspiration may be either raised too much because of underrating the complexity or lowered too much because of the lack of challenge.

BECOMING FAMILIAR WITH A NEW SYSTEM: SOME EMPIRICAL DATA ON SOCIAL AND ORGANIZATIONAL CONDITIONS OF ADVANCED LEARNING

Some empirical evidence on the progress, the conditions, and constraints of learning while carrying out one's job was obtained in an interview study. A sample of 15 female users (22 to 57 years old) of a text processing and text communication systems was asked in a structured interview to report their way of becoming familiar with the system. All of them had been working in their jobs (secretary, secretarial assistant, commercial clerks) for more than four years but had no former experiences with computers. They had to learn using a text processor which has an additional facility to communicate texts via TELEX or TELETEX. The device can also be used as an ordinary typewriter. The system is operated by function keys and menus. Experts judge it as not a very complex system. Most of the subjects (13) reported that they did not make use of the device the whole working day. On average, they worked less than four hours a day with the system. During the rest of their working time they were occupied with activities similar to those before the introduction of the new system. Obviously their situation was characterized by the above mentioned "sneaking" introduction of a "small-scale system". On the average the interviews took place 9 1/2 months after the introduction of the system.

Although the 15 persons reporting were employed by the same business firm and were users of the same system they were not given the same introductory training. The decision on the introductory training obtained depended mainly on the situation in the different departments, their current work load and available resources. Table 1 shows the different ways of taking the first steps in the learning process.

	Subjects														
	1	2	3	4	5	6	7	8	9	10	11	12	13	14	15
Reading the brochure	X							X							
Practising alone	X	X	X	X	X	X	X		X	X			X	X	
Practising together with colleagues	X	X	X		X			X		X	X	X			
Practising with the help of the manual		X											X		
Practising together with colleagues + manual ...		X						X							
Receiving a short introduction (2 hours)	X	X	X	X	X	X	X	X	X	X	X	X		X	
Taking part in a seminar (about 6 hours)	X	X	X												

Table 1: Sources of Initial Skill

The most frequent combination was to attend a short introduction and then practicing alone. This introduction had predominantly the character of a demonstration because there was usually not very much time for working at the device itself. The other important method was trying and practicing together with colleagues in the department. Only three persons took part in a seminar of about six hours. These seminars con-sisted of instruction as well as of active training. However, these seminars were explicitly dedicated to the communication facility but not to the text processing functions.

Each user was provided with a manual. The quality of print and graphic layout were attractive features of the manual. It presented the functions of and the main procedures to be executed with the system in a user-oriented style. Although designed to become a complete source of information the manual played only a minor role. Five subjects reported that they did not use the manual at all during the first week of their work with the system. The remaining ten persons used it once or twice during the first week. This ratio hardly changed after months. Another remarkable fact was that one of the colleagues wrote instructions herself on how to use the system for specific tasks in her department. Thereupon her colleagues worked more often with these instructions exactly adapted to their needs than with the original manual.

As in the early hypothesis we found some indications for a continued need for learning: (1) All subjects reported having severe problems in operating the system once or twice a week which were undue to technical defects. As the range of experience with the system varied from 1 1/2 up to 24 months this result is probably not related to special temporary demands. (2) The fact that the self-made instructions were more frequently used than the original manual is another indication for a continued need for learning. Obviously the original manual was not used because it did not support the user. Nevertheless the users still need some support as shown by the acceptance of the task-oriented material. (3) After the interviews the subjects received a questionnaire about the type of tasks that were supported by the system. The questions concerning the possible scope of tasks that could be accomplished with the system were incorrectly answered on an average of 18%. That means that nearly a fifth out of 21 questions such as "With this system you can store texts", "... receive a TELEX", "... print a received TELETEX ..." were incorrectly answered. Overratings and underratings of the system's versatility were nearly balanced. This result showed no relation to the time of experience the users had with the system. There were also no differences between users working daily with the system or only temporarily. But a correlation of +.52 was found between this error score and the self-reported working time at the system per day: the longer the users worked at the system per day the more errors they made in assessing the functional capabilities. This unexpected correlation can be explained by the different scopes of vocational activity among the subjects (Figure 1). Those who worked for the longest amount of time with the system were secretaries or secretarial assistants encountering a small range of different tasks. Those who used the device for a shorter time per day were commercial clerks whose activities were more versatile. This shows that a limited scope of activity may lead to a limited knowledge of the system's functional facilities, irrespec-

tive of the time of experience. However, a restricted set of highly prac-
tised tasks does not protect the user from unexpected events. In this case,
the chance to solve the problem by one's own resources is low because of
an impoverished knowledge of alternative functional facilities.

Figure 1: Self-reported Working Time at the System per Day (hours)

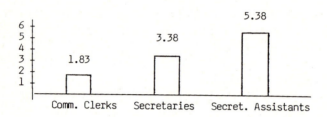

After stating the necessity of learning going beyond the period of
instruction and of first attempts of surveying the system's operational
structure, some features of this learning phase have to be discussed. Both
cognitive and motivational demands to the advanced user differ substantially from the user's situation in the introductory period.

KNOWLEDGE ACQUISITION AFTER THE INITIAL INTRODUCTION: EXPERIENCES FROM TWO LABORATORY STUDIES

Whereas in the instructional period mainly declarative knowledge is
imparted to the user he is later engaged in the application of this knowledge to his job demands. In that phase it is essentially performance which
matters. The following model (Figure 2) presents some ideas concerning
the user's knowledge as related to his or her performance.

First of all, two areas of knowledge are distinguished: knowledge
about the task and about the system. Each area is split into two levels:
knowledge about facts and about actions. The combination of both forms a
2 x 2 table. So far there is no relation between the two areas. Therefore, a
third level is assumed where knowledge from both areas and both levels is
integrated so that the knowledge about the system can be used to accomplish a certain task with the help of the device. Concerning the different
levels there is a sequential structure: There has to be a representation of a
certain fact (level I) before the knowledge of changing that fact can
emerge (level II). In the same way, the user must have the knowledge of
procedures before he or she is able to use this knowledge for dealing with

a specific task (level III). This model simply predicts that deficits in factual and action-oriented knowledge will cause shortcomings in the execution of those subactions which require the deficient elements.

This assumption was investigated in two laboratory studies. In the first study the previously interviewed sample of experienced users took part, in the second study 12 computer novices learned to work with the same system in a ten-session program. The operationalization of the theoretical model, including the tasks was equal in both studies.

Figure 2: Areas and Levels of Knowledge

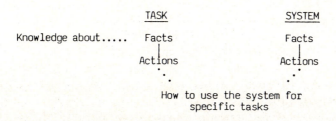

As a simple prediction model one can form 2 x 2 tables (Figure 3) with the rows standing for actual performance (level III) and the columns representing level I and II knowledge. All subactions performed were categorized according to error criteria (faultless or deficient) in both aspects, knowledge and performance.

Figure 3: Shortcomings in Knowledge and Performance for Executed Subactions

Errors on Level I and II
(Knowledge Questionnaires)

		YES	NO
Errors on Level III (Performance)	YES	cell 1	cell 2
	NO	cell 3	cell 4

Cells 1 and 2 show that there are actually two kinds of incorrectly performed subactions. For the first kind of short comings deficits on the more abstract levels of knowledge I and II could be found (cell 1). The second kind of subactions could not be explained by knowledge deficits (cell 2). In the same way we found well performed subactions with (cell 3) and without shortcomings in knowledge (cell 4). The necessity for further learning is given for subactions in cells 1, 2, and 3. But the demands differ substantially: For cell 1 the model's assumption may be correct that complete knowledge of the meaning of the necessary function keys as well as complete knowledge of the sequence of operators to attain the given subgoal are necessary presuppositions to execute this subaction correctly. A lack of this basic knowledge has to be filled before correct execution and appropriate application to a real task can be expected. Regarding the subactions in cell 2 it becomes clear that complete background knowledge alone does not warrant correct usage of this subaction in the context of a task. It is clear that the application of abstract knowledge to a practical problem is not successful in these cases. The success in performance for subactions in cell 3 cannot be explained by complete knowledge of the subaction's elements but may be due to situational or random factors. In spite of successful performance in a special case deficient knowledge restricts a potential generalization.

Prediction analysis (Hildebrand, Laing & Rosenthal, 1977) reveal that errors of type 1 decreased according to the learning progress in the sample of the longitudinal study, but the overall differences between the novice and expert samples were not significant. The number of entries in cell 4 increased.More important was the result that the portion of type-3 error configurations decreased whereas the portion of type-2 configuration increased in the course of the learning process. Both developments were significant. As the data from both knowledge questionnaires showed a substantial increase in manifest knowledge these developments can be explained as follows: In the very beginning of the learning process the subjects find solutions for the tasks partly by trial and error or by chance. Although this initial skill does not need to have an immediate effect on generalized abstract knowledge, as measured on level I and II, performance may be quite good (cell 3). As abstract knowledge becomes more elaborate the portion of subactions in cell 3 decreases. On the other hand, an increased body of generalized knowledge also augments the entries in cell 2 - on the condition that the application of this knowledge to new problems fails. Again, this seems to be an important feature of advanced learning.

LEARNING WHEN TO LOOK FOR MORE INFORMATION: MOTIVATIONAL PROBLEMS

One lesson the advanced learner should learn is that there is more information available than he or she retains in memory permanently. Therefore she or he should acquire a notion of what kinds of sources of information are at his or her disposal and which are the occasions when this additional information should be accessed. This feature puts cognitive demands on the learner which are considered in the preceding section. This section is devoted to motivational problems in active information search. According to the above mentioned model, occasions for further learning are distinguished on two dimensions: (1) with or without an overt problem in operating the system and (2) with or without deficits in background knowledge (cp. Figure 3). Knowledge deficits which do not immediately cause shortcomings in performance have to be detected or at least anticipated by the user himself. In order to complete his or her knowledge in a certain area she or he has to put up with additional costs such as search of information or additional time consumption although these costs cannot be justified by current problems in performing his tasks. In this situation learning effort may be limited. However, in absence of situational constraints exactly this configuration can lead to actively exploratory behaviour as observed in our longitudinal study: The subjects were not prescribed how to acquire the necessary knowledge: by active exploration, reading the manual, or any combination of both. It was found that subjects who had attained a level of skill and knowledge that allowed them to manage also unknown situations, deliberately used inappropriate methods and functions exploring the system. They took the risk of committing errors and encountering uneasy situations in order to enhance their knowledge and to reduce uncertainty in the long run.

If, on the other hand, there are manifest problems in performance, further learning does not only depend on the user's epistemic curiosity but also on his intention to attain his task's goal. Such problems can arise when some sort of external incident coincides with shortcomings in factual or action-oriented knowledge. There may be e.g. changes in the type of tasks so that the user has to find another solution (Carroll & Mack, 1984). Errors in operating may lead the user into unknown system states which require new activity to leave this confusing state. The same may result from badly planned work processes.

However in practice, not all problems in operating turn into an occasion for further learning. It depends on attributive processes whether such an incident is appraised as a challenge to one's own problem solving abilities or not. If the user judges the task demands (including the required operating knowledge) as appropriate with respect to his or her state of knowledge and experience, he or she may define the situation as a problem that has to be tackled by him or her self (cf. Meyer & Hallermann, 1977). On the other hand the users may believe that the demands are too high as compared to their abilities and feel overloaded. In this case they may reject the problem as one to be solved by others. What kind of appraisal results depends not only on the individual's personality but also on very subtle aspects of the work atmosphere (Schneider, 1985). In the latter case, attempts originate to delegate the solution of the problem or even its future prevention and most probably, due to this, no learning will take place. Several strategies have been reported: some users called the technical service declaring that the device was not working properly. Another possibility was to state that those tasks could not be accomplished with that system. If the task could not be rejected on the whole, some users tried to solve the task by other conventional means, returning e.g. to their typewriter.

SUPPORT IN KNOWLEDGE ACQUISITION: EXTERNAL SOURCES OF INFORMATION

The features of advanced learning while carrying out one's job outlined above show that there are many situations where the user needs information from an external source. It has already been stated that these situations are mostly due to adapting initial knowledge to the demands of changed tasks related to daily work. Searching for an appropriate source of information and making proper use of it are key problems in advanced learning as contrasted with the initial training. It was shown (Schönpflug, 1986a,b; Linde & Bergström, 1986) that the user needs "both internal representation of external sources, and internal representation of the information to which the sources refer" (Schönpflug, 1986a, p. 129). During the first instruction the users are more engaged in processing the abundant amount of new information given to them than with the choice between different external sources of information. Therefore, the efficient use of sources of information has to be an important goal of advanced training.

Three potential sources of information for the advanced learner should be discussed: (1) As a most direct source of information the responses of the system itself can be regarded. For example, errors in operating the device effect messages informing the user. Responses to syntactically correct user input also contain some information about internal functional features of the system. (2) Manuals and implemented help systems are a more comprehensive source of information. With regard to our system under investigation we confine ourselves to manuals although some of their features may apply to passive help systems, too. (3) Finally colleagues or other persons familiar with the system play an important role. The following three aspects are chosen to compare the three sources of information listed above: contents of information, accessibility, and feedback mechanism.

Contents of Information

System responses such as error messages can only provide information regarding the syntactic or semantic level of interaction (Jorgensen & Barnard, 1986) but not regarding the task level. Even if it is possible to implement a knowledge-based help facility which is able to keep track of high-level task goals it should be thoroughly discussed whether such a system is desirable. Information on the syntactic and semantic level can also be found in manuals (Rupietta, 1983). But in addition, the manual has the potential to describe comprehensive examples concerning task level knowledge. Of course these examples are inflexible and not necessarily related to the user's actual tasks. A colleague, skilled in the use of the same system is potentially able to give information on the syntactic, semantic, and task level.

Accessibility of Information

Concerning system responses the user does not have to take active measures to receive them. In many cases, timing and kind of appearance are totally determinated by the software. But regarding all other sources of information this is up to the user's own initiative. Gaining access to an external source of information requires active search by the user and therefore an interruption of the primary task. Solving problems with the help of a manual or a passive help system can only be successful if the user is able to define the problem (cp. Miyake & Norman, 1979). He or she must be able to ask useful questions in order to find further information from the manual. This information may be used to create new hypotheses, which can be tested in practice (Carroll & Mack, 1984). Of course, an ap-propriate problem definition does not warrant success but it is a necessary precondition. Asking a colleague or any other qualified person for help can dispense the user from this additional task. In direct social contact he or she has the chance to demonstrate the problem or simply to show what is displayed at the screen. In this way the problem's definition is delegated to the helper.

Especially in practice, the formal aspect of accessibility of information and help should not be neglected. Though it sounds trivial one has to be aware of the possibility that there is no other person who can be involved in the problem solving process. This is often the case when persons have to work individually in their own rooms with few work-related contacts to others. Furthermore, there may not only be a factual but some kind of social isolation which impedes contact with prospective helpers. Sometimes this is even intended in order to avoid complications in inter-personal relationships which may be caused by an unbalanced proportion of helping and being helped (cf. Jones & Nisbett, 1971). Accessing a help system requires further manipulation of the system which is a demand additional to the original problem. On the contrary, using a manual or asking a colleague leaves the problematic system state unchanged and requires no further device manipulation.

Feedback Mechanism

Error messages and other system responses serve as a feedback with respect to the user's previous operation. It depends on the system's design to what extent this feedback yields information the user needs for further learning (Carroll & Mack, 1984; Nievergelt, 1982). Our system under investigation frequently gives just the information that some thing did or did not work. In a smaller number of cases it informed the users exactly what did not work, and in a few cases not only some information was given about what had happened but also about the measures that could be taken to solve the problem.

Using the manual or a passive help system for whatever reasons unsuccessfully, creates a negative feedback relating to the user's tendency to use it again. Whether the organization of the manual or his or her own abilities are supposed to be responsible for this failure, does not influence the growing preference to use other sources of information. The possibility that the user will employ the manual again is diminished if there are other sources of support. In the second laboratory study we found a rate of unsuccessful uses of the manual between 43.2 and 64.6 per cent with the highest value in tl. The drastic decrease of the number of uses (Figure 4) may be due to this negative feedback.

Figure 4: *Frequencies of Using the Manual per Person with Growing Experience*

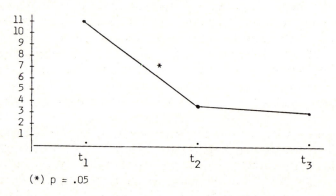

(*) p = .05

On the other hand, in a social situation the feedback mechanisms are more flexible. The helper has several options of giving positive feedback even if he or she cannot offer a complete solution of the user's problem. Instead of a factual solution the user might receive information on other potential strategies. For example, the helper can encourage the user to circumvent the problem by using other technical equipment or to reject the task officially. In any case, social support itself may be positive reinforcement. A social situation does not only offer actually a better chance to solve the problem because of a new joint problem definition but also a higher possibility of reinforcement for choosing a social source of information, irrespective of the factual outcome.

Another reason for the preference of social support are attribution processes. Unsolved problem situations differ considerably to the extent that they are based on social interaction or not. Finding no solution in a manual or not being able to interpret a system's message leaves the question of attribution open. It is up to the user's history of learning, his personality, and social psychological variables to whether or not he attributes the failure to himself or to the system and its documentation. But when the situation develops into a social one, the chances of attributing the failure to the system or the manual increases. The higher the number of persons unable to find a solution e.g. in the manual, the less likely it is that the user would attribute this to his or her own lack of knowledge or abilities (cf. Kelley, 1973). The responsibility for the unsolved problem is distributed to more than one person (Ross & Sicoly, 1979). This again effects positive reinforcement for the choice of a social source of information although no factual solution has been found. If, on the other hand, social interaction and common efforts lead to the problem's elimination, this solution itself may serve as positive reinforcement. This way an unsuccessful as well as a successful attempt can have positive effects on the user's self-perceived abilities within the social comparison.

Flexibility regarding the contents of information and the conditions of feedback and attribution seem to favour the choice of social sources of information in advanced learning. The subjects in the field study were asked what they usually do in case of problems operating the system (Table 2). The majority (13) of this small sample usually tries to solve the problems together with colleagues. This is in line with the above reasoning.

On the other hand, frequently asking colleagues for help may have consequences on work organization, atmosphere, and work load (Battmann & Schönpflug, 1986). Furthermore, social learning in the work place creates another problem: Whereas a manual or a help system represents a standardized and invariant body of knowledge (Schnotz, Ballstedt & Mandl, 1981) socially mediated knowledge changes. Misunderstandings or inefficient strategies may proliferate among the employees. From this point of view the use of non-personal external sources of information is

Strategy	Number of Subjects
Trying alone (with the help of the manual) 2	
Asking colleagues from another department 3	
Asking colleagues from the same department 7	
Asking colleagues from any department 3	

Table 2: Preferred Source of Information

important. Theoretical reasoning as well as empirical data show that the usability of these sources often has to be improved and that their sensible and efficient use has to be trained.

CONCLUDING REMARKS

This chapter was designed to show that a considerable amount of learning takes place after the introductory training of man-computer interaction. The advanced phase of the learning process apparently involves its own characteristics calling for special attention of both practioners and researchers. Optimizing the full learning process as well as the training procedures promoting this process, should grant the competence of users to make full use of both the system's and their own potential.

FOOTNOTE

The research on which this chapter is based, has been supported by SIEMENS AG, Erlangen and München, FRG.

REFERENCES

Battmann, W., & Schönpflug, W. (1986). Kooperation an vernetzten Bildschirmarbeitsplätzen: Verhaltensökonomische Analysen. In: Optimierung geistiger Arbeitstätigkeiten. Referate des V. Dresdner Symposiums zur Arbeits- und Ingenieur-Psychologie. 11. bis 13. Februar 1986. Technische Universität Dresden (pp. 77-81).

Carroll, J. M., & Carrithers, C. (1984). Training wheels in the user interface. Communications of the ACM, 27, 800-806.

Carroll, J. M., & Mack, R. L. (1983). Actively learning to use a word processor. In W. E. Cooper (Ed.), *Cognitive aspects of skilled typewriting*. New York: Springer.

Carroll, J. M., & Mack, R. L. (1984). Learning to use a word processor by doing, by thinking, by knowing. In J. C. Thomas & M. L. Schneider (Eds.), *Human factors in computer systems*. Norwood, N.J.: Ablex.

Fischer, F. (1986). Erwerb kognitiver Fähigkeiten zur Benutzung bildschirmorientierter Textverarbeitungssysteme. In: *Optimierung geistiger Arbeitstätigkeiten*. Referate des V. Dresdner Symposiums zur Arbeits- und Ingenieur- Psychologie. 11. bis 13. Februar. Technische Universität Dresden (pp. 170-175).

Frese, M., Schulte-Göcking, H., & Altmann, A. (1987). Lernprozesse in Abhängigkeit von der Trainingsmethode, von Personenmerkmalen und von der Benutzeroberfläche (direkte Manipulation vs. konventionelle Interaktion). In W. Schönpflug, & M. Wittstock (Eds.), *Software-Ergonomie '87*. Nützen Informationssysteme dem Benutzer? Stuttgart: Teubner.

Greif, S. (1986). Neue Kommunikationstechnologien - Entlastung oder mehr Stress? Beschreibung eines Computer-Trainings zur "Stress-Immunisierung". In U.-U. Pullig, U. Schäkel, & J. Scholz (Hrsg.), *Streß*. Hamburg: Windmühle Verlag.

Helmreich, R. (1986). Planning user acceptance - a management task. In Proceedings Part II of the International Scientific Conference: *Work with Display Units*. Stockholm, May 12 - 15, 1986 (pp. 777-780).

Jorgensen, A. H., & Barnard, P. (1986). An experiment on the effect of task structure in interactive computer systems. In Proceedings Part II of the International Scientific Conference: *Work with Display Units*. Stockholm, May 12 - 15, 1986 (pp. 920-923).

Jones, E. E., & Nisbett, R. E. (1971). *The actor and the observer: Divergent receptions of the causes of behavior*. Morristown, N.J.: General Learning Press.

Kelley, H. H. (1973). The process of causal attribution. *American Psychologist, 28*, 107-128.

Linde, L., & Bergström, M. (1986). User's mental image of the content and search principles in a database. In Proceedings of the International Scientific Conference: *Work with Display Units*. Stockholm, May 12 - 15, 1986 (pp. 734-737).

Meyer, W.-U., & Hallermann, B. (1977). Intended effort and informational value of task outcome. *Archiv für Psychologie, 129*, 131-140.

Miyake, N., & Norman, D. A. (1979). To ask a question, one must know enough to know what is not known. *Journal of Verbal Learning and Verbal Behavior, 18*, 357-364.

Nievergelt, J. (1982). Errors in dialog and how to avoid them. In J.
      Nievergelt, G. Coray, J. D. Nicoud, & A. C. Shaw (Eds.), *Docu-
      ment preparation systems*. Amsterdam: North Holland.
Oborne, D. J. (1985). *Computers at work*. Chicester: Wiley.
Ross, M., & Sicoly, F. (1979). Egocentric biases in availability and
      attribution. *Journal of Personality and Social Psychology, 37*,
      322-336.
Rupietta, W. (1983). Dokumentation als Aspekt der Software- Ergonomie.
      In H. Balzert (Hrsg.), *Software-Ergonomie Tagung des German
      Chapters of the ACM am 28. und 29. 04. 1983 in Nürnberg*. Stutt-
      gart: Teubner.
Schindler, R., & Fischer, F. (1986). Effectiveness of training as a function
      of the teached knowledge structure. In F. Klix & H. Wandke
      (Eds.), *Man - Computer Interaction Research MACINTER I*.
      Amsterdam: North Holland.
Schindler, R., & Schuster, A. (1986). Benutzerschulung: Möglichkeiten,
      Probleme und Entwicklungstendenzen aus psychologischer Sicht.
      In: *Optimierung geistiger Arbeitstätigkeiten*. Referate des V.
      Dresdner Symposiums zur Arbeits- und Ingenieurpsychologie. 11.
      bis 13. Februar 1986 Technische Universität Dresden (pp. 164-
      169).
Schmalhofer, F., & Kühn, O. (1986). Die erste Stunde beim Erwerb von
      Programmierkenntnissen. Eine Computermodellierung im Ansatz.
      In M. Amelang (Hrsg.), *Bericht über den 35. Kongreß der
      Deutschen Gesellschaft für Psychologie in Heidelberg 1986*. Band
      1, Kurzfassungen. Göttingen: Hogrefe.
Schneider, B. (1985). Organizational Behavior. *Annual Review of Psycho-
      logy, 36*, 573-611.
Schnotz, W., Ballstedt, S.-P., & Mandl, H. (1981). Lernen mit Texten aus
      handlungstheoretischer Sicht. In H. Mandl (Hrsg.), *Zur Psycho-
      logie der Textverarbeitung: Ansätze, Befunde, Probleme*. München:
      Urban & Schwarzenberg.
Schönpflug, W. (1986a). Internal representation of externally stored
      information. In F. Klix, & H. Wandke (Eds.), *Man- Computer
      Interaction Research MACINTER I*. Amsterdam: North Holland.
Schönpflug, W. (1986b). The trade-off between internal and external
      information storage. *Journal of Memory and Language, 25*, 657-
      675.
Wexley, K. N. (1984). Personnel Training. *Annual Review of Psychology,
      35*, 519-551.

CONCEPTUAL ISSUES
IN THE PSYCHOLOGY
OF HUMAN-COMPUTER INTERACTION

Psychological Issues of
Human Computer Interaction in the Work Place
M. Frese, E. Ulich, W. Dzida (Editors)
© Elsevier Science Publishers B.V. (North-Holland), 1987

A THEORY OF CONTROL AND COMPLEXITY: IMPLICATIONS FOR SOFTWARE DESIGN AND INTEGRATION OF COMPUTER SYSTEMS INTO THE WORK PLACE [1]

Michael Frese

Dept. of Psychology, Ludwig-Maximilians-Universität München,
Leopoldstr. 13, D- 8000 München 40, Federal Republic of Germany

This article argues that control over one's activities and the working (system) conditions, complexity and complicatedness can be differentiated. Control refers to decision possibilities and efficient action, complexity to decision necessities, and complicatedness to those decision necessities that are difficult to control and socially and technologically unnecessary. Control should be en-hanced in software systems, complexity should be opti-mized, and complicatedness reduced. When control stands in contrast to non-complexity (ease of use) and to some "intelligent" or adaptive features of software, control should be increased at the expense of other features because control has long term positive consequences on stress-effects and performance.

INTRODUCTION

In this article, I want to discuss three concepts, control, complexity and complicatedness. I want to argue that complicatedness should be minimized, complexity optimized, and control maximized. Control should be maximal because having control over conditions and one's actions leads to positive motivational and cognitive consequences. Lack of complexity leads to boredom and monotony, too much complexity to overload. Complicatedness leads to the feeling of nuisance and loads mental capacity with processing needs that are not task oriented.

The approach taken here is in opposition to some of the literature on human computer interaction that regard as main solutions for increasing "user-friendliness" and "usability" of computer programs the reduction of their complexity (e.g. Card, Moran & Newell, 1983; Polson & Kieras, 1985; Shackel, 1985). It is interesting to see, of course, that, indeed programs that do seem to reduce complexity (e.g. the Macintosh programs) are often applauded by the users for their ease. People in their everyday life reduce the complexity of their situations as well. In work life they do this, for example, by not paying attention to things that are not quite so important (e.g., even experts only know about 25- 35% of the commands of complex systems), by chunking smaller parts into larger ones (e.g., in programming where parts are worked out as subroutines that one can worry about later), through holding open options rather than planning the whole way from the start (Oesterreich, 1981), by psychological automatization, so that one has central processing capacity free to think of other things (Hacker, 1978). Thus, people seem to be complexity-reducing beings.

On the other hand, there is a very old tradition in industrial psychology -- the job enrichment, humanization of work or industrial democracy literature -- that suggests that one should increase the complexity of the jobs (Emery & Thorsrud, 1976, Hacker, 1985, Hackman, 1977, Ulich, Groskurth & Bruggemann, 1973) (actually, they argued for higher control and higher complexity but usually did not differentiate between these two concepts). It was the promise of these job restructuring attempts that performance and well-being would be increased by giving people jobs that were appropriately complex and needed the qualifications of the workers.

Thus, these two traditions, the software ergonomics and the humanization of work protagonists, recommend very different approaches. Software ergonomists argue for a reduction of complexity; humanization of work advocates argue for an increase in complexity. Both seem to have data supporting their positions. Who is right?

It is the argument of this article that the crucial category is control and that aspects of the system that ought to be weeded out are aspects of complicatedness, but not of complexity in general. Complicatedness is that part of complexity that is difficult to control. Thus, easiness is not an important criterion for evaluating computer systems in and of itself but it is dependent on control whether easiness of computer systems leads to better or worse performance and well-being.

I shall first develop the concept of control. Then I shall develop the notions of complexity and complicatedness. The next step is to compare and contrast control, complexity and complicatedness. Then I shall argue that control at work, complexity, and complicatedness have repercussions on stress-effects and performance. Finally, I can use these concepts and apply them to software design. When developing the concepts, I shall talk about control and complexity in general, as it relates to the work situation because the design problems of computer systems are not qualitatively different from the design problems of work places in general.

THE CONCEPT OF CONTROL

Experiencing control means to have an impact on the conditions and on one's activities in correspondence with some higher order goal (Frese, 1978). This impact may be potential or it may directly influence the conditions. Potential control was studied by Glass & Singer (1972). In their experiments the subjects had a button that could turn off a loud noise (the stressor). The subjects were, however, asked not to use this button (and all of them complied). This condition produced less stress than not having such a control button. Direct control in stress situations was the issue in Seligman's (1975) experiments. When there was no control, helplessness developed.

Control at work may be applied on an individual or on a collective level. For example, if a team of two persons are able to use a certain software system but each individual alone could not have done it, they have collective control.

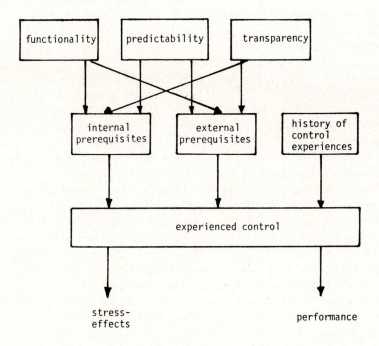

Figure 1: The conceptual framework

It is important to emphasize the goal-related nature of control. Without a goal, there is no issue of control. This concept is somewhat different from other definitions, e.g. the one by Seligman (1975) in which control is defined as non-contingency of events (an event appears or disappears regardless of a person's actions). Such a definition, not bound to the goals of a person, produces some conceptual difficulties. According to this definition, a person would have control, if he or she accidentally (contrary to the intention) produces a serious mistake (like breaking a vase). According to my concept of control, the person did not have control in this case.

Figure 1 functions to describe the theory of control that underlies this article. Experienced control has a direct influence on performance and stress effects. Experienced control is influenced by internal and external prerequisites. External prerequisites imply decision possibilities of the system and at work; internal prerequisites refer to an (appropriate) mental model and adequate skills vis-a-vis the system. These internal and external prerequisites are themselves again influenced by the functionality, the transparency, and the predictability of the system. Experienced control is also influenced by earlier experiences of control. Earlier experiences of control are a significant issue in occupational socialization (Frese, 1982) but are not important in our context here and will, therefore, not be discussed any further.

External Prerequisites

Table 1: Aspects of External Prerequisites of Control

Action sequence	Decision possibilities		
	Sequence	Timeframe	Content
Tasks (Goals)			
Plans			
Feedback (Signals)			
Conditions			

A system is controllable when a person has influence over his actions and over the conditions under which he acts. An action consists of a certain sequence (this sequence is variable, of course): goal development and goal decision, plan development and decision, execution of the action and use of feedback (Frese & Sabini, 1985, Norman, 1986). Having influence means to be able to decide what goals, what plans, what kind of feedback a person is using under what conditions. If the environment does not provide the freedom to decide, the person does not have any control. This concept is summarized in Table 1.

Decision possibilities can appear with regard to sequencing, timeframe, and content of tasks, plans, use of feedback and conditions. Decision points with regard to sequence may for example mean that people are able to determine which task they do first and which one second, in which sequence plans are being formed and executed, or in which sequence they call on signals to inform them of the success of their activities. Timeframe refers to two sets of decision possibilities: First, the decision, when a certain task is tackled or a certain plan is performed; second, deciding on how long it will take to work on a task or on a plan. Similarly, the timing of the signal alludes to when it will appear and how long it is displayed. Content refers to the substance of the decisions with regard to task, plan, signal and conditions: What particular task is done, what plan is formed, what kind of signals does one choose to use and what conditions exist for work.

Four issues are worth emphasizing in this context. First, the decisions must refer to a goal (or in the case of a task, to a superordinate goal). I decide with some goal in mind. As long as something is impertinent to the goals, non-control does not matter. For example, not being able to control the weather has few negative consequences because we usually do not develop goals in this regard. However, not being able to control the temperature in the room might have negative consequences because people have goals in this area. Similarly, if I am just trying out a new computer system without wanting to do something specific with it, control does not matter.

One implication of this reasoning is that control has dynamic properties. Computers enhance potential controllability towards a variety of objects (e.g. being able to correct errors before they appear on paper, being able to check calculations more easily, etc.). This leads to a proliferation of new goals. Using a typewriter, I cannot decide to exchange paragraphs without cutting and pasting -- non-control does not matter. But once I use a word processor, not being able to exchange paragraphs, matters. Thus, the more people know about computers and their potential and the more can be done with computers, the more goals are developed and the more important the chances to decide will become.

Second, freedom to decide has a positive quality only when the decisions do not involve high risks. If all the alternatives involve high risks, then controllability may lead to an aversive situation. This is related to the issue of goal again, because we usually do not develop goals that are very risky. Again, this has important consequences in human-computer inter-action. For example, the risk of losing the whole text with one command, may be such a high risk situation that makes the situation aversive for the novice even if there is potential control over the decision points.

Third, there is a hierarchy of goals within any one person at any one time (there may be, of course, multiple and also conflicting goals). The higher up in this hierarchy a particular goal is, the more important and central the decision becomes (e.g. life or career plan decisions). Thus, control and non-control must be weighted by the importance of the goal. However, a caveat has to be made here: For most people, higher order goals are not at their disposal any more after they have been committed to them for some time. For example, a life goal cannot be redecided at any one time. Therefore, the more practical day-to-day activities stand in the foreground of one's attention. There is actually little need to consciously think about the higher level goals. After a while, this may lead to a re-duction of their conscious "importance" and lower-level goals are in the foreground of attention and thinking and achieve high priority.

Fourth, aside from the above points about the importance of goals and goal hierarchy, it is important to ask the question, how much of the time a person is exposed to non-control or control situations. The theory predicts that exposition time is an important variable (Frese, 1984). If one is constantly under conditions of non-control (little decision making power) even in small matters, there is an impact even if the goals are not very important. The longer, one is exposed to these conditions, the stronger is their impact on experienced control, even if higher order goals (like life goals) are still to be influenced by the individual.

Internal Prerequisites of Control

The external condition represent only *potential* decision points with regard to some goal. To realize this potential, one needs to have knowledge and skills as internal requirements. The former refers to metaphors (Carroll & Thomas, 1982), conceptualizations or mental models of the system (Rouse & Morris, 1986, Norman, 1983). Skills are par-ticularly important as prerequisites of control. Skills are related to efficient actions (Volpert, 1974, Semmer & Frese, 1985), which means that goals, plans and the use of feedback must be realistic, stable-flexible and organized (compare Table 2). The goals and plans must be realistic in terms of timeframe and sequence. Stability implies that goals and plans are not immediately given up when there is some negative feedback. On the other hand, plans should for example be executed in a flexible way, i.e. they should be adjusted to the environmental conditions. Finally, organization implies that those plans that are used very often under redundant circumstances should be psychologically automatized so that one has central processing capacity free to deal with other work demands.

Table 2: Skills

Action sequence	Realistic	Stable-flexible	Organized
Goals			
Plans			
Use of feedback			

Functionality, Transparency, and Predictability

Functionality, predictability and transparence impinge on the external and internal prerequisites of control.

Functionality refers to whether a computer program allows and enhances the completion of a task. One issue of functionality is, for example, whether the computer system models real world tasks. Thus, a statistics program should calculate correctly and do what it is supposed to do. A spell program should have enough words in the dictionary. Without functionality there is no control, because the decisions are not meaningfully related to the goal (task) any more. However, a high functionality does not necessarily imply, that there are decision points available.

Transparency implies that the user can develop an internal model of the functions of the system (Maass, 1983)and that he can develop the necessary efficient skills. Thus, the system should not confuse the user by giving different commands to do the same thing under different modes or by giving explanations that are inconsistent or only half true. At each point it must be clear to what end the system is doing something and what the reasons are that the system behaves the way it does. The problem of transparency comes up particularly with so-called intelligent systems that change with the user and may thus confuse the user with ever- different procedures. Under conditions of non-transparency, the user cannot make adequate decisions referring to his goal and he cannot develop a realistic conceptualization and a flexible and stable approach. Transparency is not identical to control because it is possible to develop a system that is completely transparent, nevertheless offer little control (e.g. an expert system that perfectly explains why it is doing what, but that does not allow users' decisions).

Predictability has some overlap with the concept of transparency. If a system is not predictable, it is most likely not transparent. However, transparency refers to the present, predictability to the future. If a system's behavior cannot be foreseen it is not predictable. In the context of predictability, two issues have been discussed: predictability of what (pwhat) and predictability of when (pwhen) (Miller, 1981). Pwhat implies that one knows what happens when a certain command is typed into the machine. Pwhen implies that one knows when a certain command is executed and completed. The latter is, of course, related to the issue of system response time (Boucsein, Greif & Wittekamp, 1984). When the response time is variable, there is little predictability.

The relationship between predictability and the internal and external prerequisites of control is complex. It is possible that a system is predictable but not controllable (e.g. everything is determined by the system but there is a signal that tells what will happen next). It is also possible (although unlikely) to conceive of a system that is controllable but not predictable. For practical purposes, lack of predictability makes decisions meaningless, because when the states of a system cannot be foreseen, one cannot make adequate decisions. Similarly, it is related to the internal prerequisites of control because it is hard to develop a concept of an unpredictable system and one cannot develop an organized approach towards it.

COMPLEXITY

Our approach to the concept of complexity is shown in Table 3. Again, decisions can be related to goals, plans and signals (signifying some action, as in the case of menus) or feedback (after some action, e.g. in the case of error messages). In contrast to control, the decisions refer here not to decision possibilities but to decision necessities. There are three sets of conditions leading to complexity (Table 3) (cf. Dörner, 1976):

(1) A high number of different goals (or subgoals), plans (or subplans), and signals that need to be sequenced, put in some timeframe, or which have to be connected in terms of content.

(2) A high number of relationships (a) within each cell, e.g. relationships between different goals and (b) between cells, e.g. relationships between goals and plans. An example for (a) is that one command has implications for using another one; an example for (b) is that one has to know for which goals one can use a specific command.

Table 3: The Concept of Complexity

Decision necessities

	sequence	timeframe	content
Number of	goals / plans / signals	goals / plans / signals	goals / plans / signals
Number of relationships between	goals / plans / signals	goals / plans / signals	goals / plans / signals
Number of conditional relationship between	goals / plans / signals	goals / plans / signals	goals / plans / signals

(3) Not only the sheer number of the relationships determine complexity but complexity is increased if there are a large number of conditional relationships, e.g. that one type of command has different consequences (e.g. different error messages) in different modes or that two different plans are influenced by a third one (a kind of moderator or suppressor effect).

The various aspects of complexity are interrelated, of course. The number of goals, plans, and signals determine the potential number of relationships. The more relationships there are, the more likely it is that there are conditional relationships.

Complexity defined in this way is neither a characteristic of the environment nor of the person alone. It is a characteristic of the interaction of the person with the environment. For example, the novice still has to make decisions that are remembered facts for the expert.

In summary, complexity is determined by the sheer number of decisions that have to be made and by the relationships of these decisions. Thus, there is decision necessity.

Experienced control is similarly related to decisions, but it implies a reference to the individual's goals. Thus, there is decision freedom. One implication of this is that a person may be forced to do a complex task that he or she does not want to do -- then control is low but complexity is high.

My concept is different from Kieras & Polson's (1985) concept of complexity in several ways. Although Kieras & Polson have a similar general definition of complexity in their specific experiments, they seem to be concerned only about the number of elements in a system and not about the relationships between these elements (e.g. Polson, Muncher & Engelbeck, 1986). However, the question of relationships between the elements is important, otherwise one could not explain why delayed feedback cycles are more complex than non-delayed feedback (Dörner, 1986). Furthermore, their approach has difficulties explaining the differences between a novice and an expert. In our view, the number of elements that are acted upon are the same, but the number of decisions are different: An expert does not have to decide any more, how to delete a character: He already knows it and it is probably already automatized, i.e. no more thought (and decision) has to be wasted for doing this particular operation. (It would be possible, of course, to integrate this into their concept, as the example of Anderson's, 1983, production system shows.) The most serious problem in Kieras & Polson's formulation, however, is that it does not distinguish between complexity and complicatedness; moreover, I doubt that a low-level approach like theirs is able to make such a distinction.

COMPLICATEDNESS

Complicatedness partly overlaps with complexity. My argument here is that complicatedness is to a large extent complexity that is difficult to control. Thus, control decides whether something is just complex or additionally complicated. A system becomes complicated when it is complex and when one of the following additional conditions apply:
- when there is little functionality
- when there is high intransparency
- when there is high unpredictability
- when there are fewer decision possibilities than necessary
- when there are more decision necessities than are to be comprehended
  by the mental model or executed by the skills

- when the complexity is neither socially nor technologically necessary or adequate.

It is obvious that the first 5 reasons are related to the concept of control, as it was developed in Figure 1 (the last one has to be treated separately).

When there is lack of *functionality*, the worker has to work around the problem. Workers often experience that they have to "cheat" the system, to get the required result. In computer aided storage, they might have to cheat on how many parts are still in storage to get the computer to order them in time (Dr. Rödiger reported this example to me). Gasser (1986) has reported on the "ubiquity of anomaly" when using computer systems in office environments and how strategies of "fitting", "augmenting", and "working around" have to be used to make sure that functionality is achieved. In any case, these are complicated procedures.

When there is *intransparency*, the worker cannot develop an adequate model of the system. Intransparency can come about, when the system changes while a person is working with it. This is a problem with so called adaptive systems that change e.g. with the user's experiences (e.g., Chin, 1986). The changes may make the system intransparent, even for the designer himself (Fitter & Sime, 1980). Similar problems appear, when "intelligent" systems are able to learn new procedures -- any state is then intransparent, not controllable and, therefore, complicated to use.

When there is *unpredictability* (pwhen and pwhat), planning for the timeframe is difficult when the timing is not predictable and planning for what one is doing and forecasting what will happen is complicated. I already alluded to the problems associated with a variable (and long) system response time. Again, problems of unpredictability of what will happen can arise in adaptive and "intelligent" systems because of their changing status. The problems of imcompatibility can be seen within the framework of unpredictability as well: Incompatibility means that the expectations formed in one part of the system (or with other systems before) do not lead to the right predictions. Incompatibility may, for example, come about when a metaphor is not consistently used throughout (Rohr & Tauber, 1985) or when certain commands in one mode mean something else in a different mode.

The lack of *decision possibilities* is an external prerequisite of control (Table 1). When there are not enough control possibilities, the system is seen as complicated, because one has to work around things (see above) and because it is more exhausting (stressful) (cf. also the chapters by Ackermann & Ulich, Corbett and Spinas in this book). Hacker (1983) shows that if the sequence of a task is given, the worker shows more stress and works less planful than when the sequence can be chosen by the worker. Benbasat & Wand (1984) argue that a system-guided dialogue may be preferred by the novice but is a nuisance for the experienced user. This fits nicely into our theoretical framework. For the novice, complicatedness is related to the lack of adequate mental models and skills. Therefore, a system-guided dialogue helps the novice develop a mental model and the skills necessary. However, once the internal prerequisites are developed, further system-guidance becomes a nuisance and the added number of steps that one has to go through are interpreted as complicated. Similar problems appear with menu systems in which the experienced worker is not allowed to work with commands alone (and is, therefore, forced to plow through an endless array of menus and prompts and questions that he knows very well). In this case, the possibility to chunk information is not allowed by the system.

Whether something is seen as complicated depends on how much one has already learned of the system. These aspects are, of course, related to *mental models and skills* (cf. Table 2). If there are more decision necessities than comprehensible and if there are more elements than can be fit into the working memory, a system is seen as complicated. There is an additional distinction: (1) A system may have a high number of elements that are purely filling up memory. This is true, when e.g. the starting procedure for a system implies the execution of 10 different operations. In this case, technological automatization would increase control and reduce complicatedness. (2) Another set of a high number of elements can be reduced by thoughtful patterns. Here thinking and even creativity may be required to reduce the number of elements. While both types may be perceived by the novice to constitute complicatedness, only the former (1) will also be seen as complicated by *both* the novice and the experienced. Hacker (1983) found that the number of elements that had to be kept in working memory made for a high number of errors and fatigue while the complexity that leads to thinking and creativity decreased fatigue.

The reasons discussed so far are related to the issue of control, the following goes beyond it. Complexity is seen as complicated when it is not *socially or technologically adequate*. The notion of technological adequacy implies a dynamic property. While some people were enthused some time ago about the line editor because it gave editing possibilities (thus more control), it would now be perceived to be complicated. An implication of this is, of course, that people who know the newest technological developments will be most prone to judging older products as complicated. Similarly, something is also seen as complicated when complexity is perceived to be the product of malicious intent -- e.g. when a co-worker put into the data some complications by design so that other people cannot work with them.

Thus, a system is seen as complicated when its complexity cannot be controlled because of extrinsic aspects of the system or intrinsic reasons of having learned not enough about it. Complexity itself helps to make a system interesting and not monotonous but if this complexity leads to decision necessities that cannot be affected, then it becomes a complicated nuisance. Note that this concept of complicatedness has a social dimension -- something that is seen as "not necessary" "out of line", etc. is complicated. Thus, the same system may become complicated with social and technological advance.

This reasoning may allow to solve the above mentioned differences in recommendations given by the humanization of work school and by ergonomists. The humanization of work advocates were mainly concerned with complexity (and partly with control) enhancement but were not concerned with complicatedness. The ergonomists are often working on issues of reduction of complicatedness (rather than complexity per se). I contend that the reasoning presented here, helps to untangle these issues and develop a more sophisticated approach to software design. Before we go into this, it is necessary to discuss the effects of control, complexity, and complicatedness, however.

THE EFFECTS OF CONTROL, COMPLEXITY, AND COMPLICATEDNESS

Control has been shown to be related to stress-effects directly and as a moderator. In one group of studies, people who had little control at work showed more signs of psychological and psychosomatic dysfunctioning, e.g. depression, psychosomatic complaints, irritation/strain, exhaustion, anxiety, consumption of pills, sick days, and low self esteem (Caplan et al., 1975, Dunckel, 1985, Frese, Saupe & Semmer, 1981, Gardell, 1971, Karasek, 1979, Kohn & Schooler, 1982, Kornhauser, 1965). This also holds for studies of office workers with computerized office equipment (Cakir, 1981, Smith et al., 1981, Schardt & Knepel, 1981, Turner & Karasek, 1984). A second group of studies showed that control had a moderator effect: stress had a higher impact on psychosomatic complaints (Frese, 1984, Semmer, 1982) and on death from heart attack (Karasek et al., 1981) when control was low and a low impact when control was high.

Control also affects performance. If one is repeatedly in situations of non-control, passivity increases and an active, planful and goal-oriented approach is reduced. Non-control implies that one does not have to develop one's own goals and plans of action. There are two explanations why this afffects performance: A cognitive and a motivational account. The notion of action style (Frese, Stewart & Hannover, 1987) might give a cognitive account, why non-control leads to passivity and reduced performance. Two action styles have been studied in particular: planfulness and goal-orientation (Frese et al., 1987). These action styles function similarly to meta-cognitions (Brown, in press, Gleitman, 1985). When work does not allow long-term decisions, one gets used to not plan ahead. This may become generalized and then general planlessness ensues.

Decrements in performance appear in those tasks that require planning. A similar reasoning applies to goal-orientation and also to the use of feedback.

The motivational account is related to the concept of helplessness (Seligman, 1975). If one is repeatedly in situations of non-control, one does not care to develop goals and plans because one knows that they will not have an effect on the environment anyhow.

Not all aspects of the job are equally affected by non-control. It is useful to distinguish between officially prescribed primary tasks and other secondary tasks. The latter are affected more. The primary task of the typist is, for example, to copy the manuscript without errors. A secondary task might be to correct spelling mistakes by the author, to correct errors in grammar, and to tell the author what part of the manuscript was difficult to understand. When working with computers, it is always necessary to adapt the system to the specifics of the job. Correcting and detecting software errors (or at least to work around them, once they appear), knowing what to do when there is a breakdown and organizing one's work in an efficient way are aspects of secondary tasks. In the case of full screen editing, the typist may set the tab to move around the screen more quickly or to write tables more efficiently than to just use the cursor control keys. Often performance differences between people are due less to performance differences in the primary task than in the secondary task (Hacker, 1978, 1985). In the case of typists, correcting errors takes much longer than typing the words in the first place. Thus, preventing errors increases productivity more than simple typing speed.

Thus, there are various negative effects of non-control on performance and well-being.

Lack of *complexity* leads to boredom and has similar stress-effects as control.[2] A certain amount of complexity has to exist, to be able to use creative solutions that require intellectual capacities. If jobs provide only little complexity, this leads to a reduction of the use of intellectual resources and eventually to a sort of cognitive atrophy in which one looses one's intellectual abilities to solve problems (Kohn & Schooler, 1982). On the other hand, complexity that is too high is too difficult to deal with and produces qualitative overload (Kahn, 1974). Furthermore, performance is low because there are too many decisions involved that overload central processing capacity. Thus, in contrast to control, there is an optimal degree of complexity (I am talking about complexity that is potentially controllable). Complexity that is too high stifles performance, too low complexity does the same thing. It is known from the achievement motivation literature (Heckhausen, 1980) that people like to solve moderately complex problems and that achievement is lower with very low and very high aspiration levels. Thus, emotional and performance effects are most positive under conditions of optimal complexity.

One could argue that complexity is non-functional when it is a state of the tool and not a state of the main task (cf. Hacker in this volume). When writing an article, the word processor would be the tool (and should be as simple as possible) to be able to work on the content of my article (the main task, that should be moderately complex). There is some truth to this argument and, in fact, the complicatedness of software leads to being a nuisance when it appears as part of a tool (cf. Dzida in this volume). This nuisance is related to control, again, since the complicated tool is a kind of forced detour on the route to the main goal (solving the task). However, this view does not give the whole picture for the following reasons:

(1) The differentiation between tool and main task is difficult to uphold. What is the tool and what is the main task for a data entry typist? Here the use of the tool is the main task. Similarly, my thinking while writing an article is a tool as well. At the same time thinking the content of the article through is the main task. Again, the differentiation between tool and main task is blurred.

(2) The complexity of a system should be seen within the context of the whole job. This leads to the interesting hypothesis that people whose main task is not very complex, might be stimulated by the complexity of the system. For example, data entry workers, whose job content provides very little complexity, might profit from a complex system more than managers (note: it is more useful, of course, to mix data entry work with other activities to not have this kind of low job content).

(3) With the advent of computers in the work place, many tasks are becoming computer related. Here, the main tasks can only be solved well, when one is using the computer well. This point is driven home when newly introduced computers have to be augmented and fitted or worked around (Gasser, 1986). The tools (computer) and the main tasks are mixed more and more.

(4) Computers are different from other tools, because they are multi-purpose machines (DiSessa, 1986). Since they allow flexibility and adaptability, people develop the aspiration level of realizing these potentials. Thus, taking away artificially the whole complexity of the machine, will only lead to a less functional use of it.

(5) Complex tools may be thoroughly enjoyable as in the example of some video games (again the main task is to work on the tool). Complicatedness does have a meaning here, namely it refers to that part of the video game that cannot be influenced by increasing skills (of course, video games try to be complex but not complicated).

Thus, the differentiation between tool and main task may have some value in reconciling the ergonomists' and the humanization of work advocates' views mentioned in the introduction. But we need to search for an additional answer. This answer is, of course, that one has to differentiate between controllable complexity and one that is difficult to control

-- the latter I call complicatedness. While it is okay to increase controllable complexity, complicatedness should be weeded out.

I argue that *complicatedness* has none of the positive effects of optimal complexity and maximal control. When there is complexity that we have little control over or that we think is technologically and socially not necessary, we are typically angered by complicated systems and find them a nuisance (cf. also Osterloh, 1983). The important reason for this is that little control and complexity are combined. We are forced to make decisions, take care of processes, go detours that do not lead directly to our goals, that are not stimulating and that are not necessary. Besides these emotional effects, complicatedness also leads to lower performance (Hacker, 1983) because of the reasons specified above.

IMPLICATIONS FOR SOFTWARE DESIGN

From the discussion so far, it follows, that software design should maximize control, optimize complexity and minimize complicatedness.

Maximization of Control

One can follow the outline of Table 1 to evaluate whether a program allows control. Word processing may serve as an example. Some word processing programs use "masks" for form letters, in which the curser moves to a particular position, in which the address of a number has to be inserted. Often, the sequence and even the timing of these masks is predetermined. This is a case of little control. Even the task content is often predetermined, as well (e.g., there is a preprogrammed dictionary of paragraphs that is often used in letters of a particular industry). Plans may be related to menus. The following questions exist: Can the typists change the sequence and content of the menus (e.g., are they able to turn the menus off, or can they develop their own menus, etc.). Decision possibilities with regard to feedback may be more difficult to program into the software. But it should be possible for a typist to design certain signals themselves. A typist may, for example, often forget to use a certain command. He or she might want to program a reminder into the system (e.g., reminding to save something). If these reminders were to be included in all programs, they would be patronizing and would often disturb the train of thought and action. If the users design their own reminders, they are useful tools (and can, of course, be changed again in case they are not needed any more). The users might also want to change the sequence of the signals. And finally, users might want to determine, individually, at what point they want to get signals. For example, it has been suggested that feedback should be given if response times of the computer are long (Shneiderman, 1980) -- people may differ here and it is useful to be able to choose at what point they would like to get feedback on response times. Control over conditions may mean that users are able to turn off sounds or the blinking of the curser, as well as using different types of keyboards or programming the keyboards or certain function keys. Control over conditions of work also means, of course, that users have an influence on which system is introduced and how it is introduced, which help systems (with whom as helper) they get, whether their work can be interrupted by commands from the outside, etc.

The issue of control becomes particularly important with the introduction of "intelligent" software. When, for example, an expert system "uses" the expert only as a helper of its program instead of the expert using the expert system, control is taken away.

It may not always be possible to give control to the user in every one of the cells of Table 1. But as the examples show, it is useful to go through the cells and determine to which extent one has been able to increase users' control. Control often implies that the user is able to change (even program) parts of the software. Two points are important here: First, the user should not be forced into having to change but should have the *option* to change (this is particularly true for the novice user). Thus, the system must provide a useful default option for each of the above mentioned examples. These default options should emphasize the development of a mental model and skills (the internal prerequisites of the experience of control). That means, that here explanations on the system functions should be given. Second, it is neither useful nor desirable that every user should become a programmer. People typically use the computer as tool to accomplish some other task (e.g. producing a text). Demanding that the user acquires complicated skills to change the work place, changes the focus from the real task to the tool. Rather, changing the program should be easy and computer assisted. Changing the system should use similar strategies as in "teaching" some robots. A robot is told by example what particular movements have to be done in which sequence. One button tells the robot that this is the example that is to be done from now on. Rather than having complicated strategies of telling what kind of mask a person wants to have, or in what sequence he wants to have programs loaded, a general "example- button" should be developed that automatically stores that particular strategy that the user prefers.

One of the more exciting developments in human-computer interaction has been the concept of direct manipulation (Altmann, 1987, Hutchins, Hollan & Norman, 1986, Shneiderman, 1983). With this design users see immediately whether an action led to the goal and the system is functional and transparent. Of particular importance are the chances to control the object and task directly (Hutchins et al., 1986). Therefore the operator feels in control.

Another development in software design is related to the concept of control: the concept of management of trouble by Brown & Newman

(1985). They suggest that the design should not be oriented towards decreasing any chances for errors because many design problems, tasks that a particular program is being used for, and personal approaches cannot be anticipated. Rather, it should make the errors controllable, i.e. it should make them manageable. Making the correcting of errors and the repairing of the effects easy and reducing the risks involved are more important design requirements than error reduction (cf. also Frese & Peters, 1987).

The internal prerequisites of learning a mental model and skills are, of course, also related to control. They will not be discussed in details here. However, it is interesting to note that control over the process of learning enhances training processes, as well (Frese et al., 1987).

It needs to be clear that having control also implies that the user is actively involved in the process of introducing new technology (e.g. a new computer system). The general goal is that the user *is able to design his or her work place* -- a principle that has long been discussed in industrial psychology as desirable (Ulich, 1978) but which has become a viable alternative with the advent of personal computers.

Optimization of Complexity

A very low level of complexity leads to boredom, a very high level to overload and to the frustration of not being able to achieve one's goals. Furthermore, people choose problems of moderate complexity. This means that the complexity of the software should not be reduced to zero. This should also not be done because it would reduce control as well (since both complexity and control hinge on decisions). However, that part of complexity that is difficult to control (complicatedness) should, of course, be reduced to zero.

Minimization of Complicatedness

Complicatedness should be minimized because it is a nuisance and it impedes performance. If complexity is not functional, intransparent, unpredictable, if there are no decision possibilities and little material to develop mental models and skills from, and if there is no social and technological adequacy, it turns into complicatedness. One way to reduce complicatedness is by reducing overall complexity (decision necessities). It is argued here that this would not be a good strategy because it leads to boredom, lower well-being and lower performance (cf. Hacker this volume). The better strategy is to increase functionality, transparency, predictability and the internal and external prerequisites of control experiences.

CONCLUSION

When developing software, the designer has to make choices. Most often these choices are not of the sort 'All arguments speak for this procedure' but rather of the type 'Some arguments speak for this route, but other arguments speak against it'. In short, the designer has to make choices under trade-off conditions. Since this is so, it is important to develop explicit rules of thumb on what alternatives are more important or less important. These rules of thumb should be made theoretically plausible so that they can be tested empirically.

In this article I have argued for the importance of experienced control and have tried to develop a conceptualization of control, complexity and complicatedness. I have argued for the maximization of control, optimization of complexity and minimization of complicatedness.

This is then the answer to the contradictory suggestions of the job enrichment literature (increase control!) and of software ergonomists (make it as easy as possible!): Too little complexity is boring and leads to an atrophy of mental capacities (thinking creatively) as well as to a reduction in performance. Moreover, if there is no complexity, there is usually no control either (because there are no decisions). If complexity and control do not go together, this leads to the experience of complicatedness. It is complicatedness, that the software ergonomists want to reduce to achieve user friendly systems. And here I agree, of course. However, sometimes software ergonomists may go a little far and reduce the complexity and control as well. Therefore the warning of the job enrichment people has to be heeded that a job renders an adequate amount of complexity and control.

There is one set of design decisions that our formulation is particularly critical towards: Reducing both complexity and control. For example, software that reduces the complexity level automatically when the user makes mistakes, reduces control and transparency over the system and should be avoided.

The emphasis on control is not entirely new to the field of software psychology (Cheriton, 1976, Shneiderman, 1980, Turner & Karasek, 1984, DIN- Entwurf, 1984). However, the relations between control and complexity and complicatedness have not been spelled out before. I do not think that my proposal answers all the questions. It is necessary to develop the concepts of complexity and complicatedness a little more formally than has been done in this paper. But I do think, that these three concepts are a starting point to analyze the work situation and software systems used in the work place.

The bulk of the arguments used in this article has not been from human computer interaction literature but from traditional (European) industrial psychology. This is not surprising. The question of good design of the work place has been the prime issue in industrial psychology for quite some time. The problems have not changed completely but are only accentuated differently when talking about software design (cf. Hacker in this volume). It is important to keep in mind that software design -- although becoming more important -- is only one aspect of job design. Therefore, good job design means to incorporate concepts of good software design into a complete work place -- hopefully a work place that allows a maximum of control.

FOOTNOTES

1) Acknowledgment: This paper is based on a first draft that was written while I visited the Center for Human Information Processing, Institute for Cognitive Science at the University of California, San Diego. Particularly Don Gentner, Don Norman, Dave Owen, Paul Smolensky and Judith Stewart have influenced my thinking about human-computer interaction. The visit was made possible by a travel grant from the Deutsche Forschungsgemeinschaft (No FR 638/2-1) which is gratefully acknowledged. I am also grateful to Siegfried Greif and Helmut Peters for their critique of earlier versions of this article.

2) Complexity and control are very often related. Semmer (1984) has measured both on two levels: by observers and by subjects' responses on a questionnaire. The correlations between the two variables were .70 and .43 on the respective levels. Karasek (1979) has even combined control and complexity into one index. Additionally the literature on the job restructering, control and complexity are seen as two sides of a coin: One should increase complexity and control in order to induce job satisfaction and development of the person (Ulich, Groskurth & Bruggemann, 1973, Hacker, 1985, Hackman, 1977). But these empirical correlations do not necessary imply that complexity and control are conceptually the same.

REFERENCES

Altmann, A. (in press). Direkte Manipulation: Empirische Befunde zum Einfluß des Benutzeroberflächen-Designs auf die Erlernbarkeit von Textsystemen. *Zeitschrift für Arbeits- und Organisationspsychologie.*

Anderson, J. R. (1983). *The architecture of cognition.* Cambridge, Mass.: Harvard University Press.

Benbasat, I., & Wand, Y. (1984). A structured approach to designing human-computer dialogues. *International Journal of Man-Machine Studies, 21,* 105 - 126.

Boucsein, W., Greif, S., & Wittekamp, J. (1984). Systemresponsezeiten als Belastungsfaktor bei Bildschirm- Dialogtätigkeiten. *Zeitschrift für Arbeitswissenschaft, 38*, 113 - 121.

Brown, A. L. (in press). Metacognition, executive control, self- regulation, and other even more mysterious mechanisms. In F. E. Weinert & R. W. Kluwe (Eds.), *Metognition, motivation, and understanding.* Hillsdale, N.J.: Erlbaum.

Brown, J. S., & Newman, S. E. (1985). Issues in cognitive and social ergonomics: From our house to Bauhaus. *Human-Computer Interaction, 1,* 359 - 391.

Cakir, A. (1981). Belastung und Beanspruchung bei Bildschirmtätigkeiten. In M. Frese (Ed.), *Stress im Büro* (pp. 46 - 71). Bern: Huber.

Caplan, R. D., Cobb, S., French, J. R. P. (jr.), van Harrison, R., & Pinneau, S. R. (jr.) (1975). *Job demands and worker health.* Washinghton: NIOSH.

Card, S. K., Moran, T. P., & Newell, A. (1983). *The psychology of human-computer interaction.* Hillsdale, N.J.: Erlbaum.

Carroll, J. M., & Thomas, J. C. (1982). Metaphor and the cognitive representation of computing systems. *IEEE Transactions on Systems, Man, and Cybernetics, 12,* 107 - 116.

Chin, D. N. (1986). User modeling in UC, the UNIX consultant (*Proceedings of the CHI'86 Conference on human factors in computing systems*). Boston: 24 - 28.

DIN 66 234 (1984). Normenausschuß Informationsverarbeitungssysteme (NI) (1984 als Entwurf verabschiedet). *Bildschirmarbeitsplätze. Grundsätze der Dialoggestaltung.* Deutsches Institut für Normung e. V.

DiSessa, A. A. (1986). Models of computation. In D. A. Norman & S. W. Draper (Eds.), *User centered systems design.* Hillsdale: Erlbaum.

Dörner, D. (1976). *Problemlösen als Informationsverbeitung.* Stuttgart: Kohlhammer.

Dörner, D. (1986). Heuristisches Wissen beim Lösen einer einfachen Steuerungsaufgabe (*35. Kongreß der Deutschen Gesellschaft für Psychologie*). Heidelberg: 1986.

Dunckel, H. (1985). *Mehrfachbelastungen am Arbeitsplatz und psychosoziale Gesundheit.* Frankfurt: Lang.

Emery, F., & Thorsrud, E. (1976). *Democracy at work: The report of the Norwegian industrial democracy program.* Leiden: Nijhoff.

Fitter, M., & Sime, M. (1980). Creating responsive computers: Responsibility and shares decision-making. In H. T. Smith & T. R. G. Green (Eds.), *Human interaction with computers* (pp. 39 - 65). London, New York.

Frese, M. (1978). Partialisierte Handlung und Kontrolle: Zwei Themen der
    industriellen Psychopathologie. In M. Frese, S. Greif, & N.
    Semmer (Eds.), *Industrielle Psychopathologie* (pp. 159 - 183).
    Bern: Huber.

Frese, M. (1982). Occupational socialization and psychological
    development: An underemphasized research perspective in
    industrial psychology. *Journal of Occupational Psychology, 55,*
    209 - 224.

Frese, M. (1984). Transitions in jobs, occupational socialization and strain.
    In V. Allen & E. V. D. Vliert (Eds.), *Role transitions:
    Explorations and explanations* (pp. 239 - 253). New York: Plenum
    Press.

Frese, M., Albrecht, K., Altmann, A., Lang, J., Papstein, P. v., Peyerl, R.,
    Prümper, J., Schulte-Göcking, H., Wankmüller, I., & Wendel, R.
    (1986). *The effects of an active development of the mental model
    in the training process: Experimental results on a word processing
    system.* Manuscript.

Frese, M., & Peters, H. (1987). *Zur Fehlerbehandlung in der Software-
    Ergonomie: Theoretische und praktische Überlegungen.* München:
    Manuscript.

Frese, M., & Sabini, J. (Eds.) (1985). *Goal directed behavior: The concept
    of action in psychology.* Hillsdale: Erlbaum.

Frese, M., Saupe, R., & Semmer, N. (1981). *Stress am Arbeitsplatz von
    Schreibkräften. Vergleich zweier Stichproben.* In M. Frese (Ed.),
    Stress im Büro. Bern: Huber.

Frese, M., Stewart, J., & Hannover, B. (1987). Goal- orientation and
    planfulness: Action styles as personality concepts. *Journal of
    Personality and Social Psychology, 52* (6).

Gardell, B. (1971). Technology, alienation and mental health in the
    modern industrial environment. In L. Levi (Ed.), *Society, stress
    and disease.* London: Oxford Univ. Press.

Gasser, L. (1986). The integration of computing and routine work. *ACM
    Transactions on Office Information Systems, 4,* 205 - 225.

Glass, D. C., & Singer, J. E. (1972). *Experiments on noise and social
    stressors.* New York: Academic.

Gleitman, H. (1985). Some trends in the study of cognition. In S. Koch &
    D. E. Leary (Eds.), *A century of psychology as science:
    Retrospections and assessments.* New York: McGraw-Hill.

Hacker, W. (1978). *Allgemeine Arbeits- und Ingenieurpsychologie* (2nd ed.).
    Bern: Huber.

Hacker, W. (1983). Psychische Beanspruchung bei Text- und
    Datenverarbeitungstätigkeiten an Bildschirmgeräten: Ermittlung
    und Gestaltung. *Zeitschrift für Psychologie, Supplement 5,* 24 -
    41.

Hacker, W. (1985). Activity: A fruitful concept in industrial psychology. In M. Frese & J. Sabini (Eds.), *Goal directed behavior: The concept of action in psychology* (pp. 262 - 284). Hillsdale, N.J., London: Erlbaum.

Hackman, J. R. (1977). Work design. In J. R. Hackman & J. L. Suttle (Eds.), Improving life at work. *Behavioral science approaches to organizational change* (pp. 96 -). Santa Monica, California: Goodyear Publishing Company, Inc. (162)

Heckhausen, H. (1980). *Motivation und Handeln*. Berlin: Springer.

Hutchins, E., Hollan, J. D., & Norman, D. A. (1986). Direct manipulation interfaces. In D. A. Norman & S. W. Draper (Eds.), *User centered system design*. Hillsdale: Erlbaum.

Kahn, R.L. (1974). Conflict, ambiguity, and overload: Three elements in job stress. In A. McLean (Ed.), *Occupational stress* (pp. 47-61). Springfield, Ill.: Thomas.

Karasek, R. A. (1979). Job demands, job decision latitude and mental strain: Implications for job redesign. *Administrative Science Quarterly, 24*, 285 - 308.

Karasek, R. A., Baker, D., Marxner, F., Ahlbom, A., & Theorell, T. (1981). Job design latitude, job demands, and cardiovascular disease: A prospective study of Swedish men. *American Journal of Public Health, 71*, 634 - 705.

Kieras, D., & Polson, P. (1985). An approach to the formal analysis of user complexity. *International Journal of Man- Machine Studies, 22*, 365 - 394.

Kohn, M. L., & Schooler, C. (1982). The reciprocal effects of the substantive complexity of work and intellectual flexibility: A longitudinal assessment. *American Journal of Sociology, 84*, 24 - 52.

Kornhauser, A. (1965). Mental health of the industrial worker. New York: Wiley.

Maass, S. (1983). Why systems transparency? In T. R. G. Green, S. J. Payne, & G. C. van der Veer (Eds.), *The psychology of computer use* (pp. 19 - 28). London: Academic Press.

Miller, S. (1981). Predictability and human stress: Toward a clarification of evidence and theory. In L. Berkowitz (Ed.), *Advances in experimental social psychology*, Vol. 14. (pp. 203- 256). New York: Academic.

Norman, D. A. (1983). Some observations on mental models. In D. Gentner & A. L. Stevens (Eds.), *Mental models*. Hillsdale: Erlbaum.

Norman, D. A. (1986). Cognitive engineering. In D. A. Norman & S. W. Draper (Eds.), *User centered system design*. Hillsdale: Erlbaum.

Österreich, R. (1981). *Handlungsregulation und Kontrolle*. München: Urban & Schwarzenberg.

Osterloh, M. (1983). *Handlungsspielräume und Informationsverarbeitung.*
    Bern: Huber.
Polson, P. G., & Kieras, D. E. (1985). A quantitative model of the
    learning and performance of text editing knowledge (*Proceedings
    of the CHI'85 conference on human factors in computing systems*).
    San Francisco: 207 - 212.
Polson, P. G., Muncher, E., & Engelbeck, G. (1986). A test of a common
    elements theory of transfer (*Proceedings of the CHI'86
    Conference on human factors in computing systems*). Boston, 78 -
    83.
Rohr, G., & Tauber, M. (1975). Virtual objects and virtual places how
    people comprehend their tasks using complex application software
    (*Macinter-Workshop on "Knowledge and visual information
    representation"*). Stuttgart: Talk.
Rouse, W. B., & Morris, N. M. (1986). On looking into the black box:
    Prospects and limits in the search for mental models.
    Psychological Bulletin, 100, 349 - 363.
Schardt, L. P., & Knepel, W. (1981). Psychische Beanspruchungen
    kaufmännischer Angestellter bei computergestützter
    Sachbearbeitung. In M. Frese (Ed.), *Stress im Büro* (pp. 125 -
    158). Bern: Huber.
Seligman, M. E. P. (1975). *Helplessness: On depression, development and
    death.* San Francisco: Freeman.
Semmer, N. (1982). Stress at work, stress in private life and psychological
    well-being. In W. Bachmann & I. Udris (Eds.), *Mental load and
    stress in activity: European approaches* (pp. 42 - 55). Amsterdam:
    Elsevier.
Semmer, N. (1984). *Streßbezogene Tätigkeitsanalyse: Psychologische
    Untersuchungen zur Analyse von Streß am Arbeitsplatz.* Weinheim:
    Beltz.
Semmer, N., & Frese, M. (1985). Action theory in clinical psychology. In
    M. Frese & J. Sabini (Eds.), *Goal directed behavior: The concept
    of action in psychology* (pp. 296 - 310). Hillsdale: Erlbaum.
Shackel, B. (1985). Ergonomics on information technology in Europe - a
    review. *Behaviour and Information Technology, 4*, 263 - 287.
Shneiderman, B. (1980). *Software psychology.* Cambridge Massachusetts:
    Winthrop Publishers.
Shneiderman, B. (1983). Direct manipulation: A step beyond programming
    languages. *Computer, 16*, 57 - 69.
Smith, M. J., Cohen, B. G. F., Stammerjohn, L. W. (jr.), & Happ, A.
    (1981). An investigation of health complaints and job stress in
    video display operations. *Human Factors, 23*, 387 - 400.
Turner, J. A., & Karasek, R. A. (1984). Software ergonomics: Effects of
    computer application design parameters on operator task
    performance and health. *Ergonomics, 27*, 663 - 690.

Ulich, E. (1978). Über das Prinzip der differentiellen Arbeitsgestaltung. *Industrielle Organisation, 47*, 566-568.

Ulich, E., Groskurth, P., & Bruggemann, A. (1973). *Neue Formen der Arbeitsgestaltung. Möglichkeiten und Probleme einer Verbesserung der Qualität des Arbeitslebens.* Frankfurt: Europ. Verlagsanstalt.

Volpert, W. (1974). *Handlungsstrukturanalyse als Beitrag zur Qualifikationsforschung.* Köln: Pahl-Rugenstein.

Psychological Issues of
Human Computer Interaction in the Work Place
M. Frese, E. Ulich, W. Dzida (Editors)
© Elsevier Science Publishers B.V. (North-Holland), 1987

ON TOOLS AND INTERFACES

Wolfgang Dzida

Gesellschaft für Mathematik und Datenverarbeitung mbH
D-5205 Sankt Augustin 1, Schloss Birlinghoven

In view of the ergonomic and technological advances the phenomenon "computer" is taken as a tool. A historical study of the relationships between workers and different kinds of tools reveals the interface as becoming a more differentiated and important component in that relationship. An interface model is introduced as an essential part of the conceptual model a user needs for mastering the intangibility of a computer. The paper argues for application independent interfaces as providing a number of advantages to the user. Close to this is the hypothesis which points to the advantages which may accrue to the user, if s/he adapts to the intangibility in that some abstract action schemata become incorporated in his/her mental model of the interface. Technical trends seem to be compatible with this psychological postulate.

HISTORICAL BACKGROUND

A brief historical review is given in advance, so as to introduce the computer as a special type of tool. From the user's point of view this tool particularly differs from earlier developed types of tools in that it allows an interchange between user and tool in dialogue terms. As a consequence of this technical development, the interface between human and computer was brought into the focus of psychological research.

Three Steps in the Development of Tools and Interfaces

Tools have engendered striking technological progress to take some burden off human beings. In looking at the history of tools and the development of their interfaces to users three steps may be identified.

Firstly, the amount of physical effort to get things done could be reduced. Later, when tools became more complex and took the functionality of machines the user was relieved of sensori-motor activity.

Finally, modern machines like computers reduce the burden of some mental activities, such as calculating, reasoning and decision making.

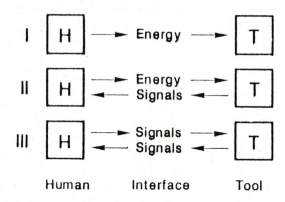

Figure 1: *Three steps in the development of tools and interfaces*

Figure 1 illustrates the historical development of interfaces in terms of three steps. In the beginning it was the user's physical energy, his/her dexterity and deftness which made him/her superior in handling a tool. It was the user, who was in control of the function embodied in a tool. During performance s/he always kept a vivid imagination of the work flow and the results created. Various sensations provided feedback so as to enable the user to control the course of action. The user acquired skills and habits allowing him/her to react automatically to specific work situations. Rapidity and precision of muscular action was substantial in doing that.

At an early stage in the history of our tools the "interface" between user and tool was characterized by poperties of handiness. The interface characteristics changed in the course of further developments. Machines became more suitable for a precise treatment of objects. The amount of precision achieved by machines was no longer achievable by human experts, particularly in the short machine processing time. The user, of course, was still urgently needed to initiate an action and to control its accomplishment. At the interface the machine process was initiated, for instance, by the manipulation of a lever arm. Feedback, however, was no longer received via sensations from muscles and tendons. Typically, the operator received some feedback by means of (symbolic) signals, for instance, on a scale. With the implementation of this symbolic and abstract kind of feedback we can observe rudimentary dialogues between man and machine. Nevertheless, a real *dialogue* was not yet introduced. The control of the machine process still required input engendered by the operator's physical energy.

A dialogue with conventional tools is unknown. One cannot enter into a dialogue with a camera or a pencil, unless even the flashing of a LED triggered by the user is perceived as dialogue with the tool "camera". The sensorimotor feedback experienced on writing with the pencil should not be regarded as a dialogue, since dialogue in the narrower sense presupposes a return as part of the output of the tool which is language like, at least similar to an artificial language.

Human-machine dialogue started when a certain kind of computing machinery was developed which required input of symbols in order to control the machine. It was the exchange of signals which established an interaction between man and machine as a dialogue, although the language applied is still quite artificial. In order to come up to our common expectations about a dialogue, some additional features had to be implemented. For instance, if the computer were really capable of conducting a dialogue then the user would receive immediate response to his/her input. A "batch mode" dialogue is not really a dialogue, although symbols have to be used to control the performance of the machine.

Characteristics for dialogue systems as users perceive them have been formulated (Dzida et al., 1978). For instance, in analogy to dialogues between humans one may expect that human-comupter dialogue is error-tolerant. A dialogue is error-tolerant if the user's intended result is obtained despite obviously faulty input (cf. DIN 66 234, Part 8). Self-descriptiveness is another example of how dialogue characteristics determine the human-computer interface. This characteristic refers to the explanations a user can require from the system in the context of a certain work step. These examples may suffice to emphasize the fact that the interchange with a computer resembles a dialogue between persons, with the computer remaining a tool and not becoming a partner.

One may argue that the historical or phenomenological analysis of tools and interfaces provides some trivial results. To my experience, however, this analysis helps novice users in reflecting the nature of the strange object "computer" and to catch an idea of what is meant by an "interface" as a component of the machine.

Increasing Importance of Interfaces between Human and Tool

In the course of the historical development of tools the interface between human and tool became more important. Interface design is crucial for a user to have access to machines in a task adequate manner allowing him to exploit the technical advantages without unnecessary additional strain.

Benefits may accrue from technical progress in the development of tools and machines. However, there are disadvantages, too. It is of vital importance to compensate for disadvantages. This can be achieved by the development of ergonomic human-machine interfaces, because there are only few characteristics which cannot be compensated for by ergonomic interface design, for instance, the logical or physical malfunction of a tool or deficiencies of the material which a tool is made of.

To computer naive users, but even to specialists, problem solving by means of software tools became complicated. This is partially because the concrete visual conceptualization of what is happening in the machine has been lost. In addition, the feedback of stimulating sensations necessary for the user to handle a traditional machine is now drastically reduced and is substituted by highly *abstract modes of operation*. "Direct manipulation" of objects on a display is an interface design proposal which is intended to remedy lack of tangibility so that at least some of the objects can be perceived by touch (Card, Moran and Newell, 1983). But does this technical and ergonomic progress suffice for the user to tackle problems at his/her work station?

The more an interface becomes relevant for efficient problem solving the less a designer should rely on his/her purely engineering competence in developing an interface. S/he should ask for advice, particularly cognitive psychologists. However, one may ask whether it is possible to apply results of cognitive psychological research in a field where the success of problem solving mainly depends on the availability of problem adequate interfaces. Cognitive psychologists have been mostly concerned with areas of problem solving where the success of the solving process depends on an application of *abstract operators*, such as transformation rules in mathematical logic. One of the most striking differences between a logic operator required to perform a mental operation and a physical operator ("tool") is the fact that only the latter one has an interface that provides access to the operator in a more or less suitable manner. An application of cognitive psychological research on interface design can be concentrated on that part of a computer interface which is most common to human problem solving processes.

With the advent of dialogue systems it has now been discovered that the interface between human and machine became more differentiated. A model for user interfaces will be introduced in more detail (next paragraph), so as to point to that part of the interface which is most challenging to cognitive psychologists. This interface is called "tool interface". Other parts of the human-computer interface appear to be less relevant to human problem solving. Nevertheless the design of these parts of the interface may provide a more or less convenient context in which problem solving processes can be conducted in dialogue terms.

A MODEL FOR USER INTERFACES

An interface model is important for the user to serve as a "conceptual model". It is devised as a tool for the understanding or teaching of the physical system (the term conceptual model refers to Norman, 1983, p.12).

'Interface' as a Component of the User's Conceptual Model

The interface between user and machine is not just closely related to the designer's interest to outline an adequate architecture of the system. An interface is also an essential concept to assist the user in solving problems with the aid of machines, particularly when a user is interested in adapting the machine to his own working style. Since the interface has become a complex part of the machine, the user is faced with an additional problem: to manipulate the interface before getting a software tool to be active.

An interface may be defined as a set of rules which determine the interchange of data (information) between user and computer. A user should know most of the rules. An interface model can be a great help to the user, since it allows him/her to know which areas s/he can influence. Some parts of an interface, for instance, s/he can manipulate without altering the data; other parts provide him/her with access to the data and its processing; again other parts make it possible to influence organizational processes of his/her environment.

An International User Group within IFIP TC6, Working Group 6.5 (International Federation for Information Processing), has discussed an interface model. I suggested a definition of the model in terms of a net as illustrated by figure 2.

In figure 2 circles indicate interfaces, rectangles indicate activities (processes), arrows indicate the direction of information (data) flow. The processes P1 and P2 can be taken as pieces of interface software, with P1 governing, for instance, the presentation of symbols on the display and with P2 selecting the option in a menu according to the user input (however, without inducing the process of an application program). P1 and P2 can be regarded as technical components of an interface manager. For those who are interested in implementation details some technical papers are already available, for instance, Shaw et al. (1983). It should be emphasized that the model is neither right nor wrong. From the historical background outlined in paragraph 1 of this paper, however, one might find the model quite plausible.

The model can be regarded as a proposal for the sake of establishing a terminology. This has the advantage that it is no longer necessary to refer to "the user interface" in undifferentiated terms. Furthermore, different design aspects can be described relatively independently of each

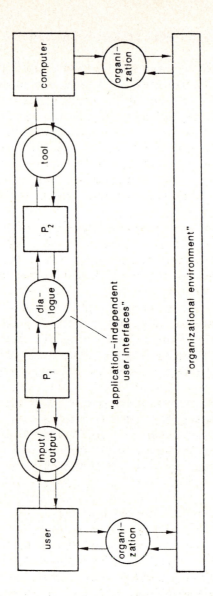

Figure 2: The IFIP WG 6.5 user interface model (cf. IFIP, 1981)

other. Thus, even the architecture of an interface may be defined in terms of the model. However, the major purpose of this paper is to discuss whether the model is suitable for the user's need to form a "mental model" of the interface.

The Interface for Input and Output

Rules for user input and software system outputs define this part of the user interface (I/O-interface). This part is sometimes called the "surface" of the system. Such a metaphor implies that there must be something behind. The model illustrated by figure 2, however, does not introduce any metaphor, in order to avoid a misleading understanding of the concept "interface". Instead, different aspects of the comprehensive interchange of data or information between a user and his/her working environment are analyzed. This model implies that for each aspect there are real physical entities in dialogue systems. The following examples may explain this:

Input rules: The manner in which characters are to be input by the user or by which the cursor is positioned on the display (for example with key, "mouse" or lightpen). Also determined are how tasks are represented and the means by which they can be submitted to the system (for example by means of soft keys or function keys on a key board).

Output rules: The manner in which data and tools can be presented to the user is established. The data output by the system should be well-grouped and presented in formated manner. Suitable forms of coding should be selected: "local coding" can be used to assign specific meanings to specific fields on the screen; "color coding" can be used to attract the user's attention.

A large amount of ergonomic literature exists from which one may derive design hints. In designing the I/O-interface, for instance, sensory limits of the user have to be considered. Most of the limits are well-known and also translated into national and international standards for VDU work stations. (Examples: Cakir, Hart & Stewart, 1979, 1980; Van Cott & Kinkade, 1972.)

The Dialogue Interface

The dialogue is a process implemented for the sake of task performance in the course of which the user inputs data in one or several dialogue steps and is given feedback with respect to the processing of these data (cf. German DIN standard, DIN 66 234, Part 8).

Certain rules determine the dialogue between user and software system, for instance, how the user can obtain explanations from the system about an input field or the purpose of a tool, how the user can issue jobs (for instance, only on request from the system or after selecting an option in a menu). The rules also determine how the user can influence (e.g. interrupt, continue or cancel) task processing by the system.

Figure 3 illustrates the definition of dialogue in terms of a net. There are three subprocesses within the feedback loop: (1) an operation of the user (O), for instance a command (c) submitted to the system, (2) an

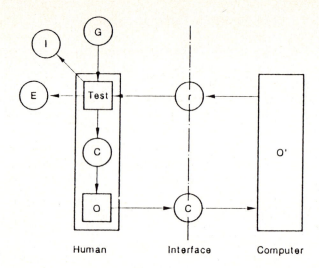

Human   Interface   Computer

Figure 3: Components of dialogue

operation of the system (O'), for instance the processing of the just submitted command as well as a feedback to the user concerning the result
(r), (3) a cognitive operation of the user, called test (Test), which implies
a decision, whether the goal (G) has been actually achieved. If this is the
case, then "exit" (E) otherwise the user's cognitive system identifies an
incongruence (I). This definition of dialogue is close to the so called
TOTE unit (cf. Miller et al., 1960).

If figure 2 and figure 3 are integrated, it is quite easy to show that
two types of dialogue steps can be distinguished (figure 4). Type one dialogue merely changes the display state that is simply what is on the screen.
Therefore, type one dialogue can be called *display related dialogue*. Type
two dialogue provides a task adequate transition from the current data
state the application program is concerned with into a new data state.
Hence, type two dialogue can be called data related dialogue or better *task
related dialogue*. The distinction between type one and type two dialogue
is important for the user's "mental model" of the system, since it is this
model that guides his/her use of the system (the term mental model refers
to Norman, 1983, p.12).

A basic ergonomic requirement is the suitability of a dialogue for
the task (DIN 66 234, Part 8). This objective can be achieved if the dialogue supports the user in the job s/he is actually doing without unnecessary additional strain being placed on him by the system itself. In terms of

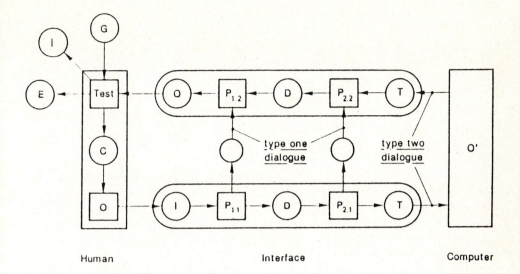

Figure 4: Two types of dialogue steps: 1. display related dialogue, 2. task related dialogue

figure 4 this means that the amount of effort necessary for type one dialoge step is reduced to a minimum. For instance, if it is quite clear from the point of view of the work process where the cursor has to be positioned in a display area, the cursor should be automatically placed in the expected position.

The dialogue is fit for the task, if it supports a user's display related dialogue steps. However, this is not sufficient. The dialogue should also support the user in his/her task related dialogue steps. This kind of support depends on the quality of the tool interface (chapter 2.4).

Dialogue with a machine is a new phenomenon in the history of man's tools. In terms of research and development, more has hitherto been invested in the interface for input and output than in the dialogue interface. Topics for research can be derived from the list of principles of dialogue design (DIN 66 234, Part 8). For example: "Self-descriptiveness" is a dialogue capability of software tools; in contrast to traditional tools, software tools can explain their internal states and their own behaviour themselves. Because of their highly abstract mode of operation, this explanation is necessary, but as yet is not adequately investigated or implemented.

The Tool Interface

A tool can be applied in a variety of ways. The design of a tool interface aims at adapting the way of application to the user's way of performance. Application of tools indispensably involves a convenient and efficient *access* to them. The access to a traditional tool is by hand. The access to a software tool is by information. What kind of information is necessary for the user's selection task? This paper argues for the hypothesis that there are advantages to the user, if he or she is able to know about the access of tools in terms of *abstract* concepts.

An example: The user is editing a paper on "user-friendliness". The word "user-friendliness" is expected to occur repeatedly in the text. The text editor provides a tool interface which facilitates the input of complicated or long or repeated words. By means of a so called STRING-SET the user defines the key "U" to be representative for the string "user-friendliness". In combination with a certain function key the user has a convenient access to a set of tools. The whole string will be produced as per default command. The user's access is supported by the supersign "U" which is a feature of the tool interface. The user may apply this interface in order to prepare for his/her typing task and to perform more easily. It is typical for this tool interface that it can only be utilized if the user can form a mental representation of the practical use of tools in terms of an *abstract* concept. An abstraction has to be made from the nitty-gritty details of the manual performance.

One may argue, however, that it is more favourable to access to computer tools by "direct manipulation mode" or by natural language. It might be that this argument holds for those tool interfaces which should provide a convenient access by occasional users. But is a convenient mode of access always efficient? There is some empirical evidence for the efficiency of formal and thereby abstract modes of access to data bases (Katzeff, 1986). Further research is necessary. This paper postulates that abstract properties of a tool interface do appear to provide an efficient performance. For an interdisciplinary cooperation between computer science and cognitive psychology, it is this characteristic of the tool interface which is most challenging.

From theory about "schematic thinking" (Schank and Abelson, 1977) one may infer that cognitive action schemata enable the user to generate knowledge about an appropriate selection of tools. An action schema generates a representation of a "prototypical action" which may fit to the task at hand. Then the user is capable of achieving the intended result, namely the access to a tool which appears to be problem adequate.

There is some empirical evidence, however, that there is no need for the user to gain direct experience in the problem space, in order to generate a proper prototypical action schema. Pollard and Gubbins (1982) demonstrated in an experiment that people were superior in solving a deductive reasoning problem when they generated an *abstract* performance schema which was applicable to the task at hand. Provided this specific kind of thinking process investigated is equivalent to the user's reasoning process when he or she selects an appropriate tool then one may conclude that users should succeed at the tool interface to the extent that they possess and can retrieve *abstract* action schemata.

Rules which govern the *scope* of application of software tools also characterize the tool interface. The user may be interested in knowing what services the tools offer and how well the tools are matched to each other, for example, whether the same editor is available for formulating and sending a message as for formulating a monthly report. This example can be taken to explain another feature of a tool interface, namely the functional fixedness of a tool to a specific or a generic task. The *functional fixedness* property points to the fact (or to the pretended fact) that the familiar use of a tool precludes its use in a novel way to solve a problem. A highly specific editor is apt to fill index-cards with text, whereas a generic editor writes on objects whatever type they belong to. A generic tool acts on an information object only *in principle* which means that the same tool can be applied to a variety of objects. It is up to the user to *abstract from* specific applications and to generalize the application purpose of a tool. Chapter 3.2 of this paper provides some examples for generic tools.

For the user, the computer represents a number of independent or combined tools. *Combination* principles determine the tool interface. Some combination principles may be formulated as follows:
- elementary tools acting on the same object can be combined so as to produce a complex and thereby more powerful tool,
- elementary tools acting on different objects can be combined; the user develops a "procedure" for the sake of routine task accomplishment.

In both cases the user needs additional action schemata which represent *abstractions* from the concrete details of elementary action schemata. In applying these or other combination facilities the normal way of system use will be extended. The user can be enabled to develop a style of system use which is programming like in that the control structure of his working steps is made explicit. The gulf between the normal use and a programming like use of the system can be bridged in that adequate concepts are offered at the tool interface.

The Organizational Interface

Rules which determin the relationship of the user's work tasks to the work tasks of other users characterize the organizational interface. For example, work sharing, rules of conduct (standing orders), rules of cooperation. The tools of a software system should also be matched to the tools of the other users in an organizational environment. The rules of this relationship, which govern, for instance, the connection of an "electronic mail system" with the conventional in-house mail system, also form part of the organizational interface.

Dissatisfaction with the data processing system is sometimes due to a failure of the work organization to adapt to the new tools. Evaluation of the organizational interface it thus gaining increasing importance. Through the manufacture of software tools, developers have an influence on the organization of work which should not be underestimated. For instance, unforeseen preparatory activities arise which are time-consuming but necessary in order to work with the new tools. An "electronic mail system" can also change rules of communication within an organization in that, for instance, messages which have an undefined pragmatic status are exchanged outside the usual channels.

A deeper analysis of the features of organizational interfaces is beyond the scope of this paper. A conceptual base for designing such interfaces is outlined by Malone (1985).

APPLICATION-INDEPENDENT USER INTERFACES

Independence of interface components from application programs is regarded as a technical trend providing a number of advantages for the user. The history of this trend reveals successive independence of three parts of interfaces. Even the tool interface becomes more or less separate from specific applications, and is thereby engendering properties just outlined.

Interfaces Separated from Tools

It is apparent from the history of man's tools that the user interfaces of tools have always been adapted to man. Many interfaces have been standardized on the basis of ergonomic knowledge. This involves a protracted process of negotiation. The IFIP WG 6.5 model for user interfaces can be used to illustrate how step-by-step advances in standardization are achieved. In this process the design of interfaces becomes an independent activity, which means that it is relieved of any reliance upon any specific application software.

Figure 5 takes into account the fact that the *I/O-interface* is implemented independently of the computer. The programmer must accept the requirements of this interface as given and adapt the application accordingly. In practice, this means that, for example, with a given "bit-mapped display" graphical representation of information is possible, irrespective of the degree to which it is used in specific applications.

To achieve application-independence of user interfaces step by step, it is also expedient to design the *dialogue interface* in such a way that

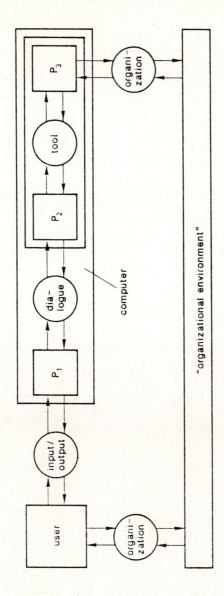

Figure 5: The IFIP WG 6.5 model for user interfaces; interface for input and output is application-independent only

applications programmers accept the dialogue requirements as standard. In figure 6 the user interfaces represented as independent of the computer can be termed "virtual terminals". The developer of application programs

can assume uniform management of the screen surface and of standard
dialogue forms.

    The last step towards standardization of user interfaces requires a
standardization of requests to the *tool interface*. If this proves successful,
the application programmer can assume that access to tools is standardized

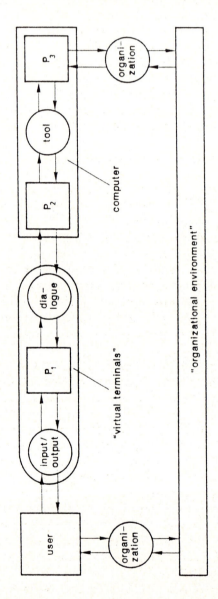

Figure 6: *The IFIP WG 6.5 model for user interfaces; I/O-interface and*
          dialogue interface are application-independent

and that the manner in which the tool can be combined or extended is pre-defined. Figure 4 illustrates the condition of computer-independent user interfaces.

Application-independent user interfaces have advantages and disadvantages. One disadvantage for example is that individual user requirements which go beyond a standard solution can incur costs. On the other hand, costs for the development of comfortable user interfaces can be distributed over a large number of customers. One advantage lies in the fact that it is easier for users to learn dialogue techniques since they can engage in similar man-machine dialogue in different application cases. Moving users between different display work stations is also facilitated. Furthermore, researching of ergonomically desirable dialogue characteristics is promoted, since it is easier to collect empirical material and critical incident reports under comparable conditions.

Technical Implementations

The route leading to application-independent user interfaces can be simulated not only on the basis of the model, but also in technical developments. All *"front-end"* processors are offered as an indispensable technical means of optimizing the user-friendliness of interfaces. A front-end processor can be regarded as a user-interface agent, sometimes called "communication agent". Each process of the agent serves for communication with a tool; relationships arising from work with tools can be dynamically reconstructed in this processor. The user can thus automate recurrent procedures in the dialogue independently of the application program. By the way, this feature pertains to the aspect of tool interface (compare with chapter 2.4).

A highly advanced development of application independent user interfaces is found in the "Xerox Star" system (cf. Xerox, 1981). Implementation of a dialogue technique which could be described as "pointing" allows the user to work in the same way in any desired application area. The user positions (i.e. points at) and selects any desired objects at the I/O-interface so that s/he can subsequently process them with an application-specific tool. The dialogue technique of "pointing" enables the user to perform job preparations for different application areas in a similar manner. Another standard technique with the "Xerox Star" ist the "set window". To define a working area on the screen, the user sets up a limited area in which the task is processed. The working area is always set up on the screen in the same way irrespective of the specific tasks. This dialogue technique is a typical contribution to the development of application-independent dialogue interfaces.

In the case of the "Xerox Star", it is also possible to study an application independent tool interface. Two conceptual considerations have probably led to this; firstly, an abstraction was made from many application-specific objects which led to the concept of "generic" objects (objects which do not have any definite characteristics referring to a specific application). Secondly, an abstraction was made from the application-specific performance of the tools, which led to the concept of "generic" tools.

"Generic objects" are for example "blank object", "blank folder", "blank record file". These objects can be used in different office areas, in the same way as a file is used wherever anything has to be stored.

"Generic tools" are "copy", "delete", "find", "repeat" and "move", which are used in different application areas. In the same way as book pages, account sheet items or salary tables can be copied with the aid of a photocopier, the tool "copy" allows the user to copy such things as letters, sentences, formulas or other display segments.

It remains to be seen which technical development will contribute to further standardization of user interfaces. The IFIP WG 6.5 model has proved its worth in helping to improve classification of developments to date.

CONCLUSIONS

In effect, computer tools have been developed to expand the efficiency of such human cognitive processes as calculating data, searching and combining information, constructing and reconstructing text structures, graphics, etc. This paper is in favour of the hypothesis that it is an abstract mode of operation of all these kinds of problems which appears to be superior.

The technical trend of human-computer interfaces, however, seems to promote the opposite direction, i.e. a display of objects commonly known from the traditional desktop and by no means being abstract or intangible representatives of our working environment.

Considering different parts of the user interface as suggested by the IFIP WG 6.5 model the controversy can easily be clarified. The quite familiar "desktop metaphor" (Cox, 1986, p.166) as well as the "direct manipulation" mode might satisfy all ergonomic requirements, so far as the *I/O-interface* or the *dialogue interface* is concerned. However, so far as the *tool interface* is concerned, progress in human-computer interface design is not due to the tangibility of the "desktop metaphor", but is due to its underlying instrumental concept which involves such abstractions as *generic* objects and tools.

REFERENCES

Cakir, A.; Hart, D.J. & Stewart, T.F.M. (1977). *The VDT Manual*. Darmstadt: IFRA.

Cakir, A.; Hart, D.J. & Stewart, T.F.M. (1980). *Bildschirmarbeitsplätze*. Berlin: Springer.

Card, St.K., Moran, Th.P. & Newell, A. (1983). *The Psychology of Human-Computer Interaction*. Hillsdale: Erlbaum.

Cox, B.J. (1986). *Object Oriented Programming. An Evolutionary Approach*. Reading: Addison-Wesley.

DIN 66 234, Part 8 (1986). *VDU work stations - Principles of dialogue design*. (Second editorial draft.) Berlin: Beuth.

Dzida, W.; Herda, S. & Itzfeldt, W.-D. (1978). User-perceived quality of interactive systems. *IEEE Transactions on Software Engineering*, SE4 (4), 270-276.

IFIP (1981). *Report of the 1st Meeting of the European User Environment Subgroup of IFIP WF 6.5*. Bonn: Gesellschaft für Mathematik und Datenverarbeitung.

Katzeff, C. (1986). *Logical reasoning, models and database query writing. The effect of different conceptual models upon reasoning in a database query writing task*. Hufacit paper No. 10, Dept. of Psychology, University of Stockholm, Sweden.

Malone, Th.W. (1985). Designing organizational interfaces. In: L. Borman and B. Curtis (eds.): *Human Factors in Computing Systems - II*. p.66-71. Amsterdam: North Holland.

Miller G.A.; Galanter, E. & Pribram, K.H. (1960). *Plans and the Structure of Behavior*. New York: Holt.

Norman, D.A. (1983). Some observations on mental models. In: D. Gentner & A.L. Stevens (Eds.): *Mental Models*. London: Erlbaum.

Pollard, P. & Gubbins, M. (1982). Content and rule manipulation on the Wason selection task. *Current Psychological Research*, 2, p. 139-149.

Schank,R.C. & Abelson, R.P. (1977). *Scripts, Plans, Goals, and Understanding*. Hillsdale: Erlbaum.

Shaw, M., Borison, E., Horowitz, M., Lane, T., Nichols, D. & Pausch, R. (1983). Descartes: A programming-language approach to interactive display interfaces. *Sigplan Notices*, 18, No.6, pp.100-111.

Van Cott, H.P. & Kinkade, R.G. (1972). *Human Engineering Guide to Equipment Design*. Washington: U.S. Government Printing Office.

Xerox (1981). *The "Xerox Star"-System*. Seybold Report 10/16.

Psychological Issues of
Human Computer Interaction in the Work Place
M. Frese, E. Ulich, W. Dzida (Editors)
© Elsevier Science Publishers B.V. (North-Holland), 1987

A CRITIQUE AND EMPIRICAL INVESTIGATION OF THE "ONE-BEST-WAY-MODELS" IN HUMAN-COMPUTER INTERACTION

Siegfried Greif & Günther Gediga

Dept. of Psychology, Work and Organisational Psychology Unit, University of Osnabrück, Knollstr. 15, 4500 Osnabrück, Federal Republic of Germany

The chapter describes and discusses theoretical, methodological and practical problems of the Cognitive Psychology of Human-Computer Interaction proposed by Card, Moran & Newell (1983), and their Model Human Processor, GOMS and Keystroke-Level Models. Results of a time series experiment on a simple task show that the assumed models of stable and additive time components are inadequate. Simple "One-Best-Way-Models" of Keystroke-Level behavior should be be replaced by "Different-Best-Way-Models" of complex and flexible human adaptation processes.

INTRODUCTION

In their book Card, Moran & Newell (1983) present a stimulating vision of the prospects for cognitive psychology to play a significant role through basic research and practical design in the growing field of human-computer interaction. The *Model Human Processor*, the *GOMS models* and the *Keystroke-Level Models* are fundamental to their influential approach to theory and practice. Together, these models offer an engineering-style theory of the user interactions with the computer, intended to form the basis for future theories and practical tools in task analysis and systems design.

In the following paper we begin with a short description of the basic models. Next, critical comments on the theoretical and methodological models will be presented followed by a summary of our own experimental research testing the validity of the basic models. Theoretical and practical alternatives are discussed in the concluding section of the paper.

DESCRIPTION OF THE BASIC MODELS

Card, Moran & Newell (1983) and Newell & Card (1985) refer to three basic models:
(1) The Model Human Processor provides a general model of human information processing.
(2) the *Goals Operations Methods and Selection rules (GOMS)* Model describes the rational problem solving strategy of the ideal user and
(3) the Keystroke-Level Model analyses observable sequences of keystrokes, button pushes and mouse moves and for each generates specific time estimates.

Together these three models are used by Card et al. to analyse and predict the error-free behavior of expert users.

The Model Human Processor

Card et al. (1983, 24 ff) try to summarise the major findings of cognitive experimental psychology through their Model Human Processor, which is conceived in terms of three interacting subsystems:
(1) the Perceptual System (P),
(2) the Motor System (M), and
(3) the Cognitive System (C).

Each subsystem is characterized by the mean speed of their elementary operations (and their ranges), called the "cycle time" following the computer analogy.

Each processor has its own memories and processors. The Perceptual Processor uses a Visual Image Store and an Auditory Image Store as their buffer or Working Memory. The parameters for these two memories are the "decay times" in msec of any individual content item, the storage capacities and the "main code types". The general Working Memory is characterized by capacities to store chunks, decay times for chunks and other items, and capacities for storing either acoustic or visual items. The Long-Term Memory is assumed to have infinite decay times and capacities and to use semantic information only.

Card, Moran & Newell (1983) derive time estimates and other parameters from their review of basic experimental findings in psychology. For example the mean and range of the cycle time of the Perceptual Processor is identified with the response time of the visual system to a very brief pulse of light (Ganz, 1975; Harter, 1967). Experiments on maximum tapping rates (Fitts & Posner, 1967; Chapanis et al., 1949), pen movements between two lines (Fox & Stansfield, 1964; Kinkead, 1975) and on the time limits of discrete micromovements of the hand are all used to derive the average cycle times of the Motor System. The parameters of the Memory Systems are derived by a more complicated averaging procedure.

The GOMS Model

GOMS Models are used to analyse and predict the behavior of the rational expert user. They are derived from the traditional Model of the General Problem Solver of Newell & Simon (1972). The components are:
(1) Goals (G),
(2) Operations (O),
(3) Methods (M) and
(4) Selection Rules (S).

(1) Card et al. (1983. p. 144 ff) describe a *Goal* (G) as "a symbolic structure that defines a state of affairs to be achieved and determines a set of possible methods by which it may be accomplished." Examples: EDIT-MANUSCRIPT, MODIFY-TEXT and EXECUTE-UNIT-TASK.

(2) *Operations* (O) are defined as "elementary perceptual, motor, or cognitive acts, whose execution is necessary to change any aspect of the user's mental state or to affect the task environment." Examples: GET-NEXT-PAGE, GET-NEXT-TASK, USE-QS-METHOD and USE-S-COMMAND.

(3) *Methods* (M): "A method describes a procedure for accomplishing a goal. It is one of the ways in which a user stores his knowledge of a task." Methods are decribed by conditional sequences of goals and operators. Example: If at end of manuscript page GET-NEXT-PAGE.

(4) *Selection Rules* (S) are the decisions between alternative methods and goals. They are based on the user's knowledge of the task environment. "The essence of skilled behavior is that these selections are not problematical, that they proceed smoothly and quickly, without the eruption of puzzlement and search that characterizes problem-solving behavior." Examples: "If-such-and-such is true in the current situation, then use method M" (or select goal G).

To predict the behavior of a user in terms of GOMS Models we have to apply an essential axiom of Card et al. (1983. p. 27) which is called the *Rationality Principle*. "A person acts so as to attain his goals through rational action, given the structure of the task and his inputs of information and bounded by limitations on his knowledge and processing ability". Implicitly Card et al. assume that the expert user makes decisions by employing the same basic efficiency criteria that they recommend for designers. Card, Moran & Newell (1983. p. 1) assume that the basic criteria of designers are "easy, efficient, error-free – even enjoyable" interfaces. The operational criteria they offer throughout their book are always minimal performance times (msec), minimal errors and minimal learning times.

With the expert user in mind, we may analyse and describe the sequence of operations of ideal users for a given task by flow diagrams or using their Command Language Grammar (CLG). A description of the ideal user's operations and keystroke times is the method of *Task Analysis* they recommend for designers. In their book they describe examples of theoretically derived GOMS Models for different tasks (mainly manuscript editing), methods, and line-editors. Card et al. (1983, p. 189) conclude, that their GOMS Models predict the observed sequence of error-free user actions "reasonably well" (matching the operator sequence 80 to 100% of the time). The error-free GOMS Model may be very simply expanded to predict typical or *routine error behavior*, if we analyse the error correction task by constructing special GOMS Models.

Their GOMS Models and their method of task analysis assume the existence of ideal expert users, who always act rationally minimizing time and errors, finding (according to their expert knowledge) and selecting at every point in the sequence of operations the shortest and safest way to the given goal. These principles are strikingly similar to Taylor's and Gilbreth's traditional Time-and-Motion-Methods which tried to identify the *"one best way"* to do a task. Therefore we may call them *"One-Best-Way-Models"* of human-computer interaction.

The Keystroke-Level Model

The GOMS Models describe, analyse and predict the *sequence* of operations or steps to reach a given goal. For the empirical description, analysis or prediction of precise *execution time* values (msecs) of a given GOMS Model, Card et al. (1983, Chapter 8) recommend their Keystroke-Level Models. As in Time-and-Motion-Studies, they are trying to find empirically based general time estimates for operations. The time parameters used in their Model Human Processor are now applied to arrive at an estimation of the *total Execution Time* (T execute) of the task by aggregating the times of six subcomponents.

Card et al. (1983) apply these six types of time components (or operators) with the aid of experimental research or their own empirical results to give time estimates for "fastman", "middleman" and "slowman". The total sum of all component time values is calculated according to their general equation predicting the mean (and range) execution time of errorless behavior for expert users. In their book they describe many examples with different tasks (mostly editing tasks), estimating theoretical execution times and comparing them with empirical data from their research. They conclude that the empirical evidence proves that their Keystroke-Level Models and time estimates are adequate for practical design. Essential to their model is the assumption of a linear equation of additive and constant time components (which should be valid at least for the major part of the phenomena, cf. Newell & Card, 1985, see below).

BASIC METHODOLOGICAL AND THEORETICAL PROBLEMS

Which models and methods of human-computer interaction are adequate is not only of theoretical importance. Psychologists have to give practical guidance how to allocate tasks and subtasks between men, computers, computer aided flexible machines or robots. The "One-Best-Way-Models" based on Card, Moran & Newell's Model Human Processor, GOMS Models and Keystroke-Level Models are being applied to hardware and software design and are becoming factual design solutions for many users. These solutions have significant consequences for the design of tasks, human efficiency and wellbeing and perhaps even the long term development of user competences. An "easy to use" design may, for example, minimize effort and therefore the required knowledge of the user to understand the complexity of the computer system. Also such models of human efficiency and difficulties may have implicit consequences for future decisions on the replacement of humans by computers or robots.

Newell & Card (1985) admit four difficulties in their vision:
1. The microscopic analysis of keystrokes is too low level. Real interface problems involve the organisational context, complex systems, multiple tasks, and the learnability of the total system.
2. The scope of the phenomena covered is too limited. There is an almost endless list of important missing problems (visual displays, the use of natural language, novices and learning, errors etc.).
3. Scientific results come too late to direct current and future technological progress.
4. The models are difficult to apply.

Their recommendation for overcoming the *problem of level* is to develop a Psychology of actions based upon the analysis of special time intervals which thereby sets the framework for Task Analysis. The *problem of scope* may be solved by adding operating principles and integrating cognitive models and experimental research on performance and error, knowledge representation, mental models and the acquisition of skill. To cope with the *problem of late science* they argue that while about every 5 years a new interface generation comes to dominate the scene, the total lifetime of an interface amounts to about 15 - 20 years. This is sufficient time for good psychological research. To bridge the *wide gap between theory and practice*, they advocate the search for good application domains, for example, intelligent tutoring systems.

Since their view is stimulating and persuasive, and potentially of fundamental relevance to the whole field of human-computer interaction, it is important to examine their models closely and evaluate their vision of its scientific and practical prospects. We will concentrate on theoretical and methodological problems and relate our evaluations later in this paper to experimental research.

The "level" of analysis - an arbitrary problem?

The question seems to elicit highly controversial debate about which level of analysis - molar, molecular, or macro - may be more important or promising for a Psychology of human-computer interaction (cf. the debate with Michael Frese at the Human-Computer Interaction Symposium of 1986 at the DGfPs Congress in Heidelberg). These controversies seem to arise from the need to decide on research strategies whilst there is continuing uncertainty about the utility of different levels of analysis.

We share Newell & Card's *vision* of a micro-level Psychology contributing to practical design solutions, but we strongly disagree with their simple restriction of the domain of Psychology to time intervals (like "below a few minutes and above tenth of seconds").

In their opinion it is the domain of social and organisational theory, to analyse the macro levels, which they acknowledge to have great relevance. But Psychology would have to give away not only Work and Organisational Psychology to other disciplines, if we follow such a restriction. The macro-levels of Learning and Educational Psychology, Personality Theories, Social Psychology, the study of longterm consequences of stress at work etc. etc. would lie outside this narrow domain.

Perhaps an alternative vision of Psychology's contribution is a move toward the *integration of micro- and macro-levels*. For example, at least theoretically it is possible to analyse general structures and processes of organisations by applying the micro-level methods of task analysis (cf. Greif, 1986).

The micro-level units of analysis below a tenth of a second are also not solely the domain of "Neural and Biochemical Theory", as Newell & Card would have us believe. A micro-level Psychology would of course not exclude the processes below the Keystroke-Level. Card et al. (1983) cite Sternberg (1975), who found an increase of mean reaction time of about 38 msec per additional item in his ET-paradigm to be consistent across different populations. Raab & Fehrer (1962) in their experiments on the dependence of reaction times on the brightness of the stimulus are discussing "great" differences of 10 - 20 msec and "mean" values of 2 - 5 msec.

The Keystroke-Level is not derived from a theoretical or measurement model. It is an arbitrary, although perhaps pragmatically useful time-standard for measurement, and therefore should not be called a "level". The theoretical and practical problems of human-computer interaction and the progress of science will not advance from arbitrary time units or overdrawn disciplinary boundaries.

Hard or soft science?

Psychology has to meet the high theoretical and methodological standards of "hard (natural) sciences" and the precise quantitative measurement standards of applied engineering sciences if it shall play a significant role in the field of human-computer interaction. To this degree we agree with Newell's & Card's (1985) general position. But the critical question is, if the models and estimates of Card et al. (1983) and Newell & Card (1985) come up with such genuine "hard standards".

Card et al. (1983, p. 27) seem to see no problem integrating an exponential function of the Power Law of Practice which says in essence, that execution times of tasks are not constant but exponentially decrease as a function of the number of trials; and, with simple linear additive time functions, which assume constant and additive time components, regardless of the number of the operations. Newell & Card (1985) demonstrate how they would simplify complex phenomena through a simple formula:

Phenomenon = Volume-part (e.g. linear part) + Difficult-part
(e.g. non-linear part)

Such a global "formula" seems liable to neglect the important differences between linear and non-linear models, as well as between the GOMS and Keystroke-Level Models, and the theory of Complexity of Polson & Kieras (1985). Newell & Card (1985) even claim to be able to integrate any new research on knowledge representation and Mental Models, Anderson's (1983) cognitive simulation models and their Model Human Processor, and Norman's (1983, 1984) theoretical taxonomy of errors.

Newell & Simon (1972) and Card, Moran & Newell (1983) also seem to be neglecting basic methodological principles and criteria of experimental psychology: sampling principles, criteria of description and operationalizing the experimental variables, experimental designs, measurement and test theory etc.. They simply are constructing ad hoc efficiency indices and comparing their numerical values.

For example in one of their so called basic "experiments" Card et al. (1983, p. 108) tested 5 different editors and a typewriter. Insufficient description of the selection of their subjects is given. For several editors they select three and for one editor and for the typewriting condition they take only one subject. They do not mention any methodological problems in calculating and comparing variances of time indices (different tasks) and ratios of the slowest to the quickest editor etc.

Failure to describe subject samples is a major deficiency of their approach, since the generalisability and practical utility of the estimates of the time parameters which they derive from their models directly depends on the population and sampling procedures. Since they are not only analysing mean values ("middle man" in their terminology) but also providing estimates for extreme groups (like their "fastman" or "slowman"), special sampling methods and particular measurement theory are needed to solve the major methodological problems of deriving unbiased estimates for extremely fast or slow subjects.

The seemingly high matches (85 - 100%, see above) between predicted and observed sequences of operations for their GOMS Models can be seen to be partly trivial, if we look critically at the matching procedure described by Card et al. (1983, p. 190 f, Appendix to Chapter 5):

Before beginning the matching, error sequences are excluded by their procedure. If the problem space of the task only allows for one single right way, this may immediately raise the matching to 100%. Since sequences of different length are difficult to match by a corresponding percentage of operations, the next step of their recommended "algorithm" is simply to insert dummy operators "in such a way as to maximize the number of matches". By such a procedure they compare the steps or operations of expert people correctly solving routine problems using the "best way" in the "problem space" to yield a model of the "most efficient" problem solver. Since for error-free solutions only detours or different correct ways cause mismatchings (in other words, dummies are constructed to compensate for detours), the set of possible detours in the objective problem space is crucial. If we now specifify the percentage of the maximum possible number of detours for a given task and problem space by x%, the minimum match will be 100 - x%. If x% is small, a high percentage of matches will be trivial. Therefore the algorithm has to be corrected by the minimum x%-value, if it is to be interpreted as an unbiased index of the matches of behavior sequences among expert users.

The testing of the execution time estimates of the Keystroke-Level Models by Card et al. (1983) can also be criticized as a "maximization procedure". Since Card et al. (1983) publish data for several tasks showing very high time values for error components, and these are omitted from the count, we know at least for these tasks and (expert) users, the sum values of errors. But Card et al. seem to overlook another basic problem, the maximization of execution time ranges. Their procedure involves the aggregation of range values for time intervals (see the formula estimating execution times below). Every additional time component (for example every keystroke- or mental-time) unduly broadens the range and reduces the discriminative power of the predicted execution time. Since they are using this range as their comparison value for the correctness of observed execution times, incorrect estimations for tasks with components with broad ranges or a large sum of range values become unlikely. Therefore, by leaving error times out of the count and overlooking the problem of summing time range values, Card et al. are not, as they claim, adopting the high standards of applied engineering sciences measurement.

Our position is not that the approach and innovative methods and models of Card et al. are devoid of theoretical and practical value. Their approach has stimulated a new type of research and application, which is more than most psychological models and methods might claim. But if we are understanding the essential message of Card, Moran & Newell correctly, we have to demand that research and the derivation of precise engineering data must be recommended with adequate experiments and descriptions of the micro-processes of "natural" human problem solving and human-computer interaction. Maybe the models of Card, Moran & Newell can be partly replicated. But from the start we need to be more careful and cautious with our samples, generalizations and ideal models.

Limited criteria of efficiency

Cognitive psychology and information-processing perspectives have stimulated laboratory research and the practical design of interactive computer systems "to be efficient and easy to use (...) so that people in our society may realize the potential benefits of computer-based tools" (Card, Moran & Newell, 1983, p. vii). But helping to design efficient tools is only one of the tasks which Psychology is facing. And perhaps there is reason to question the wisdom of designing computer systems to be easy to use. An alternative would be to design tasks and tools which embody the long term criteria that have been derived from field research for the development of human personality, action competences and health and the "Humanization of Working Life" that have been derived from field research (cf. Hacker, 1986; Ulich, Groskurt & Bruggemann, 1973; Frese, Greif & Semmer, 1978).

EXPERIMENTAL TESTS OF THE VALIDITY OF THE MODELS

There are many open questions about the general theoretical bases of the Keystroke-Level Models of Card, Moran & Newell. Applying the "hard methods" of experimental Psychology we should be able to answer the following basic questions:

1. Is it possible to reduce observable time partitionings of operations to "One-Best-Way Models" with only different speed values of the subjects ("slowman", "middleman" and "fastman") or is it necessary to construct models with completely different structures?
2. Is a simple model of stable time components sufficient or is it necessary to construct models with time values which systematically depend on attributes of the context or task?
3. Are the Card, Moran & Newells categories of time components complete or are important operators missing?
4. Can we disregard errors, the speed-accuracy conflict and other conflicting micro-goals, when we construct basic models?

To find an answer to these questions has important theoretical and practical consequences for hard- and software-design. The validity and predictive value of the models can not be tested sufficiently using only the overall sum of the time components. To construct Keystroke Models and to test basic propositions we have to apply experimental designs which apply time series and analysis of variance methods to systematically varied task attributes. Statistical tests of all discriminable time components of the Keystroke Models are required.

A simple task and a simple Keystroke Model

We used a very simple tasks called "STERZINGER LINES" (cf. Boucsein in this book).

XA WES QA WX RTZ ZDR E OKU OLIJU IK ZU

Figure 1: Example of a STERZINGER LINE.

The task is to move the cursor to any blank which has two identical letters on either side of it (e.g. the fifth blank "RTZ ZDR"). The lines are presented on the screen with a non-blinking cursor at the left margin. Target positions are randomly distributed, some lines having no target. The cursor can be moved from blank to blank by the right- and left-arrow cursor keys. The up-arrow key is used to mark the target after positioning the cursor. For non-target lines the correct position is the right margin.

Using STERZINGER LINES instead of more complex practical tasks is advantageous because subjects quickly become "experts" with the task and the number of necessary keystrokes can be varied systematically for the tasks. From this it is possible to estimate not only the keystroke times for the execution of a constant task but also the intraindividual stability of Keystroke Models with well controlled variations of target positions.

Even for this simple task it is not easy to construct a Keystroke Model by applying different procedures, models and time estimates proposed by Card, Moran & Newell (1983) in various parts and tables of their book. We test the model by using the following linear equation:

$$T = TRT + (k \times TE) + TK + TRC + ((k-1) \times TS) + TK$$

The first time component is the *system-response time for the task (TRT)* causing the user to wait before the STERZINGER LINE appears on the screen. Card, Moran & Newell assume that we simply might add the time value of the system response time, if the TRT > 1.350 msec. We used an example with TRT = 2.000 msec.

The second step is to estimate the *time it takes to examine the line (TE)*. Following Card et al. we can discriminate three different operators for this task:
(1) The time needed for eye movement.
(2) The "cycle time" of the "Perceptual Processor".
(3) The "cycle time" of the "Cognitive Processor".

The sum of these three operators is TE = 400 msec (range: 125 to 1.070 msec). TE has to be multiplied by the number (k) of the blanks which have to be examined.

The next operator *TK* is the *keystroke time* pressing down the cursor key (right-arrow key). Because it is a simple movement we can use the "cycle time" of the "Motor System", giving a value of TK = 70 msec (range: 30 to 100 msec). Pressing down the cursor key, the cursor begins to move (with negligible response time) one blank. If the cursor is steadily held down, after a *response time of the cursor of TRC* = 540 msec the cursor *"shoots" rapidly with TS* = 89 msec/blank to the next blank. If the fifth blank is the target position, the total time to reach the target without error is (k-1) x TS.

The last operation is to *mark the target* pressing the up-arrow key. Again we insert TK = 70 msec into our equation.

For the "middleman" the resulting time estimates (for TR = 2.000 msec and k=5) would be:
T = 4.536 msec = 2.000 + (5 x 300) + 70 + 540 + (4 x 89) + 70 msec

The expected range is:
T = 3.681 msec = 2.000 + (5 x 145) + 30 + 540 + (4 x 89) + 30 msec
    (Minimum or "fastman")
T = 8.446 msec = 2.000 + (5 x 1.070) + 100 + 540 + (4 x 89) + 100 msec
    (Maximum or "slowman")

Experiments

Subjects were 72 paid students, 41 were male and 31 female, with mean age of 24 years. Only 5 subjects were psychology students, the largest group (21) came from educational and teaching disciplines. Since Card, Moran & Newell do not restrict the validity of their models to non-student populations, this sample is appropriate for testing the models.

One or two weeks before the experiment a battery of pretests was administered in groups (vision test, intelligence test, personality and introspection scales, familiarity with experiments etc.). The experiment lasted for about 5 hours. After a general instruction, the introspection scales and the electrodes for physiological measurement were applicated. The major tasks were 6 blocks of STERZINGER LINES (each lasting 12 minutes) followed by two problem solving tasks. System-response times (TRT) of the STERZINGER LINES were varied experimentally (constant and variable system-response times with mean TRTs of 2.000 and 8.000 msec) and permutated systematically. Heart activity, galvanic skin response, keystrokes and times were registered continuously. The introspection scales and blood pressure measurements were administered before and after each of the 6 blocks of STERZINGER LINES and the problem solving tasks (for models and results on the psychophysiological data see Holling, in prep.). At the end of the experiment retrospective task analyses and explorations were conducted for the STERZINGER LINES and the problem solving tasks (Monecke, in prep.).

The subjects were instructed to work as quickly and accurately as possible. As an incentive the subjects were told that they could leave earlier if they worked quickly. As an incentive for accuracy the experimenter said that faulty tasks would have to be repeated (but this was not true).

Two possible methods of how to do the task were mentioned. The first method was the one described above ("screen the line - move the cursor"). The second method was to move the cursor to the next blank and check the single blank ("step by step"). Since Card et al. have constructed their models predicting the behavior of expert users, a "training period" was necessary, where the subjects could find their best method. For our simple task the training lasted for 20 min with constant response times (TRT) of 1.000 msec for all groups.

Differences between conditions were tested by robust statistical tests like Wilcoxon, Page Test of Trend, and Friedman Analysis of Variance, with a criterion of 5% or less for significance testing.

Results

(1) The first question to answer is if Card, Moran & Newell's estimates of the total execution time and the different time components are adequate.

The total execution time values of error free execution time is T = 5.402 msec for subjects using the method 1 "screen the line - move the cursor". This mean time value is about 900 msec higher than the predicted time, but Card, Moran & Newell might argue that is does not exceed their predicted range. But examining the single time components shows, that the screening component times (TE) alone give a sum value corresponding to the whole execution time predicted by the Card et al. Our subjects need about the same time for the screening phase which should be appropriate for the whole task.

(2) The second question is, if it is possible to reduce the observable time partitionings of operations to "One- Best-Way Models".

The results show, that the subjects used different methods with very different Keystroke-Level structures. The method "screen the line - move the cursor" was applied constantly by 25 subjects (Method 1) . The second "step by step" method was preferred by 17 persons (Method 2). A group of 17 subjects use mixed or variable methods. For the remaining 13 subjects a classification based on keystroke-times is difficult. The observed total execution time of method 1 is higher than the time T = 4.219 msec for the "step by step" method 2 (for k = 5 and TRT = 2.000 msec).

Comparing the partitioning of the mean time values for error free keystrokes in Fig. 2 shows the expected trivial differences between corresponding time values for the keystrokes the subjects need in method 1 to screen the line (TE), which is of course much longer than the first keystroke for method 2, where the subjects used a "step by step" method. But these longer screening times are not compensated by much shorter times taken to "shoot" the cursor.

If we take a closer look at the keystrokes after the first one, in relation to the different target positions (cf. Greif, Gediga & Holling, 1986), we find remarkable structural differences between the two methods. The time values for method 2 are independent of different target positions (time values lie on a linear regression line with a significant trend and

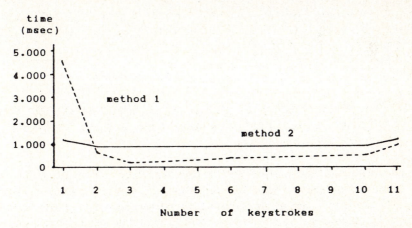

*Figure 2: Mean execution times of the keystrokes of STERZINGER tasks,
all experimental conditions, error-free beha vior (method 1:
"screen the line, find the target"; method 2: "step by step").*

strong slope for the last arrow-up key). In comparison, the execution times for method 1 (see fig. 3) show very complicated functions with significant differences depending on the target position.

The results clearly show important structural differences between the two methods studied. Additionally we have found structurally different Keystroke Models even within the group preferring the first method. Since the target position has been varied experimentally these results clearly prove a systematic dependence of time functions on the target position for the group using method 1.

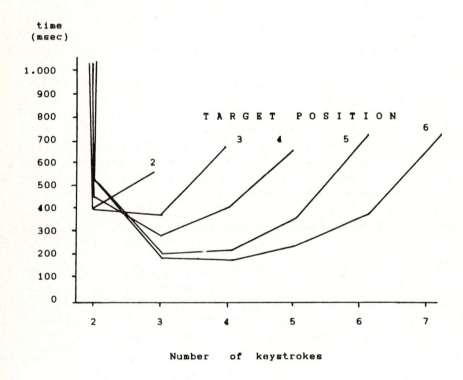

Figure 3: *Mean execution times of the keystrokes of STERZINGER tasks for method 1 ("step by step") and different target positions (1 to 6), all system-response-time conditions, error-free behavior.*

(3) Our third question is, whether a simple model of stable time components would be sufficient.

Several results show clearly, that is it necessary to construct models in which time values depend systematically on system-response times and target positions (cf. Greif, Gediga & Holling, 1986). Longer mean system-response times cause longer time values for the first keystroke. For method 2 quicker mean reaction times for keystrokes depend on longer mean system-response times. (The subjects behave as if they try flexibly to compensate the time loss through quicker reactions.) There is a small but significant (Trend Test) increase in operation times from blank to blank for method 2, independent of the target position. Subjects seem to become increasingly cautious if they do not find the target.

Our arguments and results are not new. In the last century Donders (1868) used precisely the same logic in factorizing reaction times. Our arguments also basically follow the classic critique offered by James McKeen Cattell (1886): even if it might be possible to describe the keystroke-operations of a simple task under restricted context conditions by additive factors, the general validity of the logic of a whole additive model and the elementary reaction times for other tasks (especially if they are more complex) and different context conditions (the variation of system-response times is an example) is questionable. This critique has stimulated modern experimental research (cf. the overview of Townsend & Ashby, 1983). In contrast to simple additive factor models, experimental results have to be simulated by mathematical models which predict the process by which reaction times are generated.

(4) Are the time components complete or are important operators missing?

At least one component has to be added (besides the "error-components", see below). The last keystroke (marking the target by the arrow-up key) shows much higher time values than the preceeding keystrokes (cf. Greif et al. 1986). - The subjects use much time to check their solutions before they finish a single STERZINGER task by pressing the return-key.

(5) Can we disregard errors when we construct basic models and ignore the speed-accuracy conflict or other conflicting micro-goals?

Card, Moran & Newell construct their models on the basis of error free keystroke-data from expert users ("one best or quickest way"). Of course, as they admit, speed efficiency may be reduced by losses of accuracy. Therefore they propose the keystroke-models be supplemented by special speed models or subroutines for the correction of errors. The correction of perceived errors can be described by speed models but conflicts between speed and accuracy can not be simulated by separate error-routines. Or more generally, the models do not allow one to describe processes by which people cope with multiple (conflicting) micro-goals and problems (like speed, accuracy, frustrations, monotony, personal concerns).

As the first results of investigations explorations show (see Monecke, in prep.) nearly all subjects mention conflicts between speed and accuracy. There is a substantial correlation between the individual speed and the effort the subject invests in speed after initial exploration. The significant error-differences between both methods in Analysis of Variance are very impressive (cf. Greif, Gediga & Holling, 1986). Even if method 1 were theoretically - perhaps for subjects with special perceptual and motor skills - "the quickest way", we have to explain their significantly more frequent errors and corrections (left-arrow key). If the costs of errors are high, this model would clearly be the wrong choice.

There are other important micro-conflicts which are mentioned by several subjects which have to be considered, since they are influencing the choice of methods and keystroke-behavior. The conflict between efficiency and monotony is an example. Several subjects consciously altered the preferred methods, trying to reduce the monotony of the task. Some subjects told us that they decided to work slower to reduce stress. Many examples illustrate the conflict between efficiency and wellbeing. Adequate psychological models, predicting interindividual differences in micro-goals and strategies or intraindividual changes between methods need to be much more complicated. Gediga (1986) has described formal models for such different types of conflicts which can be applied to describe the behavior of subjects who switch between methods.

THEORETICAL AND PRACTICAL PERSPECTIVES

In summary, our experimental results show that for simple STERZINGER tasks the models of Card, Moran & Newell (1983) do not fit our data. If it is possible to construct Keystroke Models we must be very careful in any generalizations from the situations in which they were derived. Individual preferences for methods, changes of task and context attributes may all imply completely different models.

Practical design consequences

Differential practical design solutions are clearly needed if, as appears, different models fit for different subjects, methods, micro-goals (speed, accuracy and perhaps wellbeing) and variations of task attributes or context conditions (like target position and system-response time). Eberhard Ulich (1983) has proposed principles of "differential job design", which could be applied to our results, with the support of field research.

He criticizes Frederic Taylor's idea of the "one best way" and advocates job design which takes account of individual differences in needs, problem solving strategies, competences and skill development. Similarly, the design of computer-systems should follow the principles of "differential hard- and software-design" (see Ackermann, Ulich & Ulich in this volume).

Premature generalizations of "One-Best-Way-Models" to computer- and software-design following simplistic Keystroke Models may have psychological dangerous consequences: human capacity and flexibility to adapt to simple tasks may give the false appearance of uniformity among users rather than reflecting the demand characteristics of the task. Thus it would be easy, but fundamentally incorrect, to infer simplistic models of the user from simple task performance and to base systems design on the predictive value of such models. The alternative approach of "Different-Best-Way-Models" and the principles of "differential job design" seem preferable as long as scientific evidence for the adequacy of the description of human capacities through simple models is lacking and when research such as ours show individual differences and flexible adaptations to tasks and context conditions to be important.

Theoretical prospects

Computer tasks can very quickly become complicated, when a person makes a mistake or if system-response time interrupts the execution of a sound problem-solving strategy. Of course people are able to behave like computers, given computer-like tasks. You may even find people who simulate a computer-model in their everyday planning and execution of activities. But it is a particular human strength that we do not break down if the system of goals, plans and operations is logically dissonant. Unlike a computer, we do not need consistently to edit and assemble our goals and plans like a computer before we are able to operate. Indeed, it even seems to be quite normal for us to be unaware of dissonance between our tasks, goals, plans, methods and actions.

Systematic Exploration and Human Flexibility

Precise studies of human micro-styles of action using the computer may help to resolve empirically the old historical controversy between Thorndike and "Gestaltpsychology" (esp. Wertheimer and partly Köhler) about the role and function of "trial and error" in learning and problem solving. Wertheimer (1945, see Woodworth 1949, p.149 ff) insisted that "trial and error" has no positive function in productive thinking. He claimed that it only interferes with or disturbs the process of problem solving. He reports examples of his own solutions to two mathematical problems. He classifies his problem solving strategy as "viewing the whole", "never getting lost in petty details, in detours", no "trial and error" and "no trying of hypotheses".

The results of several human-computer interaction studies show seemingly chaotic exploratory processes and keystroke-behavior amongst both learners and professionals (Carroll & Mack, 1983; Janikowski, 1985; Tränkle, 1985; Waern, 1986). It is remarkable that Card (1984) also, describing two experiments on visual search of command menus, concludes that the users behavior can best be described by an unsystematic search model. But what seems to be chaotic and unsystematic, may be the result of complex or unknown functional strategies of human activities. In our opinion Woodworth was right, when he stressed the need to integrate the models of "trial and errror" and reasoning strategies. Following Carroll (1984), the user who is actively exploring the computer system is facilitating his own learning. Errors may be helpful to "eliminate possibilities". Systematic trial and error does not exclude reasoning.

By "systematic trial and error" or "systematic exploration" we refer to a micro-style of action or a rational strategy for reducing the complexity of multiple tasks and goals (by elimination of "possibilities") or for actively exploring a task or "problem space" which is at least partially unknown to the subject. This type of action style (for empirical research on different action styles see Frese, Stewart & Hannover, in press) should be (significantly) different from chance paths in the "problem space" (chance zig-zag-paths). In other words, it is not "blind" trial and error behavior. But on the other hand it is not thinking and planning ahead without trials (and possible errors). Spontaneous "explorative activities", guided by stimulus properties, internal goals and intermediate plans are necessary for a stepwise approach to the solution of the problem and for the development of a partial cognitive map of the problem space.

Flexible human problem solvers might combine systematic exploration, rational planning and habitual reactions if the task, its context and the long term consequences seem to demand it. That means we need a *Theory of Human Flexibility* which describes, explains the function and predicts the inter- and intraindividual differences of human action-styles and adaptation processes to practically relevant attributes of discrete and multiple tasks. To construct and test such a theory will be a difficult and long term task for Psychology. Barnard (in press) recently has developed a promising "interacting cognitive subsystems framework", which describes capabilities for parallel processing of information. This model is an alternative and perhaps more adequate approach to the prediction of natural human information processing for specified tasks and context conditions. But we should not be surprised, if the challenge of developing a comprehensive Theory of Human Flexibility goes beyond the capabilities of currently available scientific knowledge and methods.

ACKNOWLEDGEMENTS

The project "System-Response Times" is conducted with W. Boucsein and his coworkers (Wuppertal) and is funded by the German Research Society (DFG), Grant Bo 554/2-1.

We gratefully acknowledge the support of Heinz Holling and Norbert Schnettberg in carrying out the experimental work and data processing, the collaboration of M. Lemm and K. Pezalla and the editorial help of Dr. Nigel Nicholson on an earlier version of this paper.

REFERENCES

Anderson, J.R. (1983). *The architecture of cognition.* Cambridge, Mass.: Harvard University Press.

Barnard, P.J. (in prep.). Cognitive resources and the learning of human-computer dialogs. In J.M. Carroll (Ed.). *Interfacing thought: Cognitive aspects of human-computer inter action.* Cambridge, Mass.: MIT Press.

Card, S.K. (1984). Visual search of computer Command Menus. In H. Bouma & D.G. Bouwhuis (Eds.). *Attention and performance X control of language processes.* Hillsdale, N.J.: Erlbaum.

Card, S.K., Moran, T.P. & Newell, A. (1983). *The Psychology of Human-Computer Interaction.* Hillsdale, N.J.: Erlbaum.

Carroll, J.M. (1984). Minimalist design for active users. In B. Shackel (Ed.). *Human-computer interaction - Interact '84.* Amsterdam: North Holland, 39-44.

Carroll, J.M. & Mack, R.L. (1983). Actively learning to use a word processor. In W.E. Cooper (Ed.), *Cognitive aspects of skilled typewriting.* New York: Springer, 259-283.

Cattell, J.McK. (1886). The time taken up by cerebral operations. *Mind, 11,* 220-242, 377-392, 524-538.

Chapanis, A., Garner, W.R. & Morgan, C.T. (1949). *Applied Experimental Psychology: Human Factors in Engineering Design.* New York: John Wiley & Sons.

Donders, F.C. (1868). Over de snelheid van psychische processen. Translated by W.G. Koster (1969). On the speed of mental processes. *Acta Psychologica, 30,* 412-431.

Fitts, P.M. & Posner, M.I. (1967). *Human performance.* Belmont/California: Brooks/Cole.

Fox, J.G. & Stansfield, R.G. (1964). Digram keying times for typists. *Ergonomics, 7,* 317-320.

Frese, M. (1986). *Mensch-Computer-Interaktion als arbeitspsychologisches Problem.* Paper presented to the 35th Congress of the West-German Psychological Association, Heidelberg, September.

Frese, M., Greif, S. & Semmer, N. (Eds.). (1978). *Industrielle Psycho-pathologie*. Bern: Huber.

Frese, M., Stewart, J. & Hannover, B., Goal-orientation and planfulness: action styles as personality concepts. *Journal of Personality and Social Psychology*, in press.

Ganz, L. (1975). Temporal factors in visual perception. In E.C. Carterette & M.P. Friedman (Eds.). *Handbook of perception*, Vol. V, *Seeing*. New York: Academic Press.

Gediga, G. (1986). Problemlösen als Informationsverarbeitung: Eine lern-theoretische Perspektive. *Osnabrücker Forschungsberichte, Nr. 51*.

Greif, S. (1986). *Organisational tasks, informatics design and training*. Paper presented to the CREST/SERC Advanced Course "Human Factors for Informatics Usability" (B. Shackel) Loughborough, December.

Greif, S., Gediga, G. & Holling, H. (1986). *A critical view of keystroke-level models*. Paper presented to the 21st International Congress of Applied Psychology, Jerusalem, Israel, July.

Hacker, W. (1986). Activity: A fruitful concept in industrial Psychology. In M. Frese & J. Sabini (Eds.). *Goal directed behavior: The concept of action in Psychology*. Hillsdale, N.J.: Erlbaum, 262-284.

Harter, M.R. (1967). Excitability and cortical scanning: A review of two hypotheses of central intermittency in perception. *Psychological Bulletin, 68*, 47-58.

Hick, W.E. (1952). On the rate of gain of information. *Quarterly Journal of Experimental Psychology, 4*, 11-26.

Holling, H. (in prep.). *Wahrscheinlichkeitmodelle und empirische Analysen zur Beanspruchung durch Systemresponsezeiten*. Unpubl. Manu-script, University of Osnabrück.

Janikowski, A. (1985). *Fehler beim Computer-Training*. Universität Osnabrück, unpubl. Diplomarbeit.

Kinkead, R. (1975). Typing speed, keying rates, and optimal keyboard layouts. *Proceedings of the 19th Annual Meeting of the Human Factors Society*.

Monecke, U. (in prep.). *Eine Methode der heterarchischen Aufgaben-analyse*. Unpubl. Diplomarbeit, University of Osnabrück.

Newell, A. & Card, S.K. (1985). The prospects for psychological science in human-computer interaction. *Human-Computer Interaction, 1*, 209-242.

Newell, A. & Simon, H.A. (1972). *Human problem solving*. Englewood Cliffs, N.J.: Prentice Hall.

Norman, D.A. (1983). Design rules based on analyses of human error. *Communications of the ACM, 26*, 254-258.

Norman, D.A. (1984). *Working papers on errors and error detection*. San
  Diego: Institute for Cognitive Science, University of California at
  San Diego.
Polson, P.G. & Kieras, D.E. (1985): A quantitative model of the learning
  and performance of text editing. *Proceedings of the Conference
  on Human Factors in Computer Systems* (CHI '83). New York:
  ACM.
Raab, D. & Fehrer, E. (1962). The effect of stimulus duration and
  luminance on visual reaction time. *Journal of Experimental
  Psychology, 61*, 326-337
Sternberg, S. (1975). Memory scanning: New findings and current con-
  troversies. *Quarterly Journal of Experimental Psychology, 27*, 1-
  32.
Townsend, J.T. & Ashby, F.G. (1983). *Stochastic modeling of elementary
  psychological processes*. Cambridge: Cambridge University Press.
Tränkle, U. (1985). Beobachtungen beim Erlernen der Dialogsprache CMS.
  Schriftenreihe des Rechenzentrums der Universität Münster.
Ulich, E. (1983). Differentielle Arbeitsgestaltung - ein Diskussionsbeitrag.
  Zeitschrift für Arbeitswissenschaft, 37, 12-15.
Ulich, E., Groskurt, P. & Bruggemann, A. (1973). *Neue Formen der
  Arbeitsgestaltung*. Frankfurt/M.: Europäische Verlagsanstalt.
Waern, Y. (1986). *Information used and user's models of a computer
  supported task*. Paper presented to the 21st International Congress
  of Applied Psychology, Jerusalem, Israel, July.
Wertheimer,M. (1945), *Productive thinking*. New York: Harper & Brothers.
Woodworth, R.S. (1949). *Contemporary schools of Psychology*. London:
  Methuen (revised editition, first publication 1931).

METHODOLOGICAL ISSUES
IN THE PSYCHOLOGY
OF HUMAN-COMPUTER INTERACTION

Psychological Issues of
Human Computer Interaction in the Work Place
M. Frese, E. Ulich, W. Dzida (Editors)
© Elsevier Science Publishers B.V. (North-Holland), 1987

USABILITY ASSESSMENT FOR THE OFFICE: METHODOLOGICAL CHOICES AND THEIR IMPLICATIONS

Pamela Briggs

MRC/ESRC Social and Applied Psychology Unit
University of Sheffield, Sheffield S10 2TN
England

The first part of this chapter assumes a pragmatic definition of usability in terms of four goals of office systems redesign: increased efficiency; increased user satisfaction; reduced training costs; and increased user understanding. This is followed by a critical review of related methodologies, which offer an assessment of usability in terms of the user's performance, subjective opinion, and knowledge of the system.

INTRODUCTION - A DEFINITION OF USABILITY

The terms "usable" and "user-friendly" are often used to describe those computer systems with which one can easily establish a satisfactory dialogue with a minimum training requirement. They are often associated with computers which offer multiple choice access to a variety of functions and which provide readily interpretable prompts, or systems which offer the user the capacity for "direct manipulation" (Shneiderman, 1984; Hutchins, Hollan and Norman, 1986). However, although there are plenty of emerging design principles and features which are associated with a "usable" system, there is as yet little agreement on the process by which the usability of a system can best be evaluated.

Interest in interface usability has grown because of the need to make computing power available to non-specialists. Hence usability assessment is often made in terms of the performance of novices, since experts are deemed able to cope with "hostile" systems and indeed can sometimes be heard voicing their objections to the hardware and software advances of mice and menus. Yet it is clearly nonsense to assume a definition of usability appropriate only to the novice. What is more appropriate is to establish a set of usability criteria which are relevant to the use of systems within the workplace. An argument is made here for the adoption of four main criteria, derived in the main from a consideration of issues which should, realistically, influence the design of office systems, but which are felt to be fairly generally applicable. These criteria are:

    a. increased efficiency

    b. increased user satisfaction

    c. reduced training needs, and

    d. increased user understanding.

In other words a system is considered more usable if the user can master the system more quickly, complete standard tasks more swiftly and with more enjoyment, and develop a greater understanding of the workings of the system. Some justification for this selection of criteria is given below, although clearly, while, a,b and c may be considered rather obvious goals of system redesign, d is a more unusual choice, and one which draws upon the notion of "transparency" as a design criterion (see Maass, 1983). Its inclusion here is discussed at some length, in the context of a brief study of the real problems faced by secretaries in their daily use of computerised office systems.

Performance Efficiency

The desire for increased efficiency reflects the influence of economic forces which anticipate that the time taken to create and print a document, or update a database, will decrease as a natural effect of system development. This goal of increasing the daily throughput is often seen to dictate the process of system redesign. Indeed, for office systems, Embley and Nagy (1981) state quite categorically that:

    ".. the most important general goal in editor design is to minimize

    the amount of time it takes for a user to complete an editing task."

The goal of increased efficiency is clearly relevant to systems employed within almost all work situations, but has different implications for system design, dependent upon the work context. In other words the means of increasing efficiency in, say, a software development system (intelligent editors, multiple windows for "background" compilation, etc.) would be different from that in a word-processing system, where the emphasis may be upon increasing the functionality of a system (new formatting options, style sheets etc.), while ensuring that the user fully employs the range of functions now on offer.

User Satisfaction

Clearly it is something of a sine qua non for a usable system that the user find the system satisfactory, and this condition is certainly generally applicable across all systems, in any work context. Indeed, if there is a danger in positing user satisfaction as a necessary criterion for usability assessment, it is that for some it may be seen as tautology - a simple redefinition of the vague concept "usability" in terms of an equally vague notion of "user satisfaction". This is quite clearly not the case. User satisfaction is an essential criterion for a usable system, but it is not an exhaustive one. It is easy to conceive of a system which is slow and inefficient, but which people enjoy using (some secretaries, for example, say that they prefer to use an electric typewriter because they are more "in control" of the final product). What is important, is that user satisfaction can be measured directly, as can user efficiency in a way that usability per se can not.

Training Costs

There is an implication that if a system is described as "usable" it will be mastered fairly easily. While this is a general criterion for usability, it is also the one which is most dependent upon the context of the workplace. For office systems, the amount of training required for a new machine is an important consideration. This is in part because training courses are expensive to set up, but, more importantly, it is often the case that a secretary will have to master a new system without any formal training whatsoever. This is particularly true of temporary office staff, who encounter a great number of new systems every year. However, the need to reduce training costs cannot be established as an independent goal in system design, in that it is clearly linked to the functionality or "utility" of a system (see Shackel, 1985), and in almost all cases a trade-off is necessary between the utility of a system (which in turn influences the efficiency with which a task is performed) and the cost of training a user to become proficient.

User Understanding

This is a more difficult point to argue: can we say that a system is more usable if it operates in such a way that the user comes to understand the nature of the system? In other words, is there any advantage to a system which is "transparent" rather than "opaque", in that it offers information relevant to its own structure and working? This is really an issue of just how much understanding a user needs to use a system successfully. It is possible to argue that for many jobs, users need only limited procedural information in order to complete their daily tasks. In other words users need only know *how* to carry out different functions and operations on the machine in terms of a fixed instruction sequence. Thus, for word-processing systems, a secretary need not know that information is only temporarily buffered in dynamic RAM, to know that she should save the information before switching off the machine. She only has to know that she should *always* save information before switching off.

Kieras and Polson (1982) have discussed the need for procedural/ conceptual information in the learning and operation of any system, and conclude that conceptual understanding is unnecessary, and only becomes an important issue when something goes wrong. In the normal course of events, users need only have a procedural knowledge of appropriate routines to successfully complete their work. Clearly, whether or not a user needs some conceptual understanding depends upon the extent to which they have to cope with "things going wrong".

The current author has recently completed a small study of the kind of problems secretaries face in the office, using data from the critical incident diaries of twelve university secretaries, and from a central "hot-line" for emergency problems. The severity of many of the problems reported during a two-week period was impressive. The problems fell into a number of categories: slips and mistakes made by the user; machine break-down; and problems in trying to complete someone else's work. In each of these categories severe problems could have been avoided if the user had shown greater understanding. For example, one secretary reported a winchester disc malfunction when she tried to retrieve certain files, and couldn't. It transpired that the disc had been malfunctioning for a number of weeks, with the result that considerable information had been lost, but it hadn't been detected because the secretary had thought it normal for the system to take over an hour to boot up in the mornings. Other problems occurred because secretaries misunderstood the system, particularly aspects concerned with printing, where the relationship between the text on-screen, the page size specified by the system, and the actual size of the paper caused considerable difficulties.

Clearly the user who fully understands the system is less likely to make mistakes, more likely to be able to interpret the system state, and more aware of symptoms of machine breakdown. Examples such as these provide some support for the notion that some kind of conceptual understanding be considered important for the user, whether it be achieved through training, through better manuals, or through more careful, and more "transparent" system design. For the present, I would simply like to argue that the accuracy of the model the user develops of a system is an important reflection of system usability.

THE MEASUREMENT OF USABILITY

Clearly, in the assessment of usability, there are a number of features both of the system and of the user which lend themselves to evaluation. The system itself can be rated against a checklist of good design features which are associated with more usable systems. Or some assessment can be made of the way in which knowledge of the task, and knowledge of the user is incorporated in the system design. Several sophisticated means of assessing the system against some formal description of the task exist (e.g. Kieras and Polson, 1985; Moran, 1981;

Payne, 1984), however these model the ideal process rather than reflect the real experience of the user within the workplace.

Alternatively, usability assessment can be user-centred, and can be made in terms of performance measures which provide indices of user efficiency; subjective measures which reflect the user's satisfaction with the system; and finally knowledge-based measures from which we can assess and model the user's understanding of the computer. In terms of the criteria discussed in the previous section, the latter, user-centred techniques would seem to be more direct measures of usability, hence these and their associated problems are reviewed below.

Performance Measures

If, as is argued above, tasks should be completed more efficiently with a more usable system, then one component in the evaluation of usability must involve the assessment of user performance. Fundamental assessment of user performance is usually made in terms of speed and error, hence these two dependent variables are considered central to the evaluation of any system in terms of its efficiency. As we shall see, such measures can be made more complex by incorporating some qualitative analysis such as error categorization. They can also be tied to sophisticated psychophysical models of human action, which carry inherent predictions about performance limitations under certain conditions. Nevertheless, such studies are similar in that they rely primarily on externally quantified measures of user's rate and accuracy of input.

Speed and Error

Obviously, studies which rely upon fairly gross measures of speed or accuracy have advantages in that they are easily set up, and give readily interpretable, and usually reliable results. However, there is clearly a problem if measures of either speed or error are taken independently. The assumption, for example, that an expert user will always complete a task faster than a novice is not a valid one (see for example, Akin and Rao, 1985), although one would expect fewer errors under these circumstances. Clearly a combined assessment of performance based upon both speed and error would more reliably reflect the quality of the system. Indeed it is difficult to credit research findings which are based solely on a speed of response measure (Beaumont, 1985) or overall task completion time (Dumais and Landauer, 1982). Both of these studies concluded with recommendations for future interface design. Beaumont, for example suggested that a touch sensitive screen has advantages over other interface tools, and Dumais and Landauer concluded that "natural" language command names possess no advantage over their "unnatural" counterparts. This despite an oblique and unsupported reference to a post-session questionnaire in which subjects expressed "some subjective preferences" for the more natural terms. Such cases provide very clear examples in which the limitations of the methodology preclude any possibility of generalisability of results. The scope of their conclusion is simply not adequately supported by the data they provide.

Obviously additional performance information in the form of some kind of error rate would be beneficial in these studies, although here too there are problems, since it is not always clear what may constitute an error. It would be foolish, for example to take the number of simple typing mistakes as indicative of bad word-processor software (although it may reflect the quality of the keyboard). Indeed the number of errors produced, as with the number of keystrokes, or the number of commands entered, is not an adequate measure on which to base ambitious conclusions. A more advanced assessment of user efficiency would also provide some qualitative analysis of errors, or indeed of the user's entire input.

Qualitative Analysis of Performance Data

Eason (1984) describes a field study of a banking system, the various facilities of which are accessed via a series of three digit codes. An analysis of the codes actually used by the operators showed that only four of the 36 possible codes accounted for 75% of the overall use. Only 53% of queries were judged to be handled correctly; others were either successful but inefficient, or unsuccessful. Eason's work is an example of a study in which the specific content of user's responses can point to problems in the human-computer interface. In this case the problem from the user's point of view is seen as one of conceptual set (Luchins and Luchins, 1959) in that users adhered to familiar problem solving strategies even when they were inappropriate. This may in turn reflect the unacceptable memory load imposed by large numbers of three digit codes.

Clearly the value of Eason's data rests, not in the quantitative assessment of percentage correct, but in the more qualitative analysis of the responses made. Yet Eason's study involves only minimal response categorization, and there are other studies which have taken this type of evaluation much further. The nature and extent of classification of user input naturally varies from one study to another. One fairly typical categorization is provided by Allen (1983) in discussion of the composition and editing of spoken and written letters. Rather than limit his analysis to overall letter composition time and error rate, Allen makes useful subdivisions in both of these measures. Thus composition time is broken down into the time spent initially planning the letter; the time spent actually speaking the letter; and the time spent in major pauses while during composition. In addition Allen describes letter revision time, which is in turn broken down into the time taken to mark and implement edits, with the edits themselves categorised as insertions, deletions, changes or moves, with deletions being clearly the most common.

This subdivision of dependent variables provides additional information on user's performance, and enables us to pinpoint the specific areas in which one system may be said to be more or less efficient than another. Quite clearly, there are a number of ways in which this can be done. Classifications like the one above are based upon some kind of simple analysis of the functions performed during a variety of tasks. Other, more sophisticated classifications draw upon some model of the user.

One such categorization is provided by Command Language Grammar (CLG) (Moran, 1981), which uses programming notation to describe the action sequences which a user can initiate in order to solve a particular problem. The interesting feature of this grammar is that it emphasises the different cognitive levels at which human-computer interaction can occur. Thus there is a "semantic" level, where the necessary steps in solving a particular problem are calculated; a "syntactic" level, which allows these steps to be mapped onto the command facilities available on the computer, and an "interactive" level, where the fine detail - actual commands and keystrokes - is worked out.

Davis (1983) has used CLG to classify errors made with an interactive version of SPSS. The beauty of this classification is that errors can then act as pointers to specific mismatches between the users conception of the task and the facilities available on the computer. Thus errors in the format or typing of a command string would be evidence of a mismatch at the syntax/interactive level, and would not signal any fundamental conceptual problems. Errors in the actual selection of command instructions; or inappropriate or inefficient sequencing of these instructions, would reflect a more fundamental mismatch between syntactic and semantic representation. Even more seriously, an inability to perceive the task in any kind of computer-compatible structure would show a mismatch between task and semantic levels, indicative of the user's basic ignorance of the computer.

Using this type of analysis, Davis has shown how simple error data can be used to derive quite a complex account of the specific conceptual difficulties a user may encounter with SPSS. Clearly such methodology could form the basis for any evaluation of usability, in that it reflects the degree to which a system maps onto the user's conception of the task. Classification of this type, however, is dependent upon formalisms which make gross assumptions about the way in which the user perceives and structures the task. While these assumptions may provide a reasonable general description, formal analyses fail to capture many important aspects of human behaviour (see Briggs, 1987).

An alternative type of user model which can be used to make fairly sophisticated predictions concerning the effects of different interface designs upon performance efficiency is described by Card, Moran and Newell in their (1983) "The Psychology of Human Computer Interaction". They present a "keystroke" model of the user, in conjunction with a task analysis which specifies user-defined "Goals, Operations, Methods and Selections rules". These elements combined provide a model of the user as information processor, and thus governed by the psychophysical laws mapped out within cognitive-experimental psychology over the last thirty years; and a model of the task broken down into components which reflect user decision points and action sequences. The advantage in such a model is that it can be used to predict human behaviour as constrained by routine tasks such as text editing, and that it can also predict those devices (e.g. mouse, joystick, keyboard) which allow most efficient performance. The disadvantage lies in the fact that in neglecting the subjective attitude and understanding of the user, usability factors related to longer-term use of a system are ignored. This point is raised again in the conclusion, when the relative merits of these different techniques for assessing usability are discussed.

Subjective Assessment

Within an approach to the study of the human-computer interface which relies upon subjective accounts of the users themselves, a crucial distinction must be made between the subjective interpretation the user makes of a particular system, which provides his or her conceptual model of that system, and the user's subjective appraisal of the system in terms of its ease of use. The latter is clearly relevant to a study of usability, given that it is a measure of user satisfaction, and therefore, related to the second of the usability criterion discussed earlier. Studies which aim to capture the user's model of the system are related to the third and fourth of these usability criteria (training cost and user understanding), and their role in the measurement of usability will be discussed later.

There are a number of methodological choices to be made when setting up a study to assess user opinion:
(a) The study may be designed solely to gather information, or it may contain some decision making, or evaluative component; and
(b) the study may allow participants to express their views freely, selecting their own topics for discussion, and their own criteria for evaluation or it may place constraints on both the questions presented to the participant, and the answers subsequently elicited.

The first choice, that between information gathering and evaluation, is discussed by Auld, Lang and Lang in their 1981 study of University Computer Users. They draw on the concept of "illuminative evaluation" (Parlett and Hamilton, 1972) in their justification of an approach which, they argue, avoids the dangers of making decisions, or hasty conclusions based on too shallow an understanding of the issues in a new field. The need for evaluation and assessment of necessity influences the way in which facts are interpreted, and perhaps more importantly, influences the selection of information to be gathered. Clearly, unless there is an adequate understanding of the problems and difficulties faced by a computer user at work, there is a danger of targeting the wrong variables for investigation. The choices in (a) and (b) described above, must therefore be compatible; it would be impossible to be impartial in the collection of users' subjective appraisals if those users were severely constrained in the way they could express those views, just as it would be methodologically very difficult to make any adequate evaluation of a computer system using totally unstructured data.

The methodological extremes relevant to this issue are the multiple choice questionnaire, or rating scale, and the totally unstructured interview. The latter is seldom found, owing no doubt to immense problems of analysis and quantification, and is often replaced by the structured interview as a method of gathering a wide range of user views. The former appear often in studies of computer usability, used frequently in combination with some measure of user efficiency.

Several criticisms arise from such studies, although in many cases it is the way in which they are reported which constitutes the major problem. The Dumais and Landauer study has already been mentioned as an example in which conclusions are based on simple ratings of user satisfaction which are reported in an off hand manner, without reference to specific questions or statistical evidence. In other cases the data is clearly presented, but the questions remain few, and over-simplistic. Morrison et al. (1984) for example, obtained overall ratings for two versions of an editor (speech and keyboard) on a ten point scale, in terms of general preference, followed by ratings for the ease of performing each of four specific functions. Users were then given a chance to offer reasons for their ratings in structured interviews, and asked to state their preferences in terms of pleasantness, efficiency of use and ease of learning. Parton et al. (1985) also used a rating scale, this time allowing a subjective assessment of "ease of learning" of a menu selection tree. Not too surprisingly they found that the subjects own assessment correlated highly with performance variables. Certainly it is valuable to have some technique for representing the users viewpoint, but the obvious problem with these studies is that they tell us only that one system is "better" than another in very gross terms, and without pinpointing the specific advantages one has over the other. More elaborate questionnaires may be able to do this, but the problem here is that questionnaires necessarily constrain responses, and address only those issues which the questionnaire designer feels are relevant.

More useful for pinpointing particular areas of difficulty are structured interviews. This interviewing technique has been employed by the long term study being carried out at the Applied Psychology Unit in

Cambridge. John Long and his colleagues provide an elaborate account of their structured interviewing techniques in a comprehensive study of user attitudes to the installation of a new mainframe computer in a local authority office (Long, Hammond, Barnard, Morton and Clark, 1983).

This paper clearly exemplifies the costs and benefits of using such techniques. Two major problems are obvious in such work: The first concerns the imposed structure of the interview itself and the second is a problem of appropriate analysis. Stated simply, in order to impose structure upon the interview, researchers must predefine those topics which are likely to be most useful, which is reasonable in those circumstances where preliminary studies have established the relevant factors a priori. However, this is seldom the case, and many studies which purport to present the users' viewpoint simply reflect the researchers own predjudice. Alternatively, participants can be given freedom in the selection of topics for discussion, but this exacerbates the problems of analysis. This is clearly demonstrated in the Long et al. paper, where participants are given guidelines, but are free to structure the discussion themselves. The resultant analysis is complex, but can be taken as an accurate representation of the users' views.

One criticism which applies to both performance measures of the user, and to the subjective measures described above, is given by Eason (1984), in his discussion of usability assessment. He describes a vast literature in which users are given specific tasks, dependent up on the use of specific functions, and measures of both speed and error, and subjective opinion are then taken, which act as indices of usability. In pointing out the folly of such studies he states that:

> "Since a major indicator of usability is *whether* a system or facility is used, to force a person to use it and then measure speed and errors is to destroy the phenomenon in the act of assessing it",

and argues that usability is better assessed in terms of choices made freely by the user:

> "It is the act of choice which is the essence of usability which suggests that the crucial measure is the pattern of responses to options and the way they build into a learning or non-learning strategy."

The act of choice is, perhaps, the process within the interaction of human and computer which reflects the users' knowledge, and it is the ability to make the best choices which most properly marks the expert from the novice. An alternative then, in any study of human-computer interaction is to attempt to evaluate the user's knowledge of the system he or she works with, and to see how accurately the computer is perceived. This approach escapes Eason's criticism, in that it provides a means of evaluating the capacity of the user to fully utilise a system, and to anticipate and cope with problems. Unfortunately, the task of "capturing" the user's understanding is frought with problems. Some of the most promising techniques are discussed below.

Knowledge-Based Assessment Techniques

In interacting with any machine, we bring with us certain expectations about how that machine will behave, and these expectations are dependent upon some conceptualisation of just what that machine is. Thus when we start up a car engine we employ some model of what is happening beneath the bonnet. For some, this model is an accurate system description, based on competent technical understanding. For others the model is incomplete and inconsistent, based upon half formed ideas, and hazy analogies. However, both the technically expert and the technically ignorant can drive, and the accuracy of their model of a car engine will primarily affect their ability to anticipate and cope with breakdowns.

Many computer users employ a similar tactic in their day to day use of particular software packages. However, there are important aspects of the computer as a machine which mean that users who possess an impoverished model of the system may be penalised. Perhaps the most obvious point concerns the utility of a computer system. "utility" is taken here in the sense described by Shackel (1985) to mean the range of functions offered by the machine. Thus, unlike a car which performs only one function irrespective of the skill of the operator, the utility of a computer is, to a large extent, determined by the user's model.

The second point, and one which is more relevant to this discussion, is that the actual nature of the task being undertaken on a computer is dependent upon the operation of the machine itself. This is true of other machines (the car included) in only a superficial sense. Thus the task of changing gear may be superficially different in a Porsche as compared to a Citroen Dyane, and one may be considered easier to use than the other, but the operator may successfully employ the same mental model in each case. In the case of a computer, the system design and underlying conceptual model has far reaching implications concerning the way that even basic tasks should be performed. Thus, for example, the task of creating a file within a particular "window" or on a particular "desk top" is a different task to creating a file within a tree-structured directory system, and the successful completion of any one of these tasks is dependent upon the user employing an appropriate model. With more complex tasks, such as Shell manipulation on the Unix operating system, the user's dependence upon an accurate model becomes even more obvious. It is in this sense, then, that the ease with which the user can generate a suitable model can be said to reflect system usability.

If we are to assess the model that a user has of a particular system, and take this as an indicator of the usability of that system; then we must first decide what type of knowledge is relevant; secondly propose some suitable structure with which to represent that knowledge; and thirdly find an effective means of eliciting that knowledge from the user. This is clearly not a simple task.

Knowledge Type and Structure

Richard Young, in his 1983 discussion of mental models acknowledges that:

"Although it is widely accepted that people's ability to use an interactive device depends in part upon their having access to some sort of a mental model ... the notion of the 'user's conceptual model' (UCM) remains a hazy one, and there are probably as many different ideas about what it might be as there are people writing about it."

The problem is twofold, in that (a) there are many different types of knowledge a user has about a particular computer system, and this knowledge is not all at the same "level", in the sense that knowing where a particular key lies on the keyboard is a different level of understanding from knowing which command will execute a program (Hammond et al. 1982); and (b) even if we limit discussion of models to those which represent only one "level" of knowledge, there are still fundamental problems in deciding upon what type of representation best fits the user's knowledge structure.

There have been many attempts to define the different types of knowledge we employ in everyday life, with the fundamental distinction being made between procedural and declarative knowledge (see Winograd, 1975; Anderson, 1976). Within a specific context - such as the operation of a computer system, it is perhaps easier to be specific and talk in terms of a knowledge of procedures which includes knowledge of actions and command sequences; and conceptual knowledge which relates to the understanding of the principles underlying the operation of a particular system. It may help to view this particular distinction in linguistic terms, as analogous to the distinction between syntax and semantics, where procedural knowledge is akin to a rule based grammatical knowledge in that sequences of actions must follow a pattern which can usually be specified, whereas conceptual knowledge relates to the user's understanding of what lies behind a sequence of operations, in the same sense that meaning can be said to lie behind syntax.

This division between knowledge types is mirrored in the means available for their representation. Thus procedural knowledge is typically expressed in the form of production rules which follow an "if condition then action" recipe for task completion; whereas the more declarative structure which underlies the user's conceptual understanding is often represented in terms of an overlay model, in which the user's knowledge within a particular domain is seen as a network structure, with nodes corresponding to concepts within that domain (Sleeman, 1986). Indeed, a demonstration that these overlay, or network models can provide a means of modelling user expertise has been provided by Schvaneveldt et al. (1985), who have used a network model to define and measure the conceptual structures of novices and experts, in order to pinpoint those who would benefit from additional training.

To return to the problem of usability: if we wish to see whether a particular user's conceptual model of a computer system maps adequately onto the "system image" being promoted (Norman, 1986), it is necessary to represent the user's conceptual understanding and the "system image" within structures which can be directly compared; but it it also necessary to pinpoint specific gaps within the user's knowledge in terms of their actual beliefs about a system. In other words we need to determine not only the "bones" but also the "flesh" of the user's model.

Knowledge Elicitation

One of the most fundamental problems of knowledge elicitation - that people cannot give an adequate account of the structure and content of their own expertise (see Nisbett and Wilson, 1977) has become rather a cliche within the field of expert systems. Nevertheless, it is this problem which forces the division between techniques of knowledge elicitation and the techniques designed to assess user's subjective attitudes and opinions, described earlier. It is not sufficient for the expert or user to give an unstructured, introspective account of his or her understanding of a particular topic, or computer system. Instead the goal, certainly within expert systems research, is to provide an explicit structure for that knowledge appropriate to the kind of knowledge being considered (as discussed above) and then to "clothe" this structure in a fairly systematic way. This is a difficult task, given that in realistic terms, we have not progressed very far when it comes to specifying the "content" rather than the "processes" of mind. Some of the techniques which seem most relevant to this issue are described below, while those interested in a more comprehensive account of the many problems faced by knowledge engineers, and some of the more successful implementations, should seek a different source (e.g. Welbank, 1983).

Clearly the structured interview, already discussed in relation to the elicitation of user opinion, can also be used to elicit user knowledge of a particular system. In this case, however, the structure imposed upon the interview becomes even more important, and will directly reflect the underlying model selected as the means for knowledge representation within a particular case. In a study of computer users, for example, a question and answer session could be structured in procedural terms: "how would you delete paragraph x and insert line y?" or in terms of specifying links within a network: "how are the commands 'delete' and 'insert' related?".

Given the problems people face in communicating their knowledge, and the fundamental weakness of human memory in uncued recall, some means of providing a context for the elicitation of knowledge is advisable. Welbank (1983) discusses this problem and presents a number of useful questioning strategies.

1. Critical incident

We have already proposed one means of assessing usability, in terms of pinpointing the areas of mismatch between the users conceptual model and the system image. One questioning strategy relevant to this approach is Flanagan's (1954) critical incident technique, where particularly memorable events are reported and analyzed. Clearly in some cases the users can themselves account for their errors and provide an explanation in terms of the context of the disaster, whereas in other cases discussion of critical incidents may reveal more fundamental gaps in the user's knowledge which may reflect such things as lack of consistency in the system interface.

My own study of problems within the workplace, mentioned earlier, provided examples in both of these categories. Two further, striking examples from this study involved two secretaries, who independently reported that they had wiped clean a work disc, in one case containing over three weeks work, during execution of a disc backup procedure. In each case the secretary had been interrupted during the procedure, and had subsequently keyed in the wrong disc address in response to a system prompt. This example clearly shows that when the normal execution of a routine procedure is interrupted, disorientation, possibly reflecting a lack of clarity in the system prompts, may follow. It relates to the usability issue not only in terms of the extent to which a system offers protection against such errors, but also in terms of the degree to which the system conveys information as to its current state.

2. Prompted recall

An alternative questioning strategy, which provides a context for cued recall, and which is relevant to both the novice and expert user, is to provide a scenario and ask for an explanation. Within the HCI field this has been done quite successfully by Barnard (1986), using pictures of screen displays as a recall cue. Statements generated around a picture prompt were analyzed in terms of accuracy, and the kind of information they held. Not surprisingly the number of accurate statements generated by a prompt was found to increase, with greater expertise; however one interesting finding was that the number of false statements generated remained constant. In other words, even more experienced users were generating false beliefs, despite the fact that they could carry out the relevant procedures without error.

This finding possibly reflects the fact that picture prompts provide no temporal context, and that in fact many actions, particularly within a menu-based system, are understood primarily as elements with a procedure. Highlighting just one element of that procedure may produce a certain amount of disorientation analogous to that experienced by the afore-mentioned secretaries when their routine task was disrupted. Techniques of knowledge elicitation, such as this, which remove the procedural context within a task, may be useful in assessing just how easily users can free themselves from this context, and draw upon other types of knowledge of the system.

3. Protocol analysis

An alternative approach, particularly in those circumstances where one wishes to identify specific problems faced by the user in the process of performing his or her job, is to monitor the users' reasoning process through comments made while he or she interacts with the computer. This type of "stream of consciousness" study does not easily lend itself to analysis, but it can be a very informative exercise, as shown by Hammond et al. in their study of the novice use of an interactive graph plotting system (Hammond, Maclean, Hinton, Long, Barnard and Clark, 1983). This study forms something of a bridge between the elicitation of user views, described in the previous section, and user knowledge. What is gained from studies like this is a subjective account of the users' own behaviour which often often highlights areas of difficulty, and which provides some indication of the mismatches which occur between the computer and the users' perception of the computer.

In the Hammond study, novice users were asked to follow through an introductory course on an Interactive Chart Utility (ICU), a supposedly "user friendly" graph plotting system which operates predominantly through menu selection. Protocols were derived from novice users of this system by asking them simply to provide verbal comments where appropriate, and also by stopping them at selected points and asking them to describe any particular difficulties they'd experienced. Although not subject to any formal analysis, these protocols were useful in pinpointing specific problems, such as users' confusion concerning the so called "end" key, used to signal that a particular menu was no longer required. The term obviously carried the connotation that users would proceed to another menu, whereas they were taken "back" to a previous menu which formed the immediately superior node in a hierarchical tree. Hammond et al. reflect that the users' comments show a misunderstanding of the menu hierarchy principle. Such a misunderstanding is fundamental, and its elicitation reflects the strength of protocol analysis in revealing misconceptions and areas of uncertainty within the users conceptual model of the system.

4. Kelly repertory grid

A technique which is more appropriate for an approach which has knowledge represented within a network structure, is to use Kelly's repertory grid as a means to explore important concepts and the relationships between them (Boose, 1985; Easterby-Smith, 1981).

Boose has successfully implemented such a technique within his Expertise Transfer System (ETS) - a knowledge acquisition shell which primarily elicits elements which correspond to the possible "conclusions" that the host expert-system will eventually reach (e.g. specific diseases). ETS then uses several methods of analysis to structure the links between the elements (i.e. it specifies the knowledge "nodes" within a particular domain and the way in which they are interrelated. It does this by generating production rules of the form:

$$\text{IF} \qquad A = B$$
$$\text{THEN} \qquad C = D \ (p)$$

where p is the probability or certainty factor, derived from the association strengths within the grid. Production rules of this type are commonly used within expert systems implementations. The interesting point about Boose's work is the psychological (as opposed to logical) reality of the rules derived from a repertory grid. The work is cited here because the grid itself, although used by Boose to generate an accessible knowledge base, could be used as a means to evaluate knowledge. More specifically it could be used as a tool for the assessment of the user's conceptual model and thence identify those aspects of a system which are most commonly misunderstood.

It is interesting that these different techniques address different components of user understanding, and hence different aspects of usability. Prompted recall is a technique through which one can assess: (a) the extent to which a user is dependent upon the temporal context of procedures when executing some specific task; and (b) the quality of information presented on screen at any one time, i.e. the degree to which information concerning the system state is made apparent to the user.

Critical incident allows us to be specific about misconceptions the user has about the system, and to identify problems which occur in the workplace, but which are not, perhaps, obvious from any short-term testing of the system.

Protocol analyses can give some indication as to whether or not the system maps onto users prior expectation. The degree to which the system conforms to the expectation of the user closely influences the ease with which the system is learned, and would also be associated with fewer errors.

Finally, the repertory grid helps to give a more general overview of the users understanding of the system, and indicates those areas in which the user is well or poorly informed about system operation. In this it offers a means - more direct than mere error categorisation - of pinpointing aspects of the system which are poorly understood, and may be under-utilized.

SUMMARY AND CONCLUSION

In this chapter I have argued that there are two components to the assessment of usability: the first involves the definition of usability in terms which are relevant to real issues within the workplace. I have proposed that this is best achieved in terms of establishing the criteria, or "goals" of usability research, and I have argued in favour of four such criteria as being suitable for the evaluation of office systems: efficiency; user satisfaction; reduced training cost; and increased user understanding. The second component is, of course, the methodology which assessment against these criteria is made. Here I have argued that the most suitable assessment of usability, given these criteria, is dependent upon an evaluation of the way in which the user interacts with the system, and that there are three important components of this interaction: a performance component, which reflects the user's mastery of low level procedures, and is usually assessed in terms of speed and accuracy for specific tasks; a subjective-evaluative component, in which the interaction is assessed by the user, against his or her own usability criteria; and a knowledge component, based upon the user's conceptual understanding of the system, and his or her explicit recognition of procedures and the logic which governs them. The various means by which these different components can be assessed have been reviewed, but as a final comment it is worth drawing out some of the different implications of these approaches.

An approach based upon the assessment of user performance, in terms of speed and error, makes it possible to compare systems, one against the other, and also, if combined with a more qualitative analysis, allows us to make predictions concerning just what ingredients within a system lead to greater efficiency. Such an approach also allows us to assess the ease with which a user can "master" a system, in terms of being able to complete benchmark tasks speedily and with minimum error.

However, when we look at the quality of the user-system interaction in this way, we define the user's task in terms of a repertoire of procedures. To state that a computer system is "usable" in these terms is to imply that its operating procedures can be learned quickly and performed efficiently. What is omitted is any consideration of the ease with which operators can cope with atypical interactions - how well they can respond to and recover from errors, and their ability to interpret the system state when the usual temporal context of procedures is removed. This is relevant to a longer-term view of system usability: interruptions and errors may not be an integral part of an editing procedure, but they do occur relatively frequently within the office, and any realistic assessment of usability must account for them.

Assessment conducted within the design environment, as opposed to the workplace, tends to place emphasis upon the efficiency with which standard tasks are carried out, whereas it clearly takes time for users to form opinions or to develop a thorough understanding of the system, and these criteria seem often to be dropped in favour of short-term goals.

The approach taken in this chapter has been to describe only those techniques for the assessment of usability which focus upon the user within the workplace. Each has its disadvantages when applied individually, but when combined provide a fairly comprehensive set of tools for usability assessment. However, as a final caveat, when usability assessment is taken into the office or workplace, many other factors related to the usability issue, which have been ignored in this discussion, should be taken into consideration. Problems of motivation, the ease with which a new system can be integrated into an existing organisation, and the ways in which system utility and flexibility can smooth the transition to information technology are all relevant to the assessment of the usability of a particular system within a particular setting. It is unfortunately true that research driven by this organizational perspective is seldom combined with studies of the type described here, which are more representative of a cognitive ergonomics approach, but hopefully this may be rectified in the near future.

REFERENCES

Akin, O. and Rao, D.R. (1985). Efficient computer-user interface in electronic mail systems. *International Journal of Man-Machine Studies, 22*, 589-611.

Allen, R.B. (1983). Composition and editing of spoken letters. *Int J. Man-Machine Studies, 19*, 131-193.

Anderson, J. (1976). *Language Memory and Thought*. Hillsdale, N.J.: Lawrence Erlbaum.

Auld, R., Lang, K. and Lang, T.(1981). University computer users: Characteristics and behaviour. In M.J. Coombs and J.L. Alty (Eds.), *Computing Skills and the User Interface*. London: Academic Press. pp 73-114.

Barnard, P., Wilson, M. and Maclean, A. (1986). The elicitation of system knowledge by picture probes. In *Proc.CHI 86 Human Factors in Computing Systems* (Boston, April 13-17) ACM, New York, pp. 235-240.

Beaumont, J.G. (1985). Speed of response using keyboard and screen based microcomputer response media. *International Journal of Man-Machine Studies, 22*, 589-611.

Briggs, P. (1987). What we know and what we need to know: The user model versus the user's model in human-computer interaction. *SAPU memo no. 827*, University of Sheffield.

Boose, J.H. (1985). A knowledge acquisition program for expert systems based upon personal construct psychology. *International Journal of Man-Machine Studies, 5*, 495-526.

Card, S.K., Moran, T.P. and Newell, A. (1983). *The Psychology of Human Computer Interaction*. Hillsdale, N.J.: Lawrence Erlbaum.

Davis, R. (1983). Task analysis and user errors: A methodology for assessing interactions. *International Journal of Man-Machine Studies, 19*, 561-574.

Dumais, S.T. and Landauer, T.K. (1982). Psychological investigation of natural terminology for command and query languages. In A. Badre and B. Shneiderman, *Directions in Human Computer Interaction*. Norwood, N.J: Ablex. pp 95-110.

Eason, K.D. (1984). Towards the experimental study of usability. *Behaviour and Information Technology, 3* (2), 133-143.

Embley, D.W. and Nagy, G. (1981). Empirical and formal methods for the study of computer editors. In M.L. Coombs and J.L. Alty (Eds.), *Computing Skills and the User Interface*. London: Academic Press. pp 465-496.

Flanagan, J.C. (1954). The critical incident technique. *Psychological Bulletin 51*, 327-358.

Hammond, N., Morton, J., Maclean, A., Barnard, P. and Long, J. (1982). *Knowledge Fragments and Users' Models of Systems*. Hursley Human Factors Laboratory Report, #HF071.

Hammond, N., MacLean, A., Hinton, G., Long, J., Barnard, P. and Clark, I.A. (1983). *Novice Use of an Interactive Graph Plotting System*. Hursley Human Factors Laboratory Report.

Hutchins, E.L., Hollan, J.D. and Norman, D.A. (1986). Direct manipulation interfaces. In D.A. Norman and S.W. Draper (Eds.), *User-Centred System Design: New Perspectives on Human-Computer Interaction*. Hillsdale, N.J.: Lawrence Erlbaum. pp 87-124.

Kieras, D.E. and Polson, P.G. (1982). *An Outline of a Theory of the User Complexity of Devices and Systems*. (Working paper No. 1) University of Arizona and University of Colorado, Dept. of Psychology, Tucson and Boulder.

Kieras, D.E. and Polson, P.G. (1985). An approach to the formal analysis of user complexity. *Int. J. Man-Machine Studies, 22*, 365-394.

Long, J., Hammond, N., Barnard, P. and Morton, J. (1983). Introducing the interactive computer at work: The users' views. *Behaviour and Information Technology, 2* (1), 39-106.

Luchins, A.S. and Luchins, E.H. (1959). *Rigidity of Behaviour: A Variational Approach to the Effects of Einstelling.* University of Oregon Press.

Maass, S. (1983) Why systems transparency? In T.R. Green, S.J. Payne and G.C. Van der Veer (Eds.), *The Psychology of Computer Use.* London: Academic Press. pp 19-28.

Moran, T.P. (1981). The command language grammar: A representation for the user interface of interactive computer systems. *International Journal of Man-Machine Studies, 15* (1), 3-50.

Morrison, D.L., Green, T.R.G., Shaw, A.C. and Payne, S.J. (1984). Speech controlled text editing: Effects of input modality and of command structure. *International Journal of Man-Machine Studies, 21,* 49-63.

Nisbett, R.E. and Wilson, T.D. (1977). Telling more than we know: Verbal reports on mental processes. *Psychological Review, 84,* 231-259.

Norman, D.A. (1986). Cognitive Engineering. In D.A. Norman and S.W. Draper (Eds.), *User-Centred System Design: New perspectives on Human-Computer Interaction.* Hillsdale, N.J.: Lawrence Erlbaum. pp 31-62.

Parlett, M. and Hamilton, D. (1972). *Evaluation as Illumination: A New Approach to the Study of Innovatory Programs.* Occasional Paper No. 9, Centre for Research in the Education Sciences, University of Edinburgh.

Parton, D., Huffman, K. Pridgen, P., Norman, K. and Shneiderman, B. (1985). Learning a menu selection tree: Training methods compared. *Behaviour and Information Technology,4* (2), 31-91.

Payne, S.J. (1985). Task-action grammars. In B. Shackel (Ed.), *Human-Computer Interaction - INTERACT '84.* North Holland: Elsevier Science Publishers. pp 527-532.

Schvaneveldt, R.W., Durso, F.T., Goldsmith, T.E., Bean, J.J., Cooke, N M., Tucker, R.G. and DeMaio, J.C. (1985). *Measuring the Structure of Expertise.* New Mexico State University, Memorandum #MCCS 85-32.

Shackel, B. (1984). The concept of usability. In J.L. Bennet, D. Case, J. Sandelin and M. Smith (Eds.), *Visual Display Terminals: Usability Issues and Health Concerns.* Englewood Cliffs New Jersey: Prentice Hall. pp 45-88

Shneiderman, B. (1984). The future of interactive systems and the emergency of direct manipulation. In Y. Vassiliou (Ed.), *Human Factors and Interactive Computer Systems.* Norwood, N.J.: Ablex. pp 1-28.

Sleeman, D. (1985). UMFE: A user modelling front end subsystem. *International Journal of Man-Machine Studies, 23,* 71-88.

Wellbank, M. (1983). *A Review of Knowledge Acquisition Techniques for Expert Systems.* British Telecom, Martelsham Consultancy, BT Research Laboratories, Ipswich.

Winograd, T. (1975). Frame representations and the declarative procedural controversy. In D.G. Bobrow and A.M. Collins (Eds.), *Representation and Understanding: Studies in Cognitive Science.* New York: Academic Press. pp 185-210.

Young, R.M. (1983). Surrogates and mappings: Two kinds of conceptual models for interactive devices. In D. Gentner and A.L. Stevens *Mental Models.* Hillsdale, N.J.: Lawrence Erlbaum. pp 35-52.

Psychological Issues of
Human Computer Interaction in the Work Place
M. Frese, E. Ulich, W. Dzida (Editors)
© Elsevier Science Publishers B.V. (North-Holland), 1987

ON METHODS OF ANALYSIS OF MENTAL MODELS AND THE EVALUATION OF INTERACTIVE COMPUTER SYSTEMS

Thomas Moll

Work and Organizational Psychology Unit Swiss Federal Institute of Technology (ETH) Nelkenstr. 11, CH-8092 Zürich

The contribution of psychology to software design discussed here is controversial. Central to the discussion is the question of research methods. This article will demonstrate which methods psychologists and computer scientists may jointly use to improve the 'informational model' of the software user. As there are advantages and disadvantages to single techniques in psychology and computer science, a combination of techniques will be described here. Examples will show how further development of software design may be positively affected as a result of the data gathered through this combination of techniques.

INTRODUCTION

A growing number of blue collar workers (e.g. tool and die makers) with no prior computer experience are now working with computers in the field of computer-aided manufacturing. It has been reported to us by systems programmers that those users with no previous data processing experience requiring computers to execute their work do not take full advantage of the possibilities and scope of the system to the degree expected. This coincides with results from the area of word processing: "In sum, these data provide an important lesson about the experienced users of powerful computing systems: not all will learn to use the system as imagined by the designer" (Rosson, 1984, p. 229).

With this in mind, the systems programmers of the system under discussion have implemented several functions which are supposed to facilitate the user's familiarity with the possibilities and scope of the system as well as his mastery of problem situations. These functions include a context-sensitive help system. How the users view the help system and whether the help system supports the users in problem situations cannot be specified.

Therefore, a software house is now financing an interdisciplinary project to study the behavior and mental models of the real end users. This research is being conducted by a team of psychologists and systems programmers. Our experience is based on field study observation of 24 end users during 8-day training courses.

THE SYSTEM

MECANIC is an interactive numerical control programming system developed specifically for toolmaking and moldmaking. Various tool-making machines can be readily programmed, either for milling, turning, grinding, or wire-cut electro discharge machining. The MECANIC soft-ware system runs on a work station, with typically 2MB of memory and 20 MB of disc storage. MECANIC is not a computer-aided design system, i.e. not intended for design and drafting in the mechanical engineering office. MECANIC is an interactive system which offers questions to the user to be answered or menus to make a selection. MECANIC offers a number of fixed and constantly active support-functions which can be called up with a single keystroke. For further details, see Sauter and Weydert (1985).

THE SIGNIFICANCE OF MENTAL MODELS TO THE COMPUTER USER AND SYSTEMS PROGRAMMER

An increasing number of investigations with respect to mental models in calculator usage (Halasz & Moran, 1983; Mayer & Bayman, 1981; Young, 1981), programming languages (Du Boulay, O'Shea & Monk, 1981; Jones, 1984; Mayer, 1981) and computing systems (Bennett, Parasuraman & Howard, 1984; Card, Moran & Newell, 1983; Carroll, Mack, Lewis, Grischkowski & Robertson, 1985; Carroll & Thomas, 1982; Halasz & Moran, 1983; Moran, 1981; Rumelhart & Norman, 1981) clearly show the particular importance attached to the mental models of computer users. (A survey of state-of-the-art mental model research may be found in Carroll, 1984).

The significance of mental models or "operative images" (as referred to by Oschanin, 1966) has been described in great detail in other areas of application, e.g. assembly, machine operation and control activities (Matern, Lehmann & Uebel, 1976; Hacker & Clauss, 1976; Skell, 1972; Triebe, 1981).

Proceeding from Oschanin's description of mental models (1976), a detailed description of the features, substance and characteristics of mental models may be found in Hacker (1978). Mental models are "relatively constant psychological structures which regulate the working activity" (p.

82). They regulate work activity through predictions and expectations. Mental models are incomplete, inconsistent, unstable in time, oversimplified, and often rife with superstition. They "need not be technically accurate (and usually are not), but they must be functional" (Norman, 1983, p. 7). However, descriptions of "models for searching" (Duncker, 1935) or "problem space" models (Newell & Simon, 1972) require that the acting person have a certain knowledge from which he may derive his predictions regarding his analysis, valuation, and problem solving. A computer user needs knowledge of the possible states of the system, understanding of the goals which the system can help him to attain, and the respective necessary operations. Users demonstrate various strategies of problem-solving as a function of this knowledge. When working toward their goals, they derive hypotheses based upon their mental models with respect to the solution of their problems - "model-based problem space search" - or unsuccessfully attempt operations (though successful in other situations) without having sufficiently analysed the conditions of their current situation - "methods-based problem space search" (c.f. Halasz & Moran, 1983).

The user's mental model is of particular significance to the systems programmer. As Moran wrote (1981, p. 4) "to design the user interface of the system is to design the user's model". Oschanin's distinction between informational and conceptional models is important in this context; the informational model being the "illustration of the real dynamic of an object" and the conceptional model being the "target-value conception" (Oschanin, 1976, quoted from Ulich, 1980, p. 401).

A systems programmer must have a conceptional model of the product manufactured with the aid of his program as well as an informational model of the user's practical application of his program. If he has no knowledge of how the user uses his system, he has no basis upon which to improve the system. Ulich (1980) described this problem with respect to engineers in another context: "On the other hand the development of operative images in relation to the transformation relationships between the existing and target conditions of the products is, as a rule, not possible for the constructor, as here the informational model, which only arises through practical work, - the image of real dynamics - is necessary" (pp. 401-402).

EVALUATION METHODS

Different approaches are described for testing and evaluating interactive computer systems. One important aspect of user centered design is to study the actual use of the computer system in the field.

Logfile recording

One of the most popular techniques used by the computer community to study the user's behavior is the logfile recording (Gaines, 1981; Sondheimer & Relles, 1982). Logfile recordings can be used e.g. to identify the way the system is used, the errors are made, the use of on-line assistance, and personal reactions to the system. All input and menu selections of the user and all questions and messages of the system can be stored in the memory together with the time of execution. Unconscious regulating processes which one is normally unable to process consciously cannot be verbalized. The great advantage of the logfile recording is that these processes can be recorded and thus made readily available for analysis. The type of particularly frequent novice errors can be identified this way, as well as those untapped possibilities of the system. The question remains, however, what sort of conscious cognition leads to the operations recorded with this technique.

Logfile Recording and Verbal Data: Thinking Aloud and Video Self-Confrontation

Several techniques well-known in cognitive psychology were developed with the objective of registering conscious cognition. The most famous are interviews, questionnaires, "thinking aloud" and video self-confrontation. A great number of investigations in the area of human-computer-interaction have since been conducted using "thinking aloud" (Carroll & Mack, 1983; Carroll et al., 1985; Halasz & Moran; 1983; Jones, 1984).

Duncker's technique of "thinking aloud" (1935) was and is the subject of extensive methodological discussion (cf. Nisbett & Wilson, 1977). Ericsson and Simon (1980, 1984) have developed a model which can determine under what conditions (task, instruction, time lapse between verbalization and execution) this technique may be successfully employed. Some investigations (cf. Deffner, 1984) confirm their assumptions and show no significant differences between "loud" and "silent thinkers". Even if subject's cognitions can be accurately reproduced, attention must be directed to the following potential effects when using this technique: increased concentration, better task structuring, improved problem-solving ability and preference toward a "sound strategy" in problem-solving. Finally, the "inherent problematic nature" of self-observation (Rohracher 1976) must be taken into account with regard to the use of this technique. Since the 'simultaneous' observation process always occurs after the fact, the psychological process under observation is interrupted by the observation process itself. The "degree of conscious clarity" influences self-observation: In affect situations (e.g. rage, anxiety), a considerable decrease in the verbalization of conscious cognition is to be expected.

Our investigations have shown, however, that the technique of "thinking aloud" can only be used effectively when combined with the logfile recording technique, as there are subjects who indicate that they have carried out operations which cannot be found in the logfile. This combination of techniques presents the possibility of analysing whether the causes of execution errors lie in the failure to make use of the objective available information or in the objective lack of necessary information (Hacker, 1978). Failure to make use of objective available information occurs:

1) when an insufficient spatiotemporal conditions classification of elementary movement patterns can be observed (keybord slips, writing slips);
2) when orientation operations (oversights, forgetting) are lacking; or
3) in the event of incorrect execution of orientation and construction operations (e.g. confusion, bad planning).

On the basis of the information contained in the mental model, errors of this kind are corrected immediately after they have been recognized.

Table 1 : Action Errors Despite Objectively Available Information

System's prompt	User input	Thinking aloud
Name of element ?	---= L2	
Definition ?	---= CC	
Ci ?	---= C1	
Cj ?	---= C2	
rel to Ci (r/l/u/d/) ?	---= d	" Up " "That's wrong. I'll go back"
rel to Ci (r/l/u/d/) ?	---= u	

An objective lack of necessary information exists when the cause of an error cannot be identified due to a non-functional mental model and/or when subsequent operations are a result of trial and error.

The disadvantage of this technique is that subjects who are less practiced in formulating their thoughts (in contrast to those recruited for laboratory experiments, e.g. students) verbalize only a small amount of their thought processes. Our main investigations show less verbalization in our toolbuilder and mechanic sample than in the subjects of the pilot study who were teachers and psychologists. Our investigations have further

Table 2: Action Errors Due to an Objective Lack of Information

```
Name of element ?                          ---= 15
Definition ?                               ---= CC

"I've only used this function once before. That's
why I'm not sure if it'll work. When I look
from c1 to c2, I'd assume that I have to go
to the right."

rel to Ci (r/l/u/d) ?                         ---= r


"I'm proceeding on the assumption that I'm in the center
and have to draw the line from this reference point."

rel to Ci (r/l/u/d) ?                         ---= r
rel to Cj (r/l/u/d) ?                         ---= l

"Okay, that can't be right. So I assume that I
must be looking out from the opposite circle. So
I have to enter left here and right there."


rel to Ci (r/l/u/d) ?                         ---= l
rel to Cj (r/l/u/d) ?                         ---= r

"Yes, that's also impossible. Then I'd say that it
borders on c1 below, and on c2 below, too.
Now it's got to work."

rel to Ci (r/l/u/d) ?                         ---= d
rel to Cj (r/l/u/d) ?                         ---= d

"That's something that you just have to try..."


...?   System's prompt
---=   User input
"..."  Thinking aloud
```

shown the inherent problematic nature of self-observation: In particular difficult problem situations, subjects stop thinking aloud. On the other hand, video self-confrontation with the subject's performance serves nonetheless to identify the hypotheses which underlie the operations under investigation immediately upon completion of the task without disturbing the thought process. The objective of video self-confrontation is to ascertain action accompanying and steering cognition. The fundamental idea of this technique is personal confrontation with one's own previously recorded behavior (Nielsen, 1962; Elstein, Kagan, Shulman, Jason & Loupe,1972). On the basis of "objective self awareness (Duval & Wicklund, 1972) and data (including that from other areas) gathered with this technique (see Meichenbaum & Butler, 1980) it may be concluded that this technique is helpful in clarifying differences in mental models and in shedding light on human-computer-interaction. An overview of the current research with this technique may be found in Dowrick and Biggs (1983) and some methodological problems and how to overcome them in Kalbermatten (1982). The data gathered with this technique should be interpreted in conjunction with concrete actions. Similarly, significant statements can be made only in conjunction with the data on the logfile recording when using this technique. As the advantages and disadvantages of single techniques show, a combination of techniques is essential.

Table 3: Logfile Recording and Video Self-Confrontation

```
    ---= gt p0
    ---= gl p10
    ---= gl c1
    ---= gf 14,c2,c3,15

[ERROR: Geo element required]

"It says,'Geo element required'. Then I thought, what does it
mean by 'Geo element required'? I gave the Geo element c2 and
everything that comes after it. At the moment I don't know
why I'm getting an error message. Now I've tried it again. A
while ago I went from a line to a circle and from a line to a
circle again, and I thought, that doesn't work. Now I'm
trying to see if going from one circle to another circle will
work."


    ---= gf c2,c3

[ERROR: Geo element required]

"Now I'm thinking, if it doesn't accept it this way, I'll
write them all under each other."

    ---= gf 14
    ---= gf c2
    ---= gf c3
    ---= gf 15
```

```
    ---=    User input
    "..."  Video self-confrontation
    [...]  Error messages
```

Our main investigations show that this combination of techniques (which can offset several disadvantages attributed to the use of a single technique) and a similar combination developed and tested by Hietala (1985) can offer several suggestions toward the improvement of software. For example, Table 3 shows that feedback pertaining to the problems of the user have led to improved error messages. The error message "Geo element required" now reads "Put a blank as separator (in line...) : , ".

EVALUATION OF A HELP SYSTEM

The following will describe suggestions regarding human-computer-interaction as well as recommendations toward the further advancement of help systems which stem from the aforementioned combination of techniques. Contrary to the general prerequisite that a computer must have a help function (e.g. DIN 66234 Part 8), some articles remark that help systems are the least useful parts of software. (For review of the state-of-the-art in help systems, see Borenstein, 1985; Carroll & McKendree, 1986; Houghton, 1984; Sondheimer & Relles, 1982). As a result, comprehensive investigations into the actual use of help systems as well as into the advantages and disadvantages of help systems are in order.

The Context-Sensitive Help System

When systems programmers implement help functions in a menu-driven dialog, the users are expected to either make a menu selection (module, task) or answer a question (operation). The help system under study has been implemented so that a specific help message exists for every module, task and operation.This is referred to as a "context-sensitive help system". The help message in each error situation is supplemented with a help-to-error message. The advantage of this help system is that the user immediately receives context-related help at each step without a difficult dialog.

Questionnaire Results

A general assessment of the context-sensitive help function may be found in the responses to on-line multiple-choice questions. The responses of training course participants (N=6) show that explanations in the help mode were assessed as "too general" at the end of the course (Day 8), as opposed to at the beginning of the course (Day 3). Whereas at the beginning of the course the majority felt that one could "correct one's errors after reading the help information", the majority agreed at the end of the course that one could "rarely correct one's errors". On the basis of this results, the question arises whether the help system under investigation does indeed support the user when he engages the computer in a problem-solving dialog.

Logfile Analysis Results with Thinking Aloud and Video Self-Confrontation

Initial analysis of help situations show that the help function is employed in various situations and, depending upon the situation, supports the user in different ways.

Situation I : Call for Help with Regard to Loss of Orientation in an Error Situation

The help function is frequently first activated when the user finds himself in an error situation and the system sends him an error message.

Table 4: Call For Help with Regard to Loss of Orientation

```
"Now I want to draw this line.
I'm not getting anywhere here, so I'll just try it in
'Machining'"

---= MACHINING
---= Edit the program
    Program name ?
---= test1
---= Enter or modify

"So I gave a name, but then I saw that I wasn't getting
anywhere. That's why I went back again"

---= GEOMETRY
---= Handle
---= Create
---= Help Mode

"Now I don't know what I'm supposed to do anymore. And
why I'm getting 'Handle', I don't know that either."

[You have no idea how to continue?]

"No."
```

```
...?   Questions of the System
"..."  Video self-confrontation
---=   Selection or Input of the User
[...]  Questions of the  Interviewer
```

Frequently he has already made decisions before his input or selection which preclude the attainment of his goal. Not only does he have an incomplete image of the possibilities of his input in this case, but also of the situation in which he finds himself. In this case, he does not receive the necessary information in the help mode (cf. Table 4). Should the user in such a situation accept the suggestions, subsequent errors are not unusual.

Non-context-related basic knowledge of the fundamental concepts of the system are not conveyed. A goal-oriented tutorial must therefore be developed in order to convey this basic knowledge.

Table 5: Call For Help in a Familiar Situation

```
Name of element ?          ---= 18
Definition ?               ---= SYM

[Here you say 'Symmetry']

"Yes, I tried that too, I didn't know that".

[Haven't you ever worked with 'Symmetry before ?]

"No, never. But one can. 'Reflection'. That's how I do it.
I just tried it. Maybe it'll work like this.
How else can you do it ?"...

Li ?                       ---= 17
Axis of Symmetry ?

[Now don't you know what 'Axis of Symmetry' means ?]

"Yes, right. And now I think I've called for help."

---= Help Mode

"Yes, reflected. And now I know that it's this axis.
```

```
...?    System's prompt
"..."   Video self-confrontation
---=    Selection or user input
[...]   Questions of the  interviewer
```

Situation II: Call for Help in a Familiar Situation When Single Operations Are Unfamiliar

Help situation analysis showes, that the context-sensitive help system supports users whose goals are quite clear and who know exactly what state of the system they are in. It also supports those whose problems relate purely to unfamiliarity with the input mode or who simply do not comprehend the questions in situations otherwise clear to them (cf. Table 5).

CONCLUSIONS

There are several techniques in Computer Science and Psychology which can be applied in the evaluation of interactive computer systems. Among these are logfile recordings, questionnaires, thinking aloud and the technique of video self-confrontation. With the help of examples, it was demonstrated that these techniques have specific advantages and disadvantages.

With on-line questionnaires the user's software knowledge can be tested economically. It is possible to divide the users into different subgroups and compare their handling of the computer . Whether the user makes use of his knowledge while working with the computer cannot be determined when using this single technique.

Logfile recordings are very helpful here. In our investigation, all user input and sytem prompts are stored in a file. Unconscious operations that one is normally unable to verbalize are registered with the execution time. Novice errors, as well as the untapped potential of the system, can be identified. We were able to give feedback on the main problems of the majority of the users to the software house. The systems programmers were then able to modify and improve the dialog according to these results.

No information regarding the action regulating processes can be obtained by using this technique. The reason for the same user's input can be an action slip or an incorrect mental model of the system.

We can gain information about these cognitions by using the technique of "thinking aloud". Our subjects were asked to report ongoing conscious cognitions while working with the computer. Because the subjects directly reported their conscious thoughts, we gain information about the goals, subgoals and hypotheses of the user. There are, however, some important disadvantages with regard to this technique. Sometimes people are sure that they have performed operations which we were never able to find in the logfile. Another disadvantage of this technique is that of simultaneous action: the subjects are required to perform a task and think aloud about this process at the same time. Furthermore, there is a wide range in ability of verbalization, which is somtimes inhibited in affect situations. Because we did not wish to disturb the problem solving process we didn't insist on this technique. When our subjects stopped thinking aloud, we let them perform their task silently.

As a result, our verbal protocols are sometimes full of gaps. We supplemented this technique with video self-confrontation. Immediatly after performing the task, the videotape was presented. Personal confrontation with one's previously recorded behavior supports the memory. We gain a great deal of information about the thoughts of the user relating to concrete operations.

This method combination supports the systems programmers in that a user-specific informational model as it applies to the programmer's software can be devised. They receive concrete feedback regarding the problems of the user of their software and can, for example, improve error messages or determine in which problem situations their help system supports the user and in which situations this system is inadequate.

REFERENCES

Bayman, P. & Mayer, R.E.(1984). Instructional manipulation of users' mental models for electronic calculators. *International Journal of Man-Machine Studies, 20*, 189-199.

Bennett, K.B., Parasuraman, R. & Howard, J.H.(1984). Mental models in interface design: The role of graphic displays. In A. Mital (Ed.), *Trends in Ergonomics/Human Factors I*. Amsterdam: North-Holland.

Borenstein, N.S.(1985). *The Design and Evaluation of On-line Help Systems*. Unpublished doctoral dissertations, Carnegie-Mellon University, Pittsburgh, Pennsylvania.

Card, S., Moran, T. & Newell, A.(1983). *The Psychology of Human-Computer Interaction*. Hillsdale, N.J.: Lawrence Erlbaum Associates.

Carroll, J.M.(1984). *Mental Models and Software Human Factors: An Overview*. IBM Research Report.

Carroll, J.M. & Campbell, R.L.(1986). *Softening up Hard Science: reply to Newell and Card*. IBM Research Report.

Carroll, J.M. & Mack, R.L.(1983). Actively learning to use a word processor. In W. Cooper (Ed.), *Cognitive Aspects of Skilled Typewriting* (259-281). New York: Springer.

Carroll, J.M., Mack, R.L., Lewis, C.H., Grischkowsky, N.L. & Robertson, S.R.(1985). Exploring Exploring a Word Processor. *Human-Computer Interaction, 1*, 283-307.

Carroll, J.M. & McKendree, J.E.(1986). *Interface design issues for advice-giving expert systems*. IBM Research Report.

Carroll, J.M. & Thomas, J.C.(1982). Metaphor and the cognitive representation of computing systems. *IEEE Transactions on Systems, Man, and Cybernetics, SMC-12*, 107-116.

DIN 66234 Teil 8 (1984). *Bildschirmarbeitsplaetze. Entwurf der Grundsaetze der Dialoggestaltung*. Deutsches Institut f. Normung.

Dowrick, P.W. & Biggs, S.J. (Eds.). (1984). *Using Video*. Chichester: John Wiley.

DuBoulay, B., O'Shea, T. & Monk, J.(1981). The black box inside the glass box: presenting computing concepts to novices. *International Journal of Man-Machine Studies, 14*, 237-249.

Duncker, K.(1935). *Zur Psychologie des Produktiven Denkens*. Berlin: Springer

Duval, S. & Wicklund, R.A.(1972). *A Theory of Objective Selfawareness*. New York: Academic Press.

Elstein, A.S., Kagan, N., Shulman, L.S., Jason, H. & Loupe, M.J.(1972). Methods and Theory in the Study of Medical Inquiry. *Journal of Medical Education, 47*, 85-92.

Ericsson, K.A. & Simon, H.A.(1980). Verbal Reports as Data. *Psychological Review, 87*, 215-251.

Ericsson, K.A. & Simon, H.A.(1984). *Protocol Analysis: Verbal Reports as Data*. Cambridge,MA.: MIT Press.

Deffner, G.(1984). *Lautes Denken - Untersuchung zur Qualitaet eines Datenerhebungsverfahrens*. Frankfurt/M.: Peter Lang.

Gaines, B.R.(1981). The technology of interaction-dialogue programming rules. *International Journal of Man-Machine Studies, 14*, 1, 137-150.

Hacker, W.(1978). *Allgemeine Arbeits- und Ingenieurpsychologie*. Bern: Huber.

Hacker, W. & Clauss, A.(1976). Kognitive Operationen, inneres Modell und Leistung bei einer Montagetaetigkeit. In W. Hacker (Ed.), *Psychische Regulation von Arbeitstaetigkeiten*. Berlin: Deutscher Verlag der Wissenschaften.

Halasz, F.G. & Moran, T.P.(1983). Mental Models and Problem Solving in Using a Calculator. *CHI'83 Conference Proceedings: Human Factors in Computing Systems*. Boston, Ma., 212-217.

Hietala, P.(1985). *Combining Logging, Playback and Verbal Protocols: a method for analyzing and evaluating interactive systems*. Unpublished Paper, University of Tampere, Department of Mathematical Sciences.

Houghton, R.C.(1984). Online help systems: A conspectus. *Communications of the ACM, 27*, 126-133.

Jones, A.(1984). How Novices Learn to Program. *INTERACT'84 Conference Papers: First IFIP Conference on 'Human-Computer Interaction'*. London, 50-56.

Kalbermatten, U.(1982). *The Self-Confrontation Interview (Research Reports No. 3)*. Bern: University of Bern, Department of Psychology.

Mayer, R.E.(1981). The psychology of how novices learn computer programming. *Computer Surveys, 13*, 121-141

Matern, B., Lehmann, B. & Uebel, H.(1976). Zur Ermittlung von inneren Modellen für Taetigkeiten der Prozessregulation als Voraussetzung zur Optimierung von Arbeits- und Anlernverfahren in der Betriebspraxis. In W. Hacker (Ed.), *Psychische Regulation von Arbeitstaetigkeiten*. Berlin: Deutscher Verlag der Wissenschaften.

Mayer, R.E. & Bayman, P.(1981). Psychology of Calculator languages: A framework for describing differences in users' knowledge. *Communications of the ACM, 24*, 511-520.

Meichenbaum, D. & Butler, L.(1980). Cognitive Ethology. Assessing the Streams of Cognition and Emotion. In K.R. Blankstein, P. Pliner & J. Polivy (Eds.), *Assessment and Modification of Emotional Behavior* (139-163). New York: Plenum Press.

Moran, T.(1981), The command language grammer: A representation for the user interface of interactive computer systems. *International Journal of Man-Machine Studies, 15*, 3-50.

Newell, A. & Card, S.K.(1985). The prospects for psychological science in human-computer interaction. *Human-Computer Interaction, 1*, 209-242.

Newell, A. & Simon, H.A.(1972), *Human Problem Solving*. Englewood Cliffs,N.J.: Prentice Hall.

Nielsen, G.(1962). *Studies in Self-confrontation*. Kopenhagen: Munksgaard.

Nisbett, R.E. & Wilson, T.D.(1977). Telling more than we can know: Verbal reports on mental processes. *Psychological Review, 84*, 231-259.

Norman, D.A.(1983). Some Observations on Mental Models. In D. Genter & A.L. Stevens (Eds.), *Mental Models*. Hillsdale,N.J.: Lawrence Erlbaum Associates.

Oschanin, D.A.(1966). *Das operative Abbild eines gesteuerten Objekts*. Vortrag am 18. Intern. Kong. f. Psychologie. Moskau.

Oschanin, D.A.(1976). Dynamisches operatives Abbild und konzeptionelles Modell. *Probleme und Ergebnisse der Psychologie, 59*, 37-48.

Rohracher, H.(1976). *Einführung in die Psychologie* (11th ed.). München: Urban & Schwarzenberg.

Rosson, M.B. (1984). The Role of Experience in Editing. *INTERACT'84 Conference Papers: First IFIP Conference on 'Human-Computer Interaction'*. London, 225-230.

Rumelhart, D.E. & Norman, D.A.(1981). Analogical processes in learning. In J.R. Anderson (Ed.), *Cognitive Skills and Their Acquisition*. Hillsdale,N.J.: Lawrence Erlbaum Associates, 335-360.

Sauter, R. & Weydert, J.(1985). Die Entwicklung einer Mensch-Maschine-Schnittstelle und ihr Einfluss auf das Benutzermodell. In H.G. Klopic, R. Marty & E.H. Rothaus (Eds.), *Arbeitsplatzrechner in der Unternehmung* (248-266). Stuttgart: Teubner.

Skell, W.(1972). Analyse von Denkleistungen bei der Planung und praktischen Durchführung von Produktionsarbeiten in der Berufsausbildung. In W. Skell (Ed.), *Psychologische Analysen von Denkleistungen in der Produktion*. Berlin: Deutscher Verlag der Wissenschaften.

Sondheimer, N.K. & Relles, N.(1982). Human Factors and User Assistance in Interactive Computing Systems: An Introduction. *IEEE Transactions on Systems, Man, and Cybernetics, SMC-12*, 102-107.

Triebe, J.(1981), *Aspekte beruflichen Handelns und Lernens*. Unpublished doctoral dissertation, University of Bern.

Ulich, E.(1980). Industrial Psychology - Compulsory for Engineers? In H. Boehme (Ed.), *Engineers for Tomorrow* (pp. 400-411). München: Heinz Moos Verlag.

Young, R.M.(1981). The machine inside the machine: Users' models of pocket calculators. *International Journal of Man-Machine Studies, 15*, 51-85.

Psychological Issues of
Human Computer Interaction in the Work Place
M. Frese, E. Ulich, W. Dzida (Editors)
© Elsevier Science Publishers B.V. (North-Holland), 1987

COGNITIVE OPTIMISATION OF VIDEOTEX DIALOGUES:
A FORMAL-EMPIRICAL APPROACH

John Long and Paul Buckley

Ergonomics Unit, University College London
26 Bedford Way, London WC1H OAP, United Kingdom

Psychological research intended to provide designers with information concerning the optimisation of videotex dialogues is characterised in terms of three approaches. The Formal approach offers a structure for describing completely, explicitly, and coherently, some activities of computer users. The Empirical approach provides data about users' behaviour, including their errors and difficulties. The combined Formal-Empirical approach uses both formal structures and empirical data and - unlike the unitary approaches - can show where and how user activities result in or contribute to errors and difficulties of performance. The three approaches are outlined and a research project intended to optimise the usability of videotex dialogues is used to describe the formal-empirical approach in more detail. The effectiveness of the combined approach is compared with that of the unitary alternatives. Issues arising from experience of the combined approach are discussed.

INTRODUCTION

One view of design activity is that it involves iterating between the generation of solutions to the design problem and the evaluation of their adequacy (Whitefield, 1984). The cognitive optimisation of interactive computer dialogues in general, and those of videotex systems in particular, can be similarly characterised. The dialogues need to be evaluated against appropriate criteria, and inadequacies identified. Alternative dialogues need to be generated to overcome the inadequacies. These alternative solutions in turn need to be re-evaluated for their adequacy. If the dialogues exist, the iteration begins with their evaluation; if they do not exist, it begins with their generation.

This chapter summarises the findings of a research project undertaken to help videotex designers improve the usability of computerised transaction dialogues in general and teleshopping dialogues in particular. The chapter uses this psychological research to illustrate a formal-empirical approach to the cognitive optimisation of the dialogues. The approach uses formal structures (for example, a model of the task and a model of the sources of user difficulties) to organise empirical evaluations (for example, observational studies and experiments). The resulting data are used to develop the models which are then employed in further generative and evaluative activities.

VIDEOTEX TRANSACTION SYSTEMS

The use of domestic television screens to display text and graphics is common to several types of public information services. These systems differ in their technology. For instance, the delivery methods differ. "Teletext" information is broadcast by television signals, and "Cabletext" distributed by means of switched cable networks. The focus in this chapter is on "Videotex" which normally comprises a network of computers accessed by users via the standard telephone system. Two-way communication is therefore possible. Videotex users have keypads or alphanumeric keyboards which they operate to request information and to conduct transactions.

The transactions which are currently available vary with the system. On British Telecom's Prestel system, for example, transactional services include shopping, banking, ticket booking, message sending and software downloading. Teleshopping will be the focus of the approach described here.

Although videotex services have yet to become widely popular, there are two main groups of potential users. Some services cater for specialist in-house needs of individual organisations, for example ordering spare parts or office supplies etc. The members of these so-called "Closed User Groups" may become expert or at least highly proficient. Other services, which have few or no access restrictions, cater for the needs of the general public. For example, teleshopping could be quicker and more convenient than conventional shopping, since goods can be ordered at anytime and are sent or transported by the supplier. Such a service might appeal to people without transport - for example the disabled and the aged - and to people uninterested in shopping. The focus in this chapter is on the latter group and in particular on members of the general public naive with respect to videotex transaction services. These users may have little experience of computers and little interest in learning how to use them. Such people are known to experience difficulty in operating videotex systems (Long and Buckley, 1984). The research reported here was initiated to identify sources of difficulty leading to poor usability, and to suggest how the difficulties might be eliminated, or at least reduced.

APPROACHES TO THE COGNITIVE OPTIMISATION OF VIDEOTEX DIALOGUES

There are at least three possible approaches to the cognitive optimisation of usability characterised as the evaluation and generation of alternative dialogues for computerised shopping. These are (1) a formal approach; (2) an empirical approach; and (3) a combined formal-empirical approach. Formal is here defined as explicit, well-formed and complete. It contrasts with informal. Empirical is defined as reflecting user behaviour and therefore a posteriori. It contrasts with non-empirical. As used in this chapter, formal implies non-empirical, and empirical implies informal. In terms of these definitions, the contribution of the formal approach to optimisation is by the application of abstract structures which make no explicit assumptions concerning user behaviour. In contrast, the empirical approach attempts to contribute by applying what is known about user behaviour while leaving any abstract structures implicit. The formal-empirical approach involves the use of an a priori, formal structure to acquire empirical knowledge about user behaviour, which is in turn used to modify the formal structure. Each approach will be described in terms of a framework which attempts to relate the behavioural sciences more generally to the real world of the workplace. Using the framework to model the approaches makes it possible to identify the similarities and differences between them. In addition, the framework will be used to describe, in more detail, the third approach as it was used in research conducted to help reduce difficulties in the use of teleshopping systems.

Framework

The framework has been used to model cognitive ergonomic activities and has been described in detail elsewhere (Long, in press). It is illustrated in Figure 1. The real world of work - expressed as tasks - is contrasted with the representational (or descriptive) world of knowledge-expressed as sciences and non-science. Non-scientific knowledge includes experiential knowledge, both craft and personal. The two worlds of tasks and sciences are related by means of intermediary representations, and activities which transform, that is translate, these representations. Scientific knowledge is acquired by a number of transformations, two of which - analysis and generalisation - are shown. The activity of analysing a task produces an acquisition representation, the main function of which is to support a simulation of some aspects of the real world for the purposes of data gathering. The activity of generalising the data from studies and experiments transforms the acquisition representation into the models and explanatory principles of scientific knowledge. All transformations can be iterative. Once acquired, scientific knowledge may be applied. In the framework, it is applied by a number of transformations, two of which -

particularisation and synthesis - are shown. The activity of particularising scientific knowledge produces an applications representation, for example in the form of design principles or recommendations. The activity of synthesising the applications representation with tasks effects changes in the real world of the workplace.

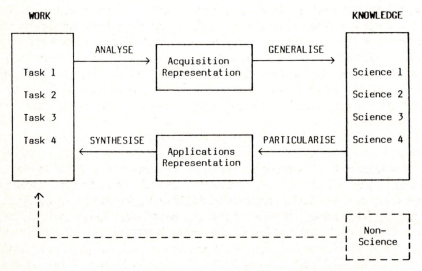

Figure 1: Framework relating the worlds of work and knowledge

Formal Approach

A formal approach to optimising the videotex dialogues of interest would have involved selecting some abstract structure within which an alternative (optimal) transaction system could have been specified. Such formalisms include state transition diagrams (Parnas, 1969); augmented transition networks (Woods, 1970); and formal grammars (Moran, 1981). For example, it would have been possible to use the representational framework offered by Moran's Command Language Grammar to model an alternative transaction dialogue. In terms of Figure 1, the Command Language Grammar is analogous to Transformational Grammar (Chomsky, 1965), which is part of the cognitive and behavioural science base of linguistics. An alternative transaction dialogue, expressed in terms of the Command Language Grammar, would have had the advantage of being explicit, well-formed and complete in terms of its own formalism. However, the model would have had no empirical content concerning users' behaviour. In other words, the formalism would have provided no grounds for assuming one dialogue optimal with respect to another. In practice, to be applicable at all for the purposes of optimisation, this "pure" formal approach would have had to be supplemented by some intuitive assumptions on the part of the researchers concerning user behaviour. Alternatively, the assumptions might have been based on some plausible explicit rationale. For example, Reisner (1981), using the formal approach in an assessment of alternative forms of a graphics system for usability, made assumptions about structural consistency (for example, which tasks are perceived by the user as similar) and the number of rules necessary to describe the system (for example, more rules make a system harder to learn). However, neither intuitions nor an explicit plausible rationale reflect user behaviour directly and were considered to be inadequate to provide the empirical content required by the acquisition and applications representations shown in Figure 1. For this reason, a formal approach by itself was considered inappropriate for the purpose of optimising videotex dialogues.

Empirical Approach

An alternative approach would have been an empirical one. For example, users might have been observed conducting transactions (Hammond, Long, Clark, Barnard and Morton, 1981), or learning to use the system (Hammond, Hinton, Barnard, MacLean, Long and Whitefield, 1984). Errors and difficulties could have been used to identify which aspects of the dialogues were causing users difficulty, and alternative versions of the dialogues constructed. In terms of Figure 1, the acquisition representation would have been reflected in the applications representation without any contribution from the science base. An alternative dialogue based on actual users' behaviour would have had much to recommend it. However, a "pure" empirical approach would not have been able to provide an explicit, well-formed and complete description of user behaviour, because no formalism would have been used to structure the empirical observations. In practice, some post hoc structure would have emerged to organise the data (for example, an error taxonomy (Hammond et al, 1981) or protocol analysis (Hammond, Jorgensen, MacLean, Barnard and Long, 1983)), but these structures are likely to have been implicit, and neither well-formed nor complete. They would not have provided an adequate set of structures for supporting the organisation and development of the acquisition and applications representations shown in Figure 1. For this reason, an empirical approach by itself was considered to be inappropriate for the purpose of optimising videotex dialogues.

Formal-Empirical Approach

A third approach was adopted which attempted to combine the strengths and avoid the weaknesses of the formal and of the empirical approaches. The formal-empirical approach, which is described in detail in the following section, used formalisms, such as models of the task, of the system and of the user, which may initially be a priori, and employed them to analyse empirical data reflecting user behaviour. The data in turn were used to refine the models further which were themselves re-used analytically. In the context of the framework for cognitive ergonomics (Figure 1), the models were either a priori or derived from the science base. In both cases, the models and their empirical content reflecting user behaviour were used to construct the acquisition and applications representations. Within the approach, it would have been possible literally to combine an extant formal structure - like Moran's Command Language Grammar - with an extant set of empirical procedures as used by Hammond et al (1981). This was not done for two reasons. First, the Command Language Grammar is complex and its application less than transparent. Second, the empirical procedures of Hammond et al (ibid) were in some cases excessive (for example, a complete machine log of every user interaction) and in some cases inadequate for the present purposes (for example, no retroactive verbal protocols). For these reasons, the approach used here employed more modest analytic structures in the form of models, and used empirical procedures which varied with their function. It remained, however, the aim of the approach to develop explicit, well-formed and complete descriptions of users' behaviour for the purpose of generating and evaluating optimised dialogues for videotex shopping services. The approach will now be illustrated in detail.

ILLUSTRATION OF FORMAL-EMPIRICAL APPROACH

Background

The illustrative project is entitled "An Evaluation of Dialogue Forms for Transaction Processing on Videotex Systems". The aims of the research were to investigate the usability of videotex for domestic transactions such as shopping and banking. At the inception of the project, it was intended that the eventual outputs would take two forms. In terms of the framework for cognitive ergonomics cited earlier, one form of output would constitute an addition to the science base and the other would be an appropriate applications representation. The work will now be described, and attempts made to relate aspects of the research to the characteristics of the formal-empirical approach.

First Stage

The first stage of the work involved specifying the scope of the research. This required an investigation of what constituted a videotex system, a user and a transaction task. Gilligan and Long (1984) report this part of the work. The various forms of text-on-television services were described and examined for their functionality with respect to informal, although explicit, categories of user and components of the transaction task. For instance, the delivery systems of these "tex" services, as described earlier, were examined for the two-way operation required by a informal characterisation of transaction processing. Specific details of the system were also related to the categories of user in terms of consequences for usability. For example, computer-like terminology in the videotex database (i.e., the use of GOTO <menu option>) was described as a potential source of difficulty for information technology unaware users while this jargon probably did not constitute a problem for those users who were aware of information technology.

The explication of the characteristics of the various categories of system, task and user facilitated the definition of the research scope, although this categorisation hardly constitutes a formal structure in the context of this chapter. Since it was intended to study the use of videotex for transaction processing in the home, users were defined as being unaware of information technology, that is naive with respect to videotex. They were, though, expected to be skilled in carrying out domestic transactions. The type of transaction task studied was shopping. It appeared that the components of this task encompassed those found in alternative choices (such as banking or messaging) and system usability for shopping had consequences equally or more critical for successful task performance. The videotex system was defined as having "Prestel characteristics". The definitions of task, user and system were used to generate an acquisition representation in the form of a simulated task performed on an extant system by approriate users. The function of the acquisition representation, as stated earlier, was to gather empirical data characterising usability.

Second Stage

The simulation defined in terms of the above analysis was used in an observational study in which empirical data concerning usability were generated and recorded. Five subjects, none with previous experience of videotex, were asked to complete eight shopping "scenarios". The scenarios each detailed a situation (e.g. a friend's birthday) and a target category of goods to be acquired (e.g. roses). The subjects used the current Prestel service to attempt to satisfy the requirements of the scenarios. They were asked to talk through their performance, and also to add retrospective comments to a replay of a muted videotape made of their earlier task activity. In this way, an empirical database of comments, difficulties and errors was produced.

Formal Structures

Before the third stage, formal structures were introduced. They each had two functions. Firstly, they expressed their domains formally, that is, as defined earlier, explicitly, coherently and fully. Secondly, and with respect to the progress of the research summarised here, more immediately, they aided the interpretation of the protocols collected in the previous (empirical) stage. The two structures will be described, and then the outcome of the protocol interpretation summarised.

Block Interaction Model

The first structure was used to interpret the sources of the difficulties expressed in the protocols and of the errors of performance made by the subjects. The structure was the Block Interaction Model (BIM) (Morton, Barnard, Hammond and Long, 1979). It is a framework that expresses user knowledge in terms of two types of knowledge source. The first type, called "ideal user knowledge" are particular and correct sources of knowledge of the current system, and they provide for error-free task performance. The other type are general (non-specific) knowledge sources. The usage of the latter can, in the model, have either of two consequences; if the general sources "overlap" with the "ideal-user" sources, then error-free behaviour can still occur; if the sources "mismatch", then recruitment of the general source (for instance, if the particular sources are incomplete) may lead to errors and misunderstanding (and therefore difficulty). The difficulties found in the protocol data could therefore be described as the (inappropriate) use of "mismatching" knowledge sources.

Task Model

The second structure was a generic model of the transaction task. This aided the interpretation of the protocols by providing a structure which helped make the subjects' goals explicit. The model, then, also made it possible to structure the difficulties. The model took a definition of a transaction, and expressed the logical requirements of a system that purported to perform the task as defined. The defining assumptions were that exchange of resources must occur and that resources are acquired to satisfy some recognised need. Since exchange includes "costs" as well as "acquisitions", two categories of information are required, that is, information about goods and information about costs. Also, for exchange to occur, at least two transacting bodies need to be involved. Because "satisfaction of need" is a defining characteristic, the two categories of information must be acquired and evaluated by both transactors to assess whether the need will be satisfied. For acquisition of information to occur, the mirror-symmetry of the system requires that the other transactor (or potential transactor) "displays" or makes available information about resources and costs.

In particular transaction systems, the task components are realised as forms determined by the task technology. The symmetry is typically disguised by naming the activities of particular transactors differently from the activities of their opposite partner, e.g. "sell" and "buy"; "barter", though, maintains a symmetrical description.

Third Stage

With the aid of these formal frameworks, the user difficulties were interpreted in terms of knowledge source interactions during attempts to achieve particular modelled task goals. A model was constructed by elaborating the BIM framework and the generic task model to produce a specific representation of the sources of user difficulty experienced while attempting to complete shopping tasks on Prestel. The data for the identification of the sources were user protocols and therefore the model produced was a result of combining formal frameworks and empirical behavioural data, a characteristic of the formal-empirical approach.

The model consisted of generalised "system" and "knowledge" variables. System variables could be considered as an expression, in terms of features of the technology, of the ideal user knowledge sources, since the technology itself defines the behaviour and therefore knowledge required for error-free performance. System variables were identified by generalising specific characteristics of the system that were associated with difficulties in the protocol. For instance, this difficulty:

> *"Right 4267, you don't leave a gap do you on the number here, I suppose you just... you can't can you 'cos it's not like a typewriter where you can leave a gap"*

while specifically attributable to a problem of entering a space with a keypad which did not support a space character, was generalised to problems associated with "input devices". "Knowledge" variables were identified by similarly generalising hypothesised mismatching knowledge sources associated with the protocol difficulties. For instance, "knowledge of typewriters" assumed to be used in the above example, was generalised to "knowledge of off-line systems". In all, fourteen system variables and seven knowledge variables were identified (Buckley and Long, 1985a; Buckley and Long, 1986b).

Fourth Stage

The reason for expressing the variables at a generalised level was to ensure the appropriateness of the variables for use in susbsequent experimental studies. Variables had to be operationalisable, that is expressible in terms of potential experimental manipulations. This requirement was made since subsequent experimentation was essential to confirm or deny the reality and importance of the effective sources of user difficulty. Protocol interpretation by itself can only lead to the generation of hypotheses and less formal suggestions.

This stage involved a specification of a second acquisition representation, this time for the purposes of generating and recording behavioural data related to effects of specific hypothesised variables concerning usability. The acquisition representation specified the requirements for a laboratory test paradigm. The task model was used again here to structure experimental studies. Particular components of the task, together with the relevant variables, were investigated separately. For instance, the response frames posed some difficulties for users in the display component but none in the acquisition and evaluation task components. Among others, experiments on the display component alone were carried out.

Fifth Stage

This stage was intended to provide confirmation of the elaborated BIM which represented hypothesised sources of user difficulty, expressed as variables. This was done by a series of experimental studies that examined the usability effects of system and knowledge variables in the various components of the task and produced empirical evidence concerning them. Only a small proportion of the possible experimental configurations could be attempted. Some of these will be briefly described below.

Evaluation

The transaction component of evaluation was examined in a laboratory simulation of this task component. For the experiments, evaluation was specified in more detail as the comparison of features of potential acquisitions with a set of "criterial" features representing the need. This definition helped the specification of the acquisition representation and also the experimental task (Buckley and Long, 1985b).

In the experiment, subjects were given a single criterion for each of a set of goods and shown various videotex representations of those goods. The goods were either (1) known or not known by the subjects. The representations (2) included or did not include a text representation of a feature clearly defining a good as adequate or not adequate with respect to the criterion; (3) included or did not include a videotex graphic which represented a feature which defined a good as adequate or not adequate with respect to the criterion. The system variable manipulated by (2) and (3) was "Extent of Description of Goods", and a knowledge variable "Knowledge of the Domain" was manipulated by (1).

The hypothesised effects of "Knowledge of the Domain" were confirmed - subjects were quicker and more accurate in deciding whether a good satisfied their criterion when they had been previously taught about the item. The inclusion of a text description also helped but not as much. The visual representation helped a little, only when subjects had to rely on the images, that is when they had no knowledge and no text representation. Although performance was above chance level, the error rate was high (35%). Given the constraints on images formed by Prestel-like visual display elements, it appeared more effective in terms of speed and accuracy to exploit user knowledge (perhaps by restricting the domain of goods to well-known branded items) or provide text descriptions of goods (although this requires a specification of users' criteria). Further experiments quantified the effects of higher resolution images and the results suggested that such images (that is similar to those found in mail order catalogues) would help, but again, only significantly when the goods are not known by users and the important evaluative features are not described by text.

Display

The display task component, which for the videotex teleshopper is the task of completing and sending response frames (RFs), was also investigated in a further set of experimental studies (Fenn, 1985; Fenn and Buckley, 1987) Subjects were given details of goods and required to complete the display task component using the experimental simulation. They were exposed to various classes of goods and various types of response frame (see Gilligan and Long, 1984, for a classification of RFs). The hypothesised effect of the system variable "Type of RF" was confirmed, and elaborated in a further experiment in which "Knowledge of Transactions" and "Instructions" were additionally manipulated. Instructions appeared to have no significant effect on the experimental task, whereas the knowledge variable did so, but only on the initial trial. The effects of knowledge were small compared with RF type, and an additional model (of "workload") was used as an alternative framework for the interpretation of the effects.

Final Version of the Sources of Difficulty Model

Many more variables could be similarly studied. Alternatively, other research could be related to the present project via the formal structures -

the models and frameworks- and substituted for specific additional experimental studies. As an example, research on database navigation via hierarchies of menus can be used to assess the likely effects of variables on the acquisition task component. The result of the incorporation of empirical data, either from new experimental studies or from other research, constitutes a confirmed and elaborated usability model. This model combines the formal frameworks of the BIM and the task model, and becomes more detailed by the incorporation of empirical data. When completed, it will express confirmed sources of user difficulty and the magnitude of time and error effects. In its present form, some sources are confirmed and quantified while others, although identified in an observational study, can be considered as potentially effective only.

Sixth Stage

While research continues to elaborate the model, it is still possible to use what is known and suggested already to generate an applications representation. This is intended to be a source of information for videotex dialogue designers, and is the result of a particularisation of scientific knowledge (for instance, the BIM model of the sources and the effects confirmed by experimental studies).

Typically, in the domain of human-computer interaction, applications representations take the form of "guidelines", "checklists" or "recommendations", and are presented to those responsible for design either by a specifically targeted report (e.g. when research is commissioned with respect to a specific question) or by publishing in trade or academic journals.

For this research, a short investigation was carried out to identify the most appropriate "vehicle" and "form" for the applications representation (Buckley and Long, 1986a).

Conclusion of Illustration

The applications representation is an expression of the appropriate science base - the models and findings of the specific research and of associated research - in terms that are useful and usable by videotex designers. Hopefully, videotex dialogues will improve as a result. In the original characterisation of design as an iterative generate-evaluate cycle, it is thought that the applications representation produced here is more effective for the generative phase. By outlining potential and actual sources of user difficulty, the designers may be directed away from those solutions that use ineffective system characteristics.

CONCLUSIONS

The illustration shows how a piece of psychologically based research generated and used formal structures and empirical evidence characteristic of the formal-empirical approach to optimising dialogues. As described earlier, in this combined approach the advantages of each single approach- formal and empirical - are integrated and the weaknesses of each counter- acted. It is suggested that only in combination can the "pure" approaches contribute effectively to assessments and optimisation of interactive dialogues.

Effectiveness of Example of Formal-Empirical Approach

In the context of this chapter, the alternatives to the combined approach are the unitary formal or empirical approaches. It is in the context of these alternatives that the relative success of the combined approach is appropriately assessed. Both the formal and the empirical approaches will be lacking with respect to the combined approach.

The formal approach in the videotex research might have taken the interacting knowledge sources concept of the BIM, and presented this to videotex dialogue designers as an optimisation tool. The BIM alone does allow statements related to design to be derived. One of these is "Don't design the dialogue so that users' knowledge mismatches with that required to operate the system". Another is "Maximise the overlap of users' know- ledge with that required to operate the system effectively". The usefulness of these statements could only be realised if designers already have an accurate idea of user knowledge, and understand what knowledge demands are imposed by the dialogue options they have available. Like Reisner's approach (ibid.), the formal expression of the interaction must be related in some way to details of user's cognitive structures and resources in order for consequences of usability to be derived.

The other alternative, the empirical approach, might in the videotex work have resulted in a corpus of information about user behaviour while teleshopping. The unstructured data set would by itself be unlikely to suggest ways to improve usability, in terms of reducing the number of difficulties. This is partly due to difficulties of interpreting behaviour (e.g. verbal protocols) without the use of a structure to explain behaviour. In addition, the generalisation from the data to the consequences of a novel dialogue design solution is difficult without a valid description of the sources of the difficulties found.

The approach, as described here in the context of videotex dialogue design, combined the formal frameworks and the empirical data. The actual behaviour of the users associated with the different acquisition representations was used to detail structures that related system and user knowledge characteristics.

Optimising the Formal-Empirical Approach

Clearly, the combination of formal structures and empirical evidence provides advantages over the unitary formal or empirical approaches to research intended to help optimise design. However, there are a number of difficulties in practice. They are presented here as matters for concern, and the suggested solutions should be regarded as speculative.

Selecting the Formal Structures

One problem is the selection of the formal structure or structures. There appear to be three areas of difficulty. Firstly, how is one to decide on the level of description that is required of the formalism? That is, what characteristics of technology, user or system should the formal structure seek to represent? This level varies greatly in current formalisms. The illustration of the videotex research involved two structures, one of which attempted to support a description of the interaction of two types of user knowledge sources. Other formalisms, e.g. the keystroke-level model (Card, Moran and Newell, 1980), describe the entire interaction of user and technology at the level of individual keystrokes. Some formalisms have a variable level, for example the Command Language Grammar (Moran, 1981).

Secondly, of all the available formalisms and potential formalisms, how can one decide their relative appropriateness? Complex knowledge based tasks might be best served by "blackboard" models like Hearsay II (Whitefield, 1984). Alternatively, production systems appear to cope adequately with the acquisition and use of cognitive skills (Anderson, 1983). The grounds for preference remain intuitive - congeneality, elegance, appropriateness and so on - no more and sometimes less than the most general of heuristics.

Thirdly, how does the functionality of one structure relate to the functionality of others? For example, blackboard models, augmented transition networks and production systems might be isofunctionate analytic structures for some purpose. At this point, neither the theoretical proof nor the empirical evidence is available to support a possible claim.

Selecting the Empirical Procedures

The selection of the appropriate procedures for collecting empirical data concerning usability will depend on a number of considerations. Firstly, behaviour should be sampled to have validity with respect to the target group and to the behaviour. The data should have the extent re-quired to be representative of the populations of users, tasks and machines, and the method of collection should not interfere excessively with the behaviour to be observed. Verbal protocols might provide extensive information about users' conscious mental processes, but at the risk of interfering with the users' normal (non-verbalised) task activity. Another consideration concerns the requirements of the "grain" of the information. Data might be observations of behaviour. Records of the lowest levels (smallest grain) could be collected by a making a detailed record of the interaction. This might result in an unwieldy data set, depending on what information is recorded. At higher levels, a compact record might be obtained, for instance, a count of videotex frame accesses. The information content of the smaller grain size record is greater than the larger. As a rule, the choice of grain should be at a level lower than any which might be required.

The appropriate level is likely to be determined by the purposes of the data collection, and these in turn are determined by frameworks and structures, except in a unitary empirical approach. The selection of the empirical procedures, then, is difficult to isolate from formal, and other non-formal structures. The following section addresses the relationship of formal structures and empirical procedures.

Relationships of Formal and Empirical Components

Given a formalism that specifies the characteristics of concern, it seems appropriate that empirical procedures should generate data compatible with these characteristics, both of level and type. If, for instance, a formal structure describes keystroke level activity, then it would seem perverse to rely on large grain empirical data such as time on task. Similarly, a time-performance model should not be associated with error data.

When a formal structure is not extant, the requirements for the empirical procedures are difficult to define, and typically, extensive and low-level records are made, for instance time-logged video recordings of behaviour at a terminal together with a record of the computer activity. Clearly, to be practical, even here some implicit taxonomy of users, tasks and technology must be made, simply to describe the situation to be recorded.

The empirical procedures will in turn affect development of the formalisms. The elaboration of the entities that the formalism attempts to represent is one such development, and in the videotex example this comprises the expression of the particular knowledge source interactions as system and knowledge variables. Also, the details of the formal framework itself may be affected by the requirements of the empirical procedures, as in the initial stages of the experimental studies in which the modelled task component of evaluation had to be expressed at a more detailed level in order to specify the requirements for the experimental task.

Sequencing the Stages

Closely associated with the relationships described in the previous section, is the problem of deciding the sequence of empirical and formal steps. The major difficulty is in choosing the first step. Is it to be a data collection procedure (on the basis of implicit assumptions), or the expression of a formal structure? In the videotex research, only an implicit and therefore informal set of criteria were used to specify the initial observational study, and so the intitial step was an empirical one, given the formal-empirical contrast.

Pragmatics

As mentioned earlier in the chapter, it was decided to construct special purpose formalisms rather than rely on extant ones, in particular the Command Language Grammar. This choice was a matter of pragmatics, associated with the difficulty of using this formalism to describe the videotex teleshoppers' behaviour. Other practical requirements that influence the choices and sequences of the combined approach are a result of the time limits within which some estimates of usability are to be made and the resources available. For instance, given that a formal-empirical approach is chosen, then the interdependence of formalisms and appropriate empirical methods means that the relevant stages should be short. Development of the formalisms and collection and examination of the empirical evidence should then proceed together, so that within the period available, the structures and data should be compatible.

Value of Approach

All of the above issues are important and some will prove to be critical. The present work hardly impacts the enormity of the problems raised. However, this should not detract from the potential of the formal-empirical approach described here for the purpose of optimising human-computer interaction.

SUMMARY

This chapter describes three possible approaches to the cognitive optimisation of interactive dialogues. Two approaches - the formal and the empirical - are described briefly. The formal approach has the advantage of being complete, explicit and coherent but not of reflecting users' interactive behaviour. The empirical approach has the advantage of reflecting users' behaviour but not of relating it to the options available for optimising design of interactive dialogues. Neither by itself is able to achieve the goal of dialogue optimisation. A third approach - the formal-empirical - is described in more detail. The approach iteratively exploits both formal structures and empirical data to relate users' interactive behaviour to sources of performance difficulty, and sources of performance difficulty to options available for optimising dialogues. The approach is illustrated by research intended to improve the usability of interactive videotex dialogues used for shopping transactions. Models of the task and of the user were constructed to relate observed behaviour (both informal and experimental) to performance difficulties expressed as system and knowledge variables. These variables once validated by experimental manipulation and evaluation constitute the de facto set of design options, which when implemented will result in the optimisation of the videotex dialogues. The combined approach, then, unlike the unitary approaches is able to achieve the goal of dialogue optimisation. Although the approach raises a number of problems, it shows promise and deserves to be pursued and developed.

ACKNOWLEDGEMENTS

The videotex work reported here was funded jointly by SERC and British Telecommunications PLC under grant GR/C/23032.

REFERENCES

Anderson, J.R. (1983). *The Architecture of Cognition*. Cambridge, Massachusetts: Harvard University Press.

Buckley, P. and Long, J. (1985a). Identifying usability variables for teleshopping. In *Contemporary Ergonomics 1985*, ed. D. Oborne. London: Taylor and Francis.

Buckley, P. and Long, J. (1985b). Effects of system and knowledge variables on a task component of teleshopping. In *People and Computers: Designing the Interface*, eds. P. Johnson and S. Cook. Cambridge, UK: Cambridge University Press.

Buckley, P. and Long, J. (1986a). Recommendations for optimising the design of videotex dialogues. In *Contemporary Ergonomics 1986*, ed. D. Oborne. London: Taylor and Francis.

Buckley, P. and Long, J. (1986b). *Using videotex for shopping: a qualitative analysis*. Paper submitted to Behaviour and Information Technology.

Card, S.K., Moran, T.P. and Newell, A. (1980). The keystroke-level model for user performance time with interactive systems. *Communications of the ACM, 23*, pp. 396-410.

Chomsky, N. (1965). *Aspects of the Theory of Syntax*. Cambridge,
      Massachusetts: M.I.T. press.
Fenn, S. (1985). *Transaction processing on videotex- an assessment of the
      response frames used in teleshopping*. Unpublished MSc disserta-
      tion, Ergonomics Unit, University of London.
Fenn, S. and Buckley, P. (1987). *Using Videotex to order goods from
      home. In Contemporary Ergonomics 1987. ed. Mewgaw*. London:
      Taylor and Francis.
Gilligan, P. and Long, J. (1984). Videotext technology: an overview with
      special reference to transaction processing as an interactive
      service. *Behaviour and Information Technology, 3*, (1), pp. 41-71.
Hammond, N., Long, J., Clark, I., Barnard, P. and Morton, J. (1981).
      Documenting human-computer mismatch in interactive systems.
      In *Proceedings of the Ninth International Symposium on Human
      Factors in Telecommunications*. Red Bank, New Jersey.
Hammond, N., Jorgensen, A., MacLean, A., Barnard, P. and Long, J.
      (1983). Design practice and interface usability: Evidence from
      interviews with designers. In *CHI 83: Human Factors in Com-
      puting Systems*. Boston, Massachusetts.
Hammond, N., Hinton,G., Barnard, P., MacLean, A., Long, J. and
      Whitefield, A. (1984). In *Interact 84*, ed. B. Shackel. North-
      Holland.
Long, J.B. (in press). Cognitive ergonomics and human-computer
      interaction. In *Psychology at Work*, ed. P. Warr. London: Penguin.
Long, J.B. and Buckley, P.K. (1984). Transaction processing using
      videotex, or: shopping on Prestel. In *Interact 84*, ed. B. Shackel.
      North-Holland.
Moran, T.P. (1981). The Command Language Grammar: a representation
      for the user interface of interactive computer systems.
      International Journal of Man-Machine Studies, 15, (1), pp. 3-50.
Morton, J., Barnard, P., Hammond, N. and Long, J. (1979). Interacting
      with the computer: a framework. In *Teleinformatics 79*, ed. E.J.
      Boutmy and A. Danthine. North-Holland.
Parnas, D.L. (1969). On the use of transition diagrams in the design of a
      user interface for an interactive computer system. In *Association
      of Computing Machinery National Conference Proceedings*.
Reisner, P. (1981). Formal grammar and human factors design of an inter-
      active graphics system. *IEEE Transactions on Software
      Engineering, SE-7*, (2), pp. 229-240.
Whitefield, A. (1984). A model of the engineering design process derived
      from Hearsay-II. In *Interact 84*, ed. B. Shackel. North-Holland.
Woods, W.A. (1970). Transition network grammars for natural language
      analysis. *Communications of the ACM, 13*, pp. 591-
      606.

AUTHOR INDEX

N

O

P

SUBJECT INDEX

A

B

C